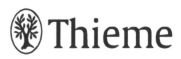

Trigger Points and Muscle Chains

Second Edition

Philipp Richter, DO
Institute of Applied Osteopathy
Burg Reuland, Belgium

Eric Hebgen DO, MRO
Founder of the Vinxel Institute of
Osteopathy
Königswinter, Germany

363 illustrations

Thieme
Stuttgart • New York • Delhi • Rio de Janeiro

Library of Congress Cataloging-in-Publication Data is available from the publisher.

This book is an authorized translation of the 4th German edition published and copyrighted 2015 by Georg Thieme Verlag, Stuttgart. Title of the German edition: Triggerpunkte und Muskelfunktionsketten in der Osteopathie und Manuellen Medizin

Translator: Johanna Cummings-Pertl, Hopland/CA, USA
Illustrator: Malgorzata and Piotr Gusta, Champigny sur Marne, France;
Christiane and Michael von Solodkoff, Neckargemünd, Germany

1st Finnish edition 2007
1st French edition 2008
1st Korean edition 2008
1st Japanese edition 2009
1st Italian edition 2010
1st Spanish edition 2010
1st Czech edition 2011
1st Chinese edition (simplified characters) 2011
2nd French edition 2013
2nd Spanish edition 2014
1st Polish edition 2014
1st Russian edition 2016

© 2019 Georg Thieme Verlag KG

Thieme Publishers Stuttgart
Rüdigerstrasse 14, 70469 Stuttgart, Germany
+49 [0]711 8931 421, customerservice@thieme.de

Thieme Publishers New York
333 Seventh Avenue, New York, NY 10001, USA
+1-800-782-3488, customerservice@thieme.com

Thieme Publishers Delhi
A-12, Second Floor, Sector-2, Noida-201301
Uttar Pradesh, India
+91 120 45 566 00, customerservice@thieme.in

Thieme Publishers Rio, Thieme Publicações Ltda.
Edifício Rodolpho de Paoli, 25º andar
Av. Nilo Peçanha, 50 – Sala 2508
Rio de Janeiro 20020-906 Brasil
+55 21 3172 2297 / +55 21 3172 1896

Cover design: Thieme Publishing Group

Typesetting by Thomson Digital, India

Printed in Germany by CPI Books

5 4 3 2 1

ISBN 978-3-13-241351-1

Also available as an e-book:
eISBN 978-3-13-241352-8

Important note: Medicine is an ever-changing science undergoing continual development. Research and clinical experience are continually expanding our knowledge, in particular our knowledge of proper treatment and drug therapy. Insofar as this book mentions any dosage or application, readers may rest assured that the authors, editors, and publishers have made every effort to ensure that such references are in accordance with **the state of knowledge at the time of production of the book.**

Nevertheless, this does not involve, imply, or express any guarantee or responsibility on the part of the publishers in respect to any dosage instructions and forms of applications stated in the book. **Every user is requested to examine carefully** the manufacturers' leaflets accompanying each drug and to check, if necessary in consultation with a physician or specialist, whether the dosage schedules mentioned therein or the contraindications stated by the manufacturers differ from the statements made in the present book. Such examination is particularly important with drugs that are either rarely used or have been newly released on the market. Every dosage schedule or every form of application used is entirely at the user's own risk and responsibility. The authors and publishers request every user to report to the publishers any discrepancies or inaccuracies noticed. If errors in this work are found after publication, errata will be posted at www.thieme.com on the product description page.

Some of the product names, patents, and registered designs referred to in this book are in fact registered trademarks or proprietary names even though specific reference to this fact is not always made in the text. Therefore, the appearance of a name without designation as proprietary is not to be construed as a representation by the publisher that it is in the public domain.

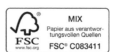

For Anja and Heike–
without whose patience and support
this book would not have been possible.
Thank you!

Preface to the Second Edition

This book was first published in German in 2006. The book's great success, also internationally, was surprising and showed us how important and necessary it was to write it. The first English-language edition of this book was published in 2008.

This second English-language edition is based on the fourth German edition, which contains two additions:

• We substantially expanded the chapter on posture. Posture problems are often overlooked as potential causes for functional problems of the locomotor system, especially of the spine. A.T. Still was convinced that locomotor system problems and especially problems involving the spine are the cause of all physical ailments. We trust that the additions to this chapter address the significance of this topic.

• We added stretching exercises to the sections on trigger points. Stretching represents the actual treatment of trigger points and provides excellent opportunities for patients to participate in their treatment by performing simple stretching exercises as "homework." One important aspect of these exercises is that they are easy to learn. This increases patient compliance with their "homework" and, with quick results, also helps patients accept the necessity to participate in their treatment success.

In this edition, we standardized the anatomical descriptions and nomenclature, which again improved the structure of the book. We extend our gratitude to Dr. Stephanie von Pfeil for editing the entire text.

Eric Hebgen
Philipp Richter

Preface to the First Edition

The idea for this book originated many years ago. Practical experiences, readings in specialized literature, attendance at seminars, and conversations with colleagues and specialists from other disciplines showed us time and again the significance of the locomotor system.

Daily clinical routine showed us in the course of years that the same lesion patterns tended to occur over and over. Years of intensive observation and investigation as well as thorough literature research confirmed that our observations agree with reality and are not just wishful thinking.

Not only osteopaths, but also posturologists and manual therapists speak of motor patterns, using different explanatory models for the development of these patterns. In a course on muscle energy techniques, both *Dr. F.L. Mitchell jr.* and *Dr. Ph. Greenman* made reference to a universal pattern. Both agree on the existence of a universal pattern, because in the case of dysfunction in the motor system other body parts always adapt with identical patterns. Similarly, the entire organism follows certain patterns in physiology; examples are processes like walking or breathing. The common embryologic origin of all tissues, the connections of the connective tissue, and the organism as a hydropneumatic system all support this theory. The endocrine system is a good example for holistic behavior as well.

The holistic principle, highly prized by the osteopath, as well as embryologic, physiologic, and neurologic axioms offer explanations for the origin of certain patterns.

In our opinion, the nervous system and the myofascial structures play key roles in this process as organizer and as executing organ respectively.

We have compared different models of muscle chains and different osteopathic working models, looking for commonalities. Consequently, we have realized that all these models share a basic premise, but from different perspectives.

In this book, we present a model of muscle chains that is based on the two motor patterns of cranial osteopathy, namely flexion and extension. Because the organism consists of two halves, it has two corresponding chains of flexion and extension.

Littlejohn's model of the "mechanics of the vertebral column" and the "Zink patterns" of the American osteopath *Gordon Zink, DO* have inspired us to divide the torso skeleton into units of movement. Much to our surprise, we realized that this division into units of movement correlated closely with the division of neurologic supply of certain organs and muscles.

We provided both chains with muscles, understanding that this can only be incomplete and theoretical. We ask the reader to keep this in mind. Nevertheless, because the organism only recognizes motor patterns, but not individual muscles, this is somewhat irrelevant.

In the second part of the book, we present a number of treatment methods for the myofascial structures.

For this purpose, we describe trigger point therapy in great detail because it is invaluable in clinic.

We have purposely limited this presentation to the mechanical aspect of osteopathy because it is significant for posture and can therefore be applied in diagnosis.

For physiologic cranial dysfunctions, we have chosen a mechanical model to attempt an explanation. We have, however, refrained from presenting visceral dysfunctions in detail, in spite of the fact that they quite clearly follow the same patterns. Structural disturbances manifest in malposture through direct fascial trains and particularly through viscerosomatic reflexes. Following the holistic principle, the organs adapt to the "container," the motor system, in the same way that static disturbances affect the location and function of the organs (adaptation of function to structure).

Our model of muscle chains is only a working model, just like many others; we do not lay claim to completeness. We were able to realize in clinic, however, that diagnosis as well as treatment of patients can become much more rational and effective when they originate in this perspective. This applies in particular to chronic and therapy-resistant cases.

Thommen and Königswinter, spring of 2006

Philipp Richter
Eric Hebgen

Table of Contents

A Muscle Chains

Philipp Richter

B Trigger Points: Diagnosis and Treatment 121

Eric Hebgen

A

Muscle Chains

Philipp Richter

1 Introduction

Role of Muscle Chains in the Body

The musculoskeletal system and **muscle chains** are the primary focus of this book. Myofascial structures participate in all somatic functions: Emotional states present as muscle tension. Physical labor requires muscle activity. Circulation, breathing, and digestion depend on an intact locomotor system.

Manual therapists—physical therapists, chiropractors, osteopaths, or Rolfing practitioners—examine and treat the locomotor system differently and with different motivations. Physical therapists and Rolfing practitioners treat the musculoskeletal system primarily to resolve discomfort (pain, tension, etc.) in the area being treated. Chiropractors and especially osteopaths view the myofascial system as a component of the body that can cause or result from dysfunction or pathology in other body systems. Another group of professionals—podologists or posturologists—are aware of the negative impact on the whole body that can result from minor shifts in weight or foot misalignments.

All somatic functions depend on well-functioning myofascial structures. The nervous system takes on the role of coordinator and controller. To avoid overloading the cortex, many activities are managed by subcortical reflexes and behavior patterns. Viscerosomatic and somaticovisceral reflexes have also been scientifically proven, which emphasize the special significance of muscle imbalances, especially of the paravertebral muscles.[79,112]

Motor and posture patterns of the human body involve the entire organism, in the same way that all physical activity results from interactions of all body systems. Osteopaths and chiropractors employ this fact in their diagnosis and therapy.

Segmental innervation of all body structures and adaptation mechanism patterns provide indications for structural involvement. Many sports injuries or musculoskeletal pain result from dysfunctions in parts of the myofascial chains. Understanding myofascial connections enables diagnosis and appropriate treatment. The osteopathic mindset provides a thought-provoking explanation for the mechanisms involved in the development and treatment of disorders.

Dr. Still's Osteopathy

When Dr. Andrew Taylor Still presented his philosophy of healing, during a phase when he rejected the medicine practiced at the time, he called it **osteopathy.** He knew full well that this term had a different meaning in the medical world at the time. His desire was to help medicine return to its origins by placing humans at the center and natural laws in the foreground. Osteopathy was the most appropriate term to illustrate that disease (pathos) results from dysfunctions in the body. Dr. Still viewed the musculoskeletal system and especially the spine as playing a central role. He recognized that all diseases and functional disorders involved mobility limitations of the spine. Osteopathy is derived from the Greek words "osteon" for bone and "pathos" for disease.[140]

Dr. Still knew from experience that treating symptoms did not bring about healing. Successful healing required expert treatment of the causes of disease. He had no doubt that disease started with circulatory disorders and that the cause was to be found in the **connective tissue.**[140] Therefore, this is where disease needed to be examined and treated. Myofascial tissue is of special importance in this process[82,140] because of its ability to serve as the following:

- Connector (connective tissue).
- Pathway for veins, lymphatics, arteries, and nerves.
- Supporting tissue (stroma, matrix) for organs and bones.
- Protective structure.

For Still, the nervous system and its surrounding fluids (**cerebrospinal fluid** [CSF]) are possibly even more significant than connective tissue. The nervous system serves as a control center and regulating organ and is responsible for all adaptation mechanisms between individual body systems. It initiates and coordinates all functions in the entire body and is responsible for all adaptation and compensation mechanisms.

Still refers to CSF as possibly "the highest known element" in the entire organism. Its composition is similar to blood and lymph serum. CSF is connected to blood via the choroid plexuses and with lymph via the peripheral nerves of the interstitium. In addition to its protective and nourishing functions for the central nervous system, Still and especially his student William Garner Sutherland attributed a special function to the CSF:[54,140,142,143] it carries the "breath of life" into all cells of the body.

Still's experience in his early years likely gave rise to the development of osteopathy. As a physician, religious believer, and son of a Methodist preacher, Still had a close connection to religion and to God. This is reflected in all his writings: God gave humans health and disease is abnormal. Still believed that the osteopath's task is to search for health in the body of patients.

In his search for true medicine, Still was inspired by two opposing directions: spirit healers and bone setters. In his view, **spirit healers** embody therapists who believe in God. They tune into tissues and, through their hands, focus energy into a pathologic area. The "breath of life" (Sutherland) then performs the healing. **Bone setters,** on the other hand, also achieve great success through physical manipulation (adjustments).

Still combined both directions in his osteopathic treatments. His special talents as a therapist derived from his precise understanding of anatomy and his excellent sense of touch, combined with his belief in the power of self-healing and his intention to help. His anatomical and physical knowledge enabled him to precisely visualize structures. His sense of touch allowed him to feel tension in tissues and apply targeted, appropriate techniques in each individual case.

As an osteopath, Still embodied both the spirit healer and the bone setter. He compared the human body to a machine and the osteopath to a mechanic who repairs the mechanics of the machine.[140]

One characteristic of Still's osteopathy was that he combined **biodynamics** with **biomechanics**. Nowadays, it seems that some of his successors have divided this duality. Some osteopaths are pure "mechanics" who emphasize the laws of anatomy and physiology and manipulate the whole body using gentle and less gentle techniques. They represent the biomechanical direction of osteopathy.

Others are more biodynamically oriented. They place less importance on biomechanics and more emphasis on their sense of touch and the body's power of self-healing. Like spirit healers, they attempt to activate the self-healing powers in tissues, with the difference being that they employ the body's rhythms in diagnosis and therapy.[8,9,72]

Of interest in this context is a statement by Viola Frymann (continuing education 2000). She says that (Sutherland's) primary respiratory mechanism (PRM) clearly manifests in healthy tissue. However, with dysfunctions, the PRM's power of expression is impeded. This means that the PRM can be employed in diagnosis and therapy. Biodynamic therapists take advantage of this phenomenon by using their hands to establish a fulcrum in the tissue.[8,72,135] After a certain period of time,

the PRM expresses itself in its various rhythms, which is an indicator that the tissue is regaining its function.

The difference between classic cranial osteopathy and biodynamics is that classical cranial osteopathy examines the tissue for motion and motion limitations and then guides the structure to be treated into unrestricted motion and holds it there. This allows the PRM to develop freely without tension and carry out its therapeutic effect.

The motions of the sphenobasilar synchondrosis (SBS) palpated and described by Sutherland correspond to motions of the head in the three planes of space, plus translations in the sagittal plane (**up and down strain**) and in the horizontal plane (**lateral strain**). Functional techniques applied to the locomotor system work according to the same principle. Therapists search for a balance point in all planes (**stacking**) and maintain the tissue in a relaxed position until automatic relaxation takes place. This shows that the principles employed in cranial osteopathy are identical to those that apply to the rest of the body.

Opinions vary about which mechanisms are ultimately responsible for tissue relaxation. Practitioners of biomechanics maintain that it involves a reflexive response originating in the tissue receptors. Biodynamic practitioners believe in the effect of the PRM.

In his therapy, Still employed a combination of so-called direct and indirect techniques. Direct techniques manipulate the segment to be treated in the corrective direction. Indirect techniques move the segment in the direction of dysfunction.

Richard Van Buskirk[23] conducted research into Still's treatment methods by asking older patients, who were treated by osteopaths in their childhood or youth, to recall the techniques used in their treatment. Some of these patients were still able to describe those techniques and Van Buskirk was surprised to find that they resembled the few techniques described by Still himself.

A short video clip still exists in which Still can be observed treating a rib. This video along with statements of patients and the limited documentation written by Still about his techniques show the following: After thorough diagnosis, the segment to be treated is placed into the lesion position until the contracted muscles relax. Then the segment is moved into the corrective position using slight pressure that is focused on the blocked joint throughout the motion.

■ Scientific Evidence

As has been mentioned, the **nervous system** plays a **central role** for Still. It forms the link between the visceral, parietal, and cranial systems. The importance of the central nervous system and especially of the spinal cord in the genesis of dysfunction and pathology has been scientifically documented in research by Korr, Sato, Patterson and others.[79,81,112]

These scientists experimentally verified the significance that Still and other manual therapists placed on the spine in the development and maintenance of pathological states. They confirmed the central, regulating role of the spinal cord. Korr[79] was able to provide scientific explanations for generally accepted phenomena observed in experiments. He referred to the locomotor system as "the primary machinery of life" and maintained that the other systems (digestion, endocrine, heart, and circulatory systems) serve the locomotor system.

The autonomic nervous system (ANS) plays a special role in this context. Both parts of the ANS are complimentary rather than antagonistic. Roughly speaking, the parasympathetic (craniosacral) nervous system (PNS) regenerates the organism. It also plays a regulating role in processes of longer duration. The sympathetic nervous system (SNS), on the other hand, adapts body system functions to current needs. It intervenes in the regulation of blood supply to active muscles, for example, by reducing blood flow to the digestive system to benefit muscles during physical activity. At the same time, the SNS increases respiration and pulse rates. The SNS enables the body to spontaneously adjust to immediate requirements.

Korr supplied neurophysiological explanations for many phenomena observed by clinicians. He coined terms such as **facilitated segment** and **neurologic lens**. A facilitated segment is a segment of the spinal cord where the stimulus threshold of all nuclei is lowered by repeated stimulation or by dysfunction of the segment due to chronic stimulation. In this condition, subliminal stimulation of the facilitated segments suffices to cause disproportional reactions. One example is acute torticollis resulting from exposure to drafts.

The term neurologic lens describes the following phenomena: If a spinal cord segment is chronically irritated, it becomes susceptible to stimuli that should normally only be able to stimulate other, more distant segments. The irritated segment is said to "attract stimuli."

In their experiments, the research team led by Korr produced other interesting results:

- Increasing the sympathetic tone (locally or generally) lowers the stimulus threshold of the segments involved and increases muscle tone for the muscles supplied by those segments.
- Blocking of vertebrae increases the sympathetic tone of the segments involved and lowers the stimulus threshold.
- Stress of all types increases muscle tone, especially in facilitated segments.
- Posture imbalances impact the muscle tone of paravertebral muscles and of muscles supplied by facilitated segments.
- Reducing the muscle tone of paravertebral muscles lowers sympathetic tone in those segments.

Taken together, research results in this area clearly illustrate two facts:

- The musculoskeletal system is one of the main agents involved in the development and maintenance of somatic dysfunctions.
- The spinal cord plays an important role as a control element and organizer in the genesis of pathological states.

Korr's characterization of the locomotor system as the "primary machinery of life" is therefore by no means an exaggeration.

Myofascial structures play a main role in all important bodily functions, from respiration (thoracic as well as cell respiration), circulation (diaphragm and muscles as venolymphatic pump), and digestion (as mobilizer of organs) to being a means to express emotions. The locomotor system enables motion, communication with others, food intake, etc.

The fact that more than 80% of all afferents originate from the locomotor system further underscores the importance of the musculoskeletal system.[79,112,158] The extreme sensitivity of muscle spindles (1 g of traction and a stretch of 1 mm cause a reaction of the muscle spindle[79]) makes the locomotor system a highly sensitive organ. This enables quick reactions, but at the same time, it increases susceptibility to dysfunctions. This results in contractions, malpositions, and coordination disorders.

Irvin [in[155]] and Kuchera and Kuchera[82] describe how a 1- to 1.5-mm tilt of the base of the sacrum suffices to change the muscle tone of the paravertebral muscles. Korr described the resulting impact on the SNS and on the entire body. However, the spinal cord as a controlling and organizing center is not influenced by only peripheral stimuli.

The emotional state of a person is a significant factor in the genesis of dysfunctions and pathologies. The limbic system plays a decisive role in this process.[158] As the body's memory, it evaluates all stimuli and impressions as either positive or negative for the person, depending on previous experience. If a stimulus is experienced as pleasant, it provides positive feedback. If the stimulus is perceived as harmful, it provides negative feedback.

The hypothalamic–pituitary–adrenal (HPA) axis controls the neuroendocrine system, which regulates hormone balance as well as the neurovegetative system. Facilitated segments are especially impacted by positive and negative emotional stimuli (e.g., weekend migraine or stress ulcers). Segments with lower stimuli thresholds remain "chronically irritated" after a certain amount of time when they are subjected to persistent stimulation.[112] **Therapy for this condition requires treatment of the entire lesion pattern to erase the imprinting of the pathological pattern at the level of the central nervous system**. In this context, Korr talked about the spinal cord as organizer of disease processes.[79]

The embryologically determined metamerism of the spinal cord leads to segmental affiliations of certain muscles, organs, vessels, skin area, bones, and joints.

Stimulating one of these structures influences the functions of all other structures associated with this segment.

Since neighboring segments are connected by interneurons, facilitation usually impacts several segments. The plurisegmental supply of organs and muscles also supports this concept. In our opinion, it is wrong to associate an organ or function with a single spinal cord segment, especially since the brain knows only motion patterns, not individual muscles. Congenital and acquired patterns are of equal importance in this context.

The digestive system has considerable autonomy due to the enteric nervous system, but it is nevertheless subordinate to overall body function, with the endocrine and neurovegetative system also providing a regulating function.

It is safe to assume that both congenital and acquired behavior patterns are found in this system, just like with the locomotor system. These patterns likely correlate with posture and locomotor system patterns and create a certain type.[151]

■ Mobility and Stability

The locomotor system consists of muscles and bones. It needs to serve two contradictory functions simultaneously: provide stability and allow movement.

The cerebellum and the vestibular system enable both functions. They both receive their information from receptors that are primarily located in myofascial structures.

Both functions are carried out by muscles: adequate basal muscle tone, ability to react quickly, and well-coordinated muscle tension enable delicate, harmonious motions as well as subtle and appropriate adjustments to ensure balance in the most efficient manner.

In its wisdom, nature (or the Creator) has provided a simple solution for this problem. Centrifugal force (expanding force of the organs) is balanced by the imploding force (inherent muscle tension) of the musculature. The extraordinary sensitivity of muscles supported by the precise coordination provided by the nervous system enables optimal and efficient stabilization of the locomotor system.

To perform harmonious motions, muscles need stable support, a central organ that coordinates activity (nervous system) and structures that guarantee their supply (metabolism). These activities are controlled by the nervous system, which activates agonists and synergists and inhibits antagonists precisely to the extent needed to perform targeted, harmonious motions.

Most motions occur unconsciously with the help of several spinal reflexes. This is necessary for humans to act anticipatorily. The cerebrum needs decision autonomy.

The spinal cord acts as a control center for all physical activities. Dysfunctions can have disastrous consequences. All afferent signals from the locomotor system reach the spinal cord and efferent signals to the muscles originate there. This is where motor and posture patterns are processed.

In the 1950s, Sherrington described several reflex actions that explain these patterns [in[21] and in[160]]. Muscles consist of different muscle fibers with different characteristics. White (fast-twitch) fibers are more suited to fast contractions, while red (slow-twitch) fibers support longer lasting tension. Both fibers exhibit different pathologic tendencies. White fibers tend toward weakness and atrophy, whereas red fibers tend toward contracture and shortening. These characteristics need to be addressed during treatment.[40,41,86,87]

■ The Organism as a Unit

At the beginning of this chapter, we pointed out that the organism always responds as a unit. We do not intend to reproduce the basic foundations of osteopathic thinking in this book, but only those concepts necessary for understanding the following chapters.

Our organism *always* acts as a unit, in physiologic as well as in pathologic states. The *entire* body participates in each physiologic process. Respiration, for example, involves all muscles. It not only activates the respiratory system muscles, but also mobilizes digestion in a certain pattern. Circulation is also supported by muscles. These activities always follow a specific process. During inspiration, the entire locomotor system, including the head, carries out a motion pattern that Sutherland called "flexion–external rotation–abduction".[101,102,142,143] Exhalation reverses this pattern: "extension–internal rotation–adduction."

Walking follows a similar pattern. Gait is a harmonious sequence of motions from the tip of the big toe to the root of nose, in the same repeating patterns. We also find this holistic behavior in pathologic states.

The best indicator of holistic behavior can be found in the embryologic development of humans. When an ovum cell is fertilized by a sperm cell, the ovum cell divides into two cells that have the same genetic code. This division continues until the cells join into cell units to form organs, muscles, bones, nervous system, etc.

This shared origin of all cells in the body supports the conclusion that all cells also jointly react to a given situation. The nervous system seems to have a special function in this process as a control and coordination center.

Sutherland bases his explanation of the human body as a unit on the membrane system and on the fluctuation of liquor.[101,102,142,143] He uses the term **reciprocal tension membrane** to describe that traction on the base of one membrane system influences all other bases. These reciprocal tension membranes consist of the cranial and spinal dura mater.

Sutherland describes the following attachment points for the dural system:

- Crista galli, in front.
- Clinoid process.
- Petrous part of temporal bone, left and right.
- Inion, in back.
- Foramen magnum.
- Cervical vertebra C2.
- Sacrum.

One practical consequence is that a position change of the sacrum, for example, automatically changes the positions of the occipitoatlantoaxial (OAA) complex and the cranial bones.

The dural system is filled with nerve tissue and fluid (CSF) and continues via the nerve sheaths to the interstitium, which is also filled with fluid. In other words, changes in the dural system exert pressure on the fluids in the dural sac. These pressure changes disperse throughout the interstitial fluid and therefore the entire body.

The PRM described by Sutherland and consisting of flexion and extension phases causes pressure changes in the entire dural system and intercellular tissue. These changes display a specific rhythmicality, and their direction and amplitude is tissue specific. The direction of movement correlates with thoracic respiration: cranial flexion corresponds to inspiration and cranial extension corresponds to expiration.

The anatomy of fasciae provides further proof of holism. Embryologically, all connective tissues originate in the mesoderm. Basically, the different layers form a single cover that divides the organism, envelopes organs and muscles, and forms the body's skin. The body's three fascia layers are connected. This continuity causes changes in one location, for example, tension or pressure, to manifest throughout all tissues. This reciprocity makes fasciae so extraordinarily important for posture, locomotion, and physical response to mechanical stress.[111]

The continuity of fasciae, the continuity of fluids, and their common origin are indicators of unity, especially since all cells share the same DNA.

The entire body will always respond as a unit, in physiology as well as in pathology. Any organ dysfunction will impact the muscles and joints that are segmentally connected to the organ. The continuity of myofascial tissue causes changes in tension and pressure ratios in the *entire* body and, via the dural system, in the cranium. Posture, cranium, and organs adapt in a specific pattern. The body endeavors to leave the functions of the entire organism undisturbed for as long as possible.

▪ Interrelation of Structure and Function

All osteopaths are familiar with the interrelation of structure and function. Structure depends on function and function impacts structure.

The most effective illustration of this concept is joint mobility. Joints need to remain mobile to prevent ankylosis. If the mobility of a joint is impaired, the synovial joint membrane produces less fluid. Lack of loading and unloading of weight on the cartilage reduces its supply. The joint capsule and the cartilage become brittle. This results in reduced joint mobility and may lead to arthrosis or ankylosis. Arthrosis results from joint dysfunction, whatever the cause.

The locomotor system provides an especially instructive example of this adaption of structure to function. Muscle dysfunctions lead to structural changes. This process happens surprisingly quickly,[2,46] but fortunately, it is partially reversible. It takes about 30 days for functional problems to cause structural changes.[41,82]

At the same time, structure determines function. For example, certain joint changes cause gait changes and impact the normal functioning of other structures. Osteopaths who work in pediatrics are especially familiar with the impact of structure on function. Still writes about the significance of osteopathic treatments for newborns.[140] Sutherland,[142,143] Magoun,[101,102] Frymann,[57] and Arbuckle[4] provide details about this topic.

Structural changes in the cranial base of newborns due to prenatal or perinatal complications are the starting point of dysfunctions in cranial nerves (X, XI, XII) and posture problems of the spine (scoliosis, kypholordosis). Magoun explains this as due to the craniosacral connection and growth impairment caused by membrane tension.[101] Korr confirms his theory.[79]

Still stated the same view 50 years earlier when he posited that circulation disorders are the beginning of disease.[140] For Still, circulation included venolymphatic and arterial circulation as well as the circulation of nerve impulses. Structural changes are subject to the laws of mechanics. The following are significant:

- Gravity.
- External forces.
- Shape and condition of joint surfaces.
- Impact of muscle traction.[107]

▪ Biomechanics of the Spine and Locomotor System

No other researcher analyzed the biomechanics of the spine in as much detail as Littlejohn[53,95,96,97,98,126] and Fryette[56] [from a different perspective]. Littlejohn takes a holistic view of the spine and attempts to provide mechanical explanations for commonly found dysfunctions. Fryette describes the behavior of individual vertebra during motion and in the presence of certain dysfunctions. Littlejohn supplies mechanical explanations for the behavior of the spine (globality).

The behavior of the spine and of the locomotor system in general is directed by mechanical laws. The spine consists of anteroposterior arches. The movement of joints is dictated by ligaments, muscles, and joint surfaces. The spine and joints respond in their own patterns to strain (tension or pressure) and this causes the remaining locomotor system to adapt accordingly.

The spine consists of two anteriorly concave arches (thoracic spinal column [TSC] and sacrum) and two posteriorly concave arches (cervical spinal column [CSC] and lumbar spinal column [LSC]). Kypholordosis develops during growth due to forces impacting the body. Congenital and acquired emotional factors should not be underestimated in this context.[25,86,141] Perinatal microtrauma[4,57,102,142,143] and childhood trauma (falling onto the buttocks) can influence this process and cause scoliosis as well as hyperkypholordosis.

Scoliosis usually develops into S-shaped curves.[4,82,145] It is as if the entire spine rotates around a vertical axis in a horizontal plane. Horizontality of the base of the sacrum plays a decisive role in this process. A tilt of 1 to 1.5 mm in the frontal plane can induce scoliosis of the spine due to the extreme sensitivity of muscle spindles.[82,155]

In the initial phase, the spine seems to adapt to a sudden tilt of the base of the sacrum by forming a global C-shaped scoliosis. However, postural factors then activate muscles to turn the C-shape into an S-shape as quickly as possible. Littlejohn's model of the mechanics of the spine provides a mechanical explanation for this process.[36,96,97] In addition to the anatomical condition of joints, muscles are the most important element as the implementers of these adaptation processes.

Scoliosis and kypholordosis impact not only the spine, but also the head, thorax, and extremities. The body as a whole participates in this process.[101]

This holistic behavior is ensured by myofascial continuity and the hydraulic system, which encompasses the CFS and interstitial fluid. Structure holistically adapts to function to ensure homeostasis.

■ Significance of Homeostasis

Homeostasis is the maintenance of a relatively constant internal milieu or balance in the organism with the help of feedback loops between the hypothalamus, the hormone system, and the nervous system.[115]

Homeostasis serves to optimize all bodily functions for the purpose of maintaining health. It is not a static state, but a constantly fluctuating process of adaptations to changing internal and external conditions. Body functions are controlled by mechanical, electrophysiological, and chemical processes. The body's metabolism is maintained by pressure gradients, polarities, temperature differences, and concentration gradients.

These processes take place in the extracellular fluid within a framework provided by the connective tissue. **Connective tissue** plays a key role in homeostasis. Every cell participates in and simultaneously benefits from homeostasis.[111] This reciprocity enables automatic regulation of all bodily functions.

When a dysfunction develops, the extracellular fluid responds to correct the problem. If this is not successful, more and more systems will be impacted. They are no longer able to contribute toward homeostasis. That is where disease begins.

The first signs of dysfunction are changes in myofascial tissue, because that is where the disease process takes place. Even minor organic disturbances cause viscerosomatic reflexes that lead to changes in myofascial structures, especially in the paravertebral muscles. This has been scientifically proven.[112] These neuromusculoskeletal reflexes are based on embryological connections. The important consideration for therapy is that the body's self-healing powers can reestablish homeostasis.

Somatovisceral reflexes as documented by Sato [in[112,82]] can be employed therapeutically to influence organ dysfunction. On the other hand, these reflexes also underscore the scope of muscle imbalances and posture disorders.

Paravertebral hypertonia is not only a sign of segmental facilitation but can also be its cause and therefore induce visceral disorders. The most frequent causes of paravertebral hypertonia are accidents (sports and work injuries), asymmetric physical activity, and differences in leg length.

■ The Nervous System as Control Center

The "primary machinery of life"[79] is powered by muscles. **The musculature is the organ of the locomotor system, and the nervous system is the control center.** Muscles need to cooperate to carry out harmonious motions. They do so by working as chains where each unit of movement supports the next one.

Example: For the biceps muscle of arm to flex the elbow, the shoulder needs to be prevented from being pulled forward. This task is carried out by the shoulder extensors and the stabilizers of the scapula.

This creates loop-shaped chains, called lemniscates (lemnisci). Since most muscles run diagonally or are fan-shaped, these lemniscates occur in the sagittal as well as in the frontal planes.

The nervous system is tasked with recruiting muscles to carry out motions. Congenital reflexes facilitate this work for the organism. Receptors in muscles, tendons, fascia, and joints provide information about motions. Together with the centers of postural and directed motility, these receptors enable finely coordinated motions and adequate adjustments to changes in balance.

■ Different Muscle Chain Models

There are several different models of myofascial chains (see Chapter 8). Rolfing therapists, physical therapists, and osteopaths have all described muscle chains. Differences in these descriptions of muscle chains result from differences in opinions and from different treatment perspectives. Rolfing therapists may not emphasize the same treatment aspects as osteopaths or physical therapists.

The model we present in Chapter 8 is based on Sutherland's theory that there are two motion patterns:
- Flexion–abduction–external rotation.
- Extension–adduction–internal rotation.

While Sutherland did not describe muscle chains, he did document the behavior of segments for both patterns. One interesting aspect of his model is that it corresponds to the motions of respiration and gait.

Since our work is based on a holistic principle of physiology and pathology, we are convinced that cranial patterns continue into the locomotor system and into the visceral domain and vice versa.

The factors described earlier (fluids, membranes, connective tissue continuity) ensure this process. In addition, physical and mechanical laws ensure that the joints of the locomotor system (including cranial sutures) carry these patterns into the entire musculoskeletal system. This is true regardless of whether the pattern was triggered by a vertebra, the ilium, an organ, or a cranial bone.

The entire organism adapts to dysfunctional and pathogenic elements to allow the body to function optimally and as free of pain as possible. This reduces tension, harmonizes pressure ratios, and maintains circulation. These factors are necessary for the body's self-healing powers to accomplish their work. According to the theory of cranial osteopathy, this maintains the primary respiration mechanism and allows the "breath of life" to reach the cells.

■ In This Book

In the first part of this book, we briefly introduce several different models of myofascial chains (Chapter 2) and then describe the physiological principles for the behavior of the locomotor system (Chapter 3).

In Chapter 4, we present the biomechanical aspects of Sutherland's cranial concept. We describe the physiologic motions of the SBS and its impact on the spine and locomotor system.

The position of the occiput above the atlas determines the location of the sacrum. This in turn determines the position of the spine, extremities, and thorax.

Chapter 5 presents the mechanics of the spine as viewed by Littlejohn. Littlejohn's concept is a functional model he developed in his practice. It explains how the individual segments of the spine relate to each other. The specific adjusting technique (SAT) developed by Bradbury and further refined by Dummer[51,52,53] represents a logical and clinically very valuable application of Littlejohn's model.

In Chapter 6, we introduce some interesting discoveries and ideas by Janda that are primarily of clinical relevance.

Chapter 7 covers a very simple type of rational diagnosis: Zink's common compensatory pattern (CCP). It examines the myofascial torsion patterns at the junctions of the spine. We employ this model to identify the dominant regions (see the "Practical Applications" section in Chapter 7). In this section, we also draw comparisons between the models of Littlejohn, Zink, and neurophysiological and anatomical facts. We show that Littlejohn's and Zink's models can be projected onto each other, and that there are neurophysiologic connections that help explain these findings. This underscores the functional and structural interrelations.

In Chapter 8, we introduce a muscle chain model that builds on Sutherland's two patterns. We describe the behavior of the various locomotor units of the body, the development of kypholordosis and scoliosis, and the muscles involved in these processes. This model exhibits some key differences compared to other models.

In our opinion, all locomotor units behave like cogwheels, similar to the cranial bones in Sutherland's cranial model. This causes counter-rotating motions between two successive locomotor units. It explains kypholordosis and scoliosis as well as counter-rotation between units (as in foot, knee, and hip position with genu valgus or genu varum).

We view **flexors** as the muscles in the concavities and **extensors** as the muscles in the convexities of the locomotor system. Dominant flexor chains automatically result in increased curvatures and dominant extensor chains result in stretching of the skeleton. Since the organism embryologically consists of two equal halves, each half of the body contains one flexor chain and one extensor chain. The nervous system directs coordination between both sides. In this book, we describe these muscle chains and explain the development of posture problems. We would like to emphasize that our model does not claim to be comprehensive and represents yet another attempt to explain phenomena found in our daily clinical practice. Our intensive research of professional literature and participation in seminars have provided us with answers to many questions and compelled us to write about this interesting topic.

The second part of this book covers practical applications. We present a diagnostic model and describe some treatment methods. We base our examination on the Zink patterns (see Chapter 7) and on simple traction tests that enable us to very quickly identify dominant structures. We focus on presenting treatments for myofascial structures. It goes without saying that organic and cranial dysfunctions must receive appropriate treatment. In this part of the book, we describe the diagnosis and treatment of trigger points in detail. This type of therapy provides rapid palliative pain relief for acute and chronic problems and normalizes structural changes in the myofascial unit.

2 Models for Myofascial Chains

2.1 Herman Kabat (1950): Proprioceptive Neuromuscular Facilitation

Dr. Herman Kabat developed the concept of proprioceptive neuromuscular facilitation (PNF) in the 1940s for treating poliomyelitis patients. Kabat was supported in his work by Margaret Knott and Dorothy Boss, who published the first book about PNF in 1956. Since then, this method has been developed further and applied successfully in patients with other disorders.

The PNF concept is based on the neurophysiologic findings of Sir Charles Sherrington:[21,160]

- Reciprocal innervation or inhibition.
- Spatial summation.
- Temporal summation.
- Successive induction.
- Irradiation (irritability).
- Postisometric relaxation (PIR; after discharge).

Kabat developed a treatment technique that integrates weak muscles into a muscle chain. The muscle chain is stimulated by targeted stimuli (visual, auditory, and tactile). This technique optimally utilizes the characteristics of nerves and muscles described by Sherrington to optimally integrate a weak muscle (or muscle group) into a motion pattern.

This technique stimulates the proprioceptive abilities of the locomotor system to strengthen weak muscles and coordinate motion sequences. The goal is to provide positive inputs to the central nervous system and to facilitate normal motion patterns via central feedback loops. This is the reason the same motion patterns are applied continuously.

Motion Patterns

PNF stimulates the following motion patterns:

■ Scapula and Pelvis

- Anterior elevation.
- Anterior depression.
- Posterior elevation.
- Posterior depression.

■ Upper Extremities

- Flexion–abduction–external rotation.
- Extension–adduction–internal rotation.
- Flexion–adduction–external rotation.
- Extension–abduction–internal rotation.

■ Lower Extremities

- Flexion–abduction–internal rotation.
- Extension–adduction–external rotation.
- Flexion–adduction–external rotation.
- Extension–abduction–internal rotation.

■ Neck

- Left flexion–right extension and vice versa.
- Flexion–lateral left flexion–left rotation and vice versa.
- Extension–lateral right flexion–right rotation and vice versa.

■ Trunk

- Trunk flexion–lateral flexion–leftward rotation.
- Trunk extension–lateral flexion–rightward rotation.

The motion pattern directions for the extremities refer to the large shoulder and hip joints adjacent to the trunk. Two antagonistic motion patterns result in a diagonal.

Application Modalities

- The initial posture of the patient can vary (supine, prone, lateral, sitting, standing).
- The segment to be treated is prestretched in a manner that stretches all muscles involved in the pattern (agonists and synergists).
- Prestretching and performing the motion must be absolutely pain free.
- Evasive motions are corrected.
- The therapist asks the patient to move into the desired direction and stimulates the motion direction through tactile contact or resistance.
- In the final position of the motion, agonists and synergists involved in the motion pattern are optimally shortened and their antagonists are stretched.
- The motion usually starts in the distal joints of the segment and then proceeds continuously toward the proximal joints.
- Special attention is paid to the rotational component, because it is important for the motion pattern.

- Intermediary joints (elbows and knees) can be stretched, remain bent, or be bent during the motion, as needed. Proximal joints (shoulder and hip) and distal joints perform the same motion.
- Patterns may be combined.
- The various Sherrington principles are taken into consideration.

Observations

- Kabat emphasizes muscle chain motions, not motion components of individual muscles.
- Kabat views musculature as a unit in the same way that Sherrington views the nervous system as a unit.
- Kabat describes different patterns for the upper and lower extremities.
- Patterns for the upper extremities associate flexion with external rotation and extension with internal rotation.
- Patterns for the lower extremities associate abduction with internal rotation and adduction with external rotation.

2.2 Godelieve Denys-Struyf

Godelieve Denys-Struyf, a Belgian physical therapist trained in osteopathy (European School of Osteopathy) and developer of the GDS method, was most likely the first to mention muscle chains in the true sense of the word.[141]

She was familiar with Kabat's PNF concept and with the Mézières method of postural re-education. Her work was also significantly influenced by Piret and Béziers, who posited that motions depend on the shape of joint surfaces and musculature disposition, especially of the pluriarticular muscles.

These two factors, according to Piret and Béziers, produce spiral motions. This creates tensions that provide shape and structure to a segment.[161] In other words, body shape is determined by motion patterns that reflect a person's emotional state. This illustrates the psychological component that is very important to Denys-Struyf.

The Mézières method restructures the locomotor system. It views posture problems as arising from impaired coordination of the muscular skeletal system. Psychological factors did not play a role for Mézières. The innovative aspect of his method at the time (1960s) was that he broke with traditional spine treatment

methods, which straightened the spine by strengthening the back muscles.

Mézières does not view kyphosis, lordosis, or scoliosis as resulting from muscular insufficiencies, but rather from tensions in the posterior muscle chain. He also determined that hypertonic posterior muscle chains are responsible for weak abdominal muscles and coordination problems. Treatment needs to focus on reducing the tonicity of posterior muscle chains from head to toe.

Denys-Struyf adopted Kabat's muscle chain principles and Mézières' principle of stretching as a form of treatment. Piret's und Beziérs' principles added a psychological dimension. Altogether, this gave rise to the first holistic muscle chain model.

Denys-Struyf describes 10 muscle chains, 5 in each half of the body. These chains normally work in coordination to carry out spiral-shaped motions. In most cases, one myofascial chain dominates this process.

The dominant chain shapes the organism and the specific gestures of each person. Denys-Struyf never doubted that it is impossible to fully neutralize the dominant chain. This would be the same as completely changing a person's character. The most we can do is to restore balance when an overly dominant chain is creating imbalance to enable coordinated movement and prevent deformities.

Denys-Struyf determined the following three causes for muscular imbalance:

- The main cause is a person's psychological state:
  - Posture, gesture, and morphology primarily reflect a person's psychological state.
- The second cause is lifestyle:
  - Not only work habits and exercise, but also lack of physical activity can lead to muscle strain and imbalanced muscle tone.
- The third factor also impacts myofascial structures via central feedback loops:
  - Stress, anger, anxiety, grief, and other emotional factors can temporarily or permanently change the tonicity of certain muscle chains.

Classification of the Five Muscle Chains

The five muscle chains in each half of the body are classified as follows:

- **Three** fundamental or **vertical muscle chains** that encompass the head and the trunk.
- **Two** complementary or **horizontal muscle chains** that encompass the upper and lower extremities.

These are relational chains that relate humans to their environment.

These five muscle chains correspond to five psychological constitutions: three fundamental and two complementary constitutions.

Interestingly, Denys-Struyf assigns each fundamental, vertical chain to an area of the cranium. The shape of this area of the cranium (convex, flat, etc.) indicates the dominance of a specific psychological predisposition. Vertical chains exhibit muscle extensions into the extremities in the same way trunk muscles connect horizontal muscle chains to the axis skeleton and the vertical chains.

Following is a list of muscle components for the five muscle chains. More information can be found in the original writings.[40]

▪ Vertical or Fundamental Muscle Chains

Anteromedian Chain (▶ Fig. 2.1)

Primary Section:
Anterior Trunk Muscles
- Pelvic floor muscles.
- Rectus abdominis.

- Lower and median parts of the greater pectoral muscle.
- Transverse muscle of thorax.
- Intercostal muscles (medial part).
- Subclavius.
- Anterior scalene muscle.
- Sternal part of the sternocleidomastoid (SCM).
- Hyoid bone muscles.

Secondary Section:
Lower Extremities
- Pyramidal muscle.
- Adductors.
- Gracilis.
- Gastrocnemius (medial part).
- Adductor muscle of great toe.

Upper Extremities
- Deltoid (anterior part).
- Brachial muscle.
- Supinator.
- Abductor muscle of thumb (pollicis).

Posteromedian Chain (▶ Fig. 2.2)

Primary Section
- Erector muscle of spine (erector spinae).
- Long neck extensors.

Secondary Section:
Lower Extremities
- Semimembranous muscle.
- Semitendinous muscle.
- Soleus.
- Toe flexors.

Upper Extremities
- Latissimus dorsi.
- Ascending part of trapezius.
- Infraspinous muscle.
- Teres minor.
- Posterior part of deltoid.
- Long part of triceps muscle of arm (triceps brachii).
- Finger flexors.
- Pronators.

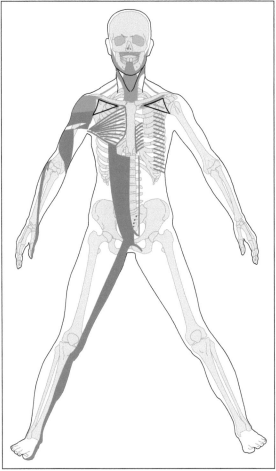

▶ **Fig. 2.1**   Anteromedian chain (as per Denys-Struyf).

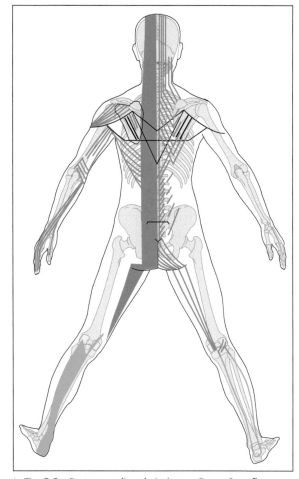

▶ **Fig. 2.2**   Posteromedian chain (as per Denys-Struyf).

Posteroanterior–Anteroposterior Chain (▶Fig. 2.3)

Primary Section
- Autochthonous or deep paravertebral muscles.
- Respiratory muscles.
- Splenius muscles of head (capitis) and of neck (cervicis/colli).
- Scalene muscles.
- Iliopsoas.

Secondary Section: Lower Extremities
- Vastus medialis.
- Rectus femoris.
- Toe extensors.

Upper Extremities
- Smaller pectoral muscle.
- Coracobrachial muscle.
- Short part of the biceps muscle of arm (biceps brachii).
- Medial part of the triceps muscle of arm (triceps brachii).
- Finger extensors.

■ Horizontal or Complementary Muscle Chains

Posterolateral Chain (▶Fig. 2.4)

Lower Extremities
- Gluteus medius.
- Biceps muscle of thigh.
- Vastus lateralis.
- Peroneal muscles.
- Lateral gastrocnemius.
- Plantar muscle.
- Lateral part of abductor muscle of little toe.

Upper Extremities
- Horizontal and descending part of trapezius.
- Supraspinous muscle.
- Median part of deltoid.
- Lateral part of triceps muscle of arm (triceps brachii).
- Anconeus.
- Ulnar extensor muscle of wrist (extensor carpi ulnaris).
- Ulnar flexor muscle of wrist (flexor carpi ulnaris).
- Abductor muscle of little finger.

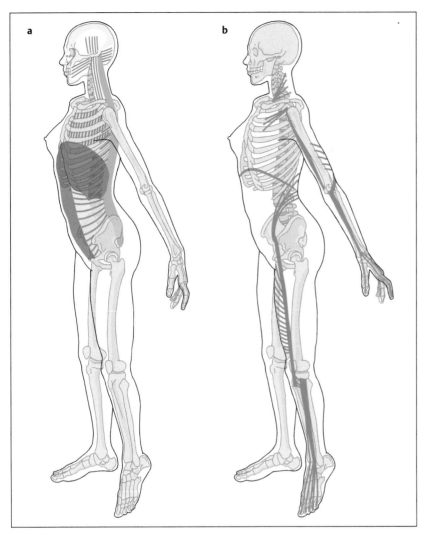

▶ **Fig. 2.3 (a, b)** Posteroanterior–anteroposterior chain (as per Denys-Struyf).

Anterolateral Chain (▶ Fig. 2.5)

Lower Extremities
- Gluteus medius.
- Tensor fasciae latae (TFL).
- Anterior tibial muscle.
- Posterior tibial muscle.
- Plantar interosseous muscles.
- Lumbrical muscles of foot.

Upper Extremities
- Clavicular part of SCM, smaller pectoral muscle, and deltoid.
- Teres major.
- Latissimus dorsi.
- Subscapular muscle.
- Long part of biceps muscle of arm (biceps brachii).
- Superficial part of supinator.
- Brachioradial muscle.
- Long and short radial extensor muscle of wrist.
- Long palmar muscle.
- Thenar muscles.
- Lumbrical muscles of hand and palmar interosseous muscles.
- Radial flexor muscle of wrist.

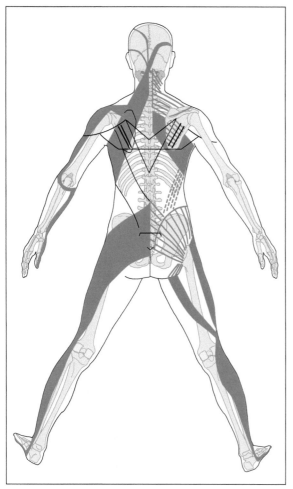

▶ **Fig. 2.4** Posterolateral chain (as per Denys-Struyf).

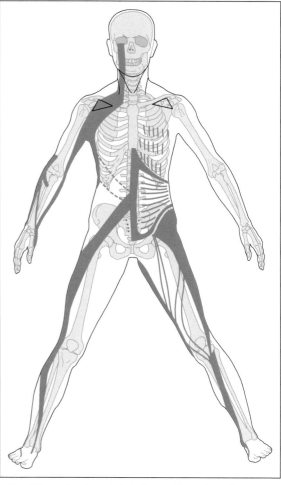

▶ **Fig. 2.5** Anterolateral chain (as per Denys-Struyf).

2.3 Thomas W. Myers

"Anatomy Trains" (Myofascial Meridians)

Thomas W. Myers, a certified Rolfing therapist at the Rolf Institute, describes a series of myofascial chains in his book *Anatomy Trains*.[108] He employs the technical language of Rolfing therapists as well as metaphors such as tracks, lines, stations, and express trains to tangibly illustrate these rather complex chains.

The book describes myofascial connections simply and comprehensibly, and with emphasis on holism and myofascial continuity. Fascial "trains" continue throughout the entire body along tracks (or myofascial meridians) that travel in the same directions. Osseous attachment sites for muscles and fasciae act as switching stations, which gives them special significance.

Myofascial meridians enable whole-body posture analysis and allow informed therapists to target specific shortened meridians for treatment.

Myers describes seven myofascial meridians that are presented here briefly.

Myofascial Chains According to T. Myers

■ **Superficial Back Line** (▶ **Fig. 2.6**)

- Plantar fascia.
- Triceps muscle of calf (triceps surae).
- Ischiocrural muscles.
- Sacrotuberal ligament.
- Erector muscle of spine (erector spinae).
- Suboccipital muscles.
- Epicranial aponeurosis (galea aponeurotica).

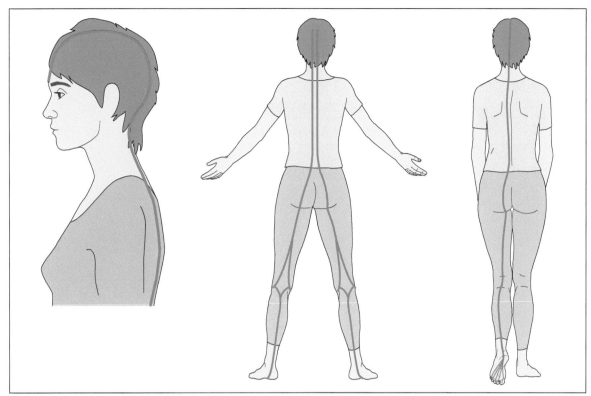

▶ **Fig. 2.6** Myofascial chains (as per Myers). Superficial back line.

■ Superficial Front Line (▶Fig. 2.7a)

- Anterior compartment muscles.
- Infrapatellar ligament and quadriceps muscle of thigh.
- Rectus abdominis.
- Sternal muscle und greater pectoral muscle.
- SCM.

■ Lateral Line (▶Fig. 2.7b)

- Sole of foot and peroneal muscle.
- Iliotibial tract, TFL.
- Gluteus maximus.
- Oblique muscles and quadratus lumborum.
- Intercostal muscles.
- Splenius muscle of head (capitis) and SCM.

■ Spiral Line (▶Fig. 2.7c–e)

- Splenius muscle of head (capitis).
- Rhomboid muscles and anterior serratus on the other side.
- Oblique muscles.
- Tensor fasciae latae and iliotibial tract.
- Anterior tibial muscle.
- Long peroneal muscle.

- Biceps muscle of thigh.
- Sacrotuberal ligament.
- Erector muscle of spine (erector spinae) back to starting point.

This line wraps around the thorax and induces torsion of the chest.

■ Arm Lines (▶Fig. 2.8)

There are four arm lines, one on each side of the arm, from the thorax or occiput to the fingers:
- Deep front arm line.
- Superficial front arm line.
- Deep back arm line.
- Superficial back arm line.

■ Functional Lines

Functional lines diagonally extend the arm lines to the pelvis on the opposite side. They connect the two sides of the body.
- Functional back line.
- Functional front line.

■ Deep Front Line

- Sole of the foot.
- Posterior leg compartment muscles.

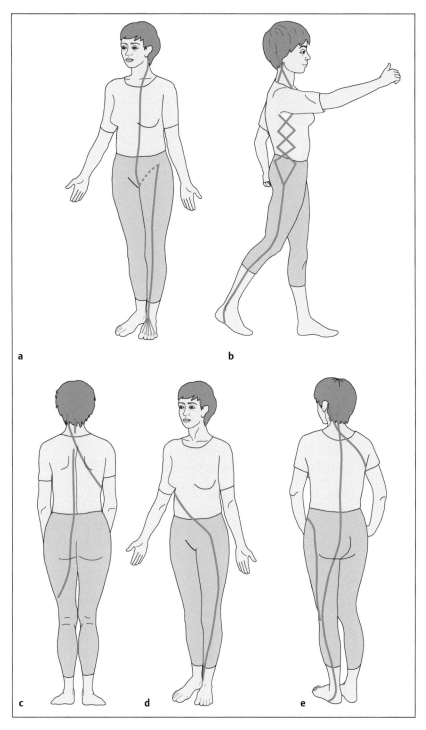

▶ **Fig. 2.7** Myofascial chains (as per Myers). **(a)** Superficial front line. **(b)** Lateral line. **(c–e)** Spiral line.

- Hip adductors.
- Iliopsoas.
- Anterior longitudinal ligament.
- Diaphragm.
- Mediastinum with pericardium.
- Pleura.

- Scalene muscles.
- Hyoid bone muscles.
- Mastication muscles.

Even though these chains are very theoretical and not always easy to understand, they do often provide explanations for the manifestation of symptoms.

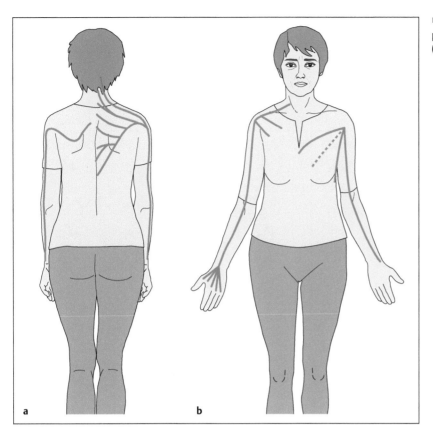

▶ **Fig. 2.8** Myofascial chains (as per Myers). **(a)** Back arm lines. **(b)** Front arm lines.

2.4 Leopold Busquet

Muscle Chains

The French osteopath, Leopold Busquet, published a series of books on muscle chains.[25–30] In the first four books, he describes the muscles chains of the trunk and the extremities. The fifth book covers cranial connections for muscle chains of the trunk. The final book of the series describes the visceral connections between abdominal organs via the suspension system (mesenteries, ligaments, omenta) and between the peritoneum and the trunk.

Busquet also wrote two other books about cranial osteopathy. It should be noted that some of his statements contradict Sutherland and other Anglo-American cranial experts. For example, his description of the palpatory signs of cranial torsion and sidebending–rotation contradicts that of Sutherland [in[102]].

Of interest are the connections that Busquet draws between organic dysfunctions (and pathologies) and posture. The author describes two groups of organ dysfunction and their impact on the locomotor system:

- Expansive (space consuming) organic dysfunctions (e.g., liver stasis) that force muscles to make room for an organ (▶ **Fig. 2.9**).

- Retractive or painful processes that recruit muscles into providing more support to an organ or to relax the painful tissue and provide pain relief (antalgic posture for inflammatory abdominal processes; ▶ **Fig. 2.10**).

Visceral dysfunctions can cause posture problems such as scoliosis, kypholordosis, pes planus (flatfoot), and pes cavus (claw foot), and can also be the starting point for muscle, tendon, and joint injuries.

Myofascial Chains According to Busquet

Busquet describes five trunk chains that extend into the extremities:
- Static posterior chain.
- Flexion chain or straight anterior chain.
- Extension chain or straight posterior chain.
- Diagonal posterior chain or "opening chain" ("open crossed muscle chain").
- Diagonal anterior chain or "closing chain" ("closed crossed muscle chain").

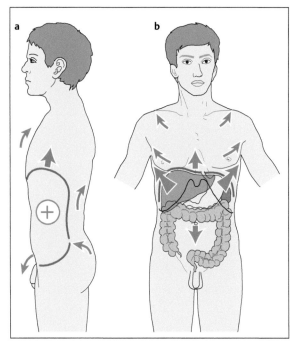

▶ **Fig. 2.9 (a, b)** "Opening tendency" for expansive processes in the abdomen.

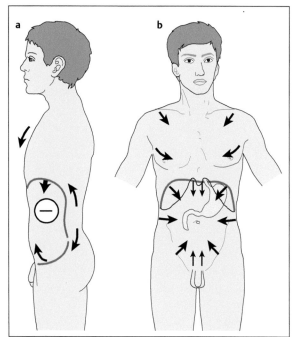

▶ **Fig. 2.10 (a, b)** "Closing tendency" (curling up) for support-seeking processes und spasms in the abdomen.

■ Static Posterior Chain (▶Fig. 2.11)

When standing, gravity tends to tilt the upper body forward. This force is countered by two passive (low-energy consuming) mechanisms:

- Pleural and peritoneal spaces that exert expansive force.
- Ligament and fascia chains that extend from the frontal bone to the sacrum.

On the lower extremities, the chain continues along the outside of the legs to the feet, and for good reason: when walking, gravity tends to tilt the body's weight toward the swinging leg.

Note: Phylogenesis provides a different explanation for these facts. During evolution, the lower (back) extremities rotated inward and this caused the posterior leg muscles to be positioned laterally. The knees and feet shifted to orient their motion plane toward the locomotor plane and the posterior structures of the leg shifted outward. This is an evolutionary example of how structure adapts to function.

The static posterior chain consists of the following structures, from superior to posterior:

- Cerebral und cerebellar falx.
- Ligaments of the vertebral arch.
- Thoracolumbar fascia.

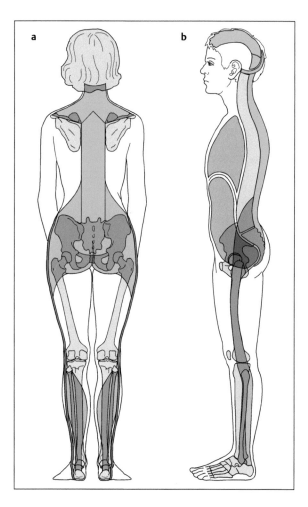

▶ **Fig. 2.11 (a,b)** Static posterior chain (as per Busquet).

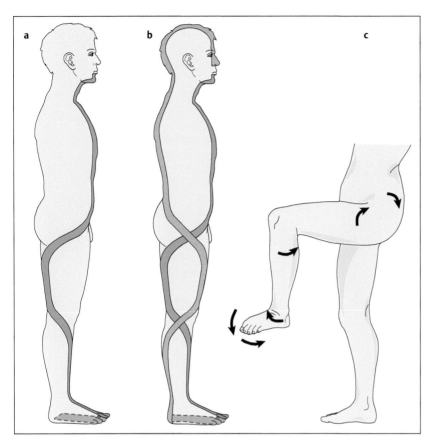

▶ **Fig. 2.12 (a–c)** Flexion chain or straight anterior chain (as per Busquet).

- Sacrotuberal and spinal ligaments.
- Fascia of the piriformis and obturator muscles.
- TFL.
- Fibula und interosseous membrane.
- Plantar fascia.

■ Flexion Chain or Straight Anterior Chain
(▶ Fig. 2.12)

Busquet assigns the following functions to this chain:
- Flexion.
- Global kyphosis of the trunk.
- Physical and psychological "curling up."
- Introversion.

This chain consists of the following muscles:

On the Trunk

- Anterior intercostal muscles.
- Rectus abdominis.
- Pelvic floor muscles.

Connection to the Shoulder Blade
- Transverse muscle of thorax.
- Smaller pectoral muscle.
- Descending part of trapezius (connects to spine).

Connection to the Upper Arm
- Greater pectoral muscle.
- Teres major.
- Rhomboid muscles.

Connection to the Cervical Spine
- Scalene muscles.
- Splenius muscle of neck (cervicis/colli).

Connection to the Head
- Subclavius.
- SCM.
- Splenius muscle of head (capitis).

Connection to the Lower Extremities
- Iliopsoas.

On the Upper Extremities

Busquet maintains that the upper extremities do not follow the standard reversal between flexion and extension. The flexor chain of the upper extremities therefore consists of the following anterior muscles:
- Anterior part of deltoid.
- Coracobrachial muscle.
- Biceps muscle of arm (biceps brachii).
- Brachial muscle.
- Hand and finger flexors.

On the Lower Extremities

The following movements result from activating the flexor chain of the leg:
* Posterior rotation of the ilium.
* Hip flexion.
* Knee flexion.
* Posterior extension in the ankle (talocrural) joint.
* Increase in foot arches.

The flexion chain of the leg consists of the following muscles:

Posterior Ilium Rotation
* Rectus abdominis.
* Smaller psoas.
* Semimembranous muscle.

Hip Flexion
* Iliopsoas.
* Internal and external obturator muscles.

Knee Flexion
* Semimembranous muscle.
* Popliteal muscle.

Posterior Extension of the Foot
* Long extensor muscle of toes.

Plantar Flexion of the Toes and Increase in Foot Arches
* Quadratus plantae.
* Short flexor muscle of great toe.
* Short flexor muscle of little toe.
* Lumbrical muscles of foot.

■ Extension Chain or Straight Posterior Chain (▶Fig. 2.13)

The extension chain encompasses the following functions:
* Extension.
* Global lordosis of the trunk.
* Opening outward.
* Communication with the environment.

It consists of the following elements:

On the Trunk

Deep Plane
* Autochthonous muscles.
* Erector muscle of spine (erector spinae).
* Iliocostal part of quadratus lumborum.

Median Plane
* Superior and inferior posterior serratus muscles.

Connection to the Shoulder Blade
* Horizontal and descending part of trapezius.
* Smaller pectoral muscle.
* Transverse muscle of thorax.

Connection to the Arm
* Latissimus dorsi.
* Teres major.
* Greater pectoral muscle.

Connection to the Cervical Spine
* Splenius muscle of neck (cervicis/colli).
* Scalene muscles.
* Spinotransversal paravertebral muscles.

Connection to the Head
* Splenius muscle of head (capitis).
* Ascending part of trapezius.
* SCM.

Connection to the Lower Extremities
* Gluteus maximus.

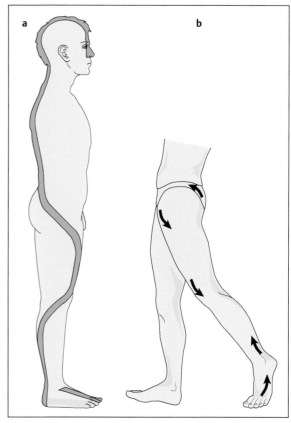

▶ **Fig. 2.13 (a, b)** Extension chain or straight posterior chain (as per Busquet).

On the Upper Extremities

The extensors of the upper extremities encompass the following posterior muscles:
* Posterior part of deltoid.
* Triceps muscle of arm (triceps brachii).
* Hand and finger extensors.

On the Lower Extremities

This extensor chain rotates the ilium forward, extends the hip and the knee, performs a plantar flexion of the ankle joint, and lowers the arch of the foot.

Forward Ilium Rotation
* Quadratus lumborum.
* Rectus femoris.

Hip Extension
* Gluteus maximus.
* Quadratus muscle of thigh.

Knee Extension
* Vastus intermedius of quadriceps muscle of thigh.
* Plantar flexion of the foot.
* Plantar muscle.

Extension of the Forefoot
* Short flexor muscle of toes (digitorum brevis).

Extension of the Toes
* Interosseous muscles.
* Short extensor muscle of toes (digitorum brevis).
* Short extensor muscle of great toe (hallucis brevis).

■ Diagonal Posterior Chain or "Opening Chain" (▶Fig. 2.14)

These diagonal chains facilitate torsion of the trunk. The anterior diagonal chains perform a forward trunk torsion and the posterior diagonal chains perform a backward trunk torsion. If both anterior chains dominate, the shoulders and both ilia are pulled medially forward. Both posterior diagonal chains pull the shoulders and ilia backward. They perform a similar function on the lower extremities.

The posterior diagonal chains abduct and rotate the legs outward. The anterior diagonal chains adduct and rotate the legs inward.

Right Diagonal Opening Chain

> *Important:* Busquet names the diagonal chains in keeping with their origin at the ilium. The right diagonal chain connects the right ilium with the left shoulder!

On the Trunk
* Iliolumbar fibers of right paravertebral muscles.
* Iliolumbar fibers of right quadratus lumborum.
* Iliocostal fibers of left quadratus lumborum.
* Left internal intercostal muscles.
* Left inferior posterior serratus.

Connection to the Left Shoulder
* Ascending part of the left trapezius.
* Left smaller pectoral muscle.
* Left transverse muscle of thorax.

Connection to the Left Arm
* Left latissimus dorsi.
* Left teres major.
* Left greater pectoral muscle.

Connection to the Cervical Spine
* Left splenius muscle of neck (cervicis/colli).
* Left scalene muscles.

Connection to the Head
* Left splenius muscle of head (capitis).
* Left SCM.
* Left trapezius.

Connection to the Right Leg
* Superficial part of gluteus maximus.

This chain causes the ilium to outflare, abduct, and externally rotate the hip; places the knee into a varus position; and supinates the foot.

The following muscles are active in the lower extremities:

Ilium Outflare
* Levator ani muscle.
* Ischiococcygeal muscle.
* Sartorius.
* Tensor fasciae latae.
* Gluteal muscles.

Abduction and External Rotation of the Hip
* Piriform muscle.
* Gluteus maximus und medius.

External Rotation and Varus of the Knee
* Biceps muscle of thigh.
* Vastus lateralis.

Varus of the Hindfoot and Supination
* Anterior tibial muscle.
* Posterior tibial muscle.
* Long extensor muscle of great toe (hallucis longus).

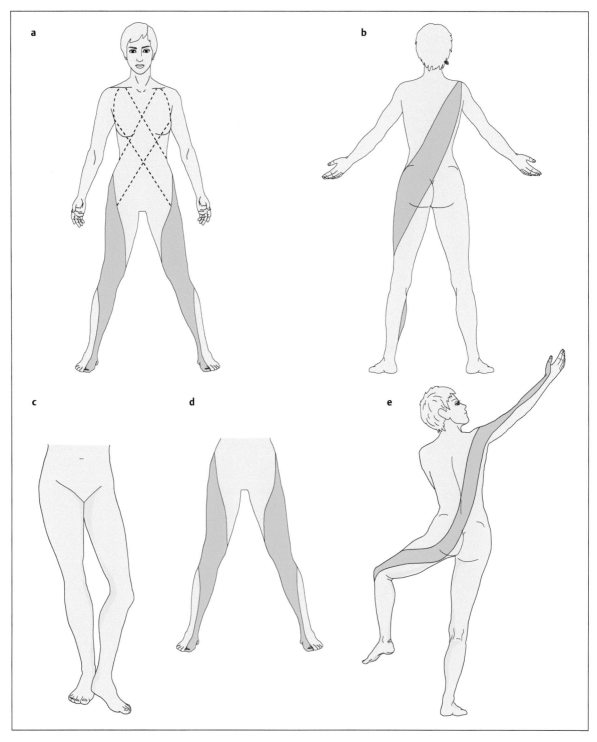

▶ **Fig. 2.14 (a–e)** Diagonal posterior chain or "opening chain" (as per Busquet).

▪ Diagonal Anterior Chain or "Closing Chain" (▶Fig. 2.15)

The left diagonal anterior chain (left ilium to right shoulder) serves as an example here.

On the Trunk
- Deep plane: left internal oblique muscle of abdomen.
- Superficial plane: right external oblique muscle of abdomen, right external intercostal muscles, right superior posterior serratus.

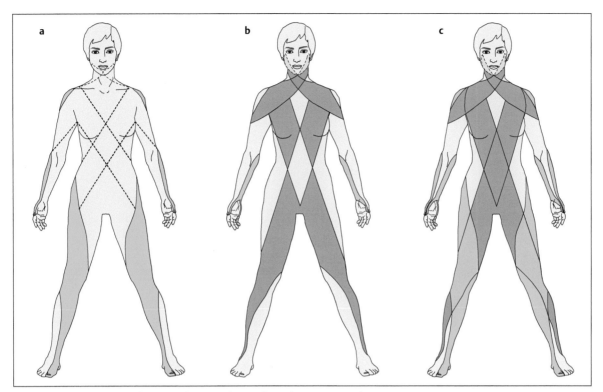

▶ **Fig. 2.15 (a–c)** Diagonal anterior chain or "closing chain" (as per Busquet).

Connection to the Right Shoulder
- Right transverse muscle of thorax.
- Right smaller pectoral muscle.
- Ascending part of right trapezius.
- Right anterior serratus.
- Right rhomboid muscles.

Connection to the Right Arm
- Right greater pectoral muscle.
- Right teres major.
- Right rhomboid muscles.

Connection to the Cervical Spine
- Right scalene muscles.
- Left splenius muscle of neck (cervicis/colli).

Connection to the Head
- Right subclavius.
- Right SCM.
- Left splenius muscle of head (capitis).
- Descending part of left trapezius.

Connection to the Lower Extremities
- Pyramidal muscle (abdominis).

Dominance of this muscle chain on the leg causes ilium inflare, internal rotation and abduction of the hip, valgus of the knee and hindfoot, and pronation of the foot and hallux valgus.

The following muscles are involved in this chain:
- Ilium inflare: internal oblique muscle of abdomen.
- Adduction and internal rotation of femur: adductors, pectineal muscle.
- Internal rotation of tibia: gracilis, semitendinous muscle, vastus medialis.
- Valgus of the knee: lateral gastrocnemius.
- Valgus of the calcaneus and pronation of the foot: peroneal muscles, abductor muscle of little toe, abductor muscle of great toe (abductor hallucis).

Functions of the Myofascial Muscle Chain

- The five muscle chains are responsible for all movements of the trunk.
- The two anterior straight chains perform flexion.
- The two posterior straight chains perform extension.
- The right anterior and the posterior straight chains perform rightward inclination.
- The left anterior and the posterior straight chains perform leftward inclination.
- The left anterior diagonal chain performs left anterior trunk torsion.
- The right anterior diagonal chain performs right anterior trunk torsion.
- The left posterior diagonal chain performs left posterior trunk torsion.

- The right posterior diagonal chain performs right posterior trunk torsion.
- The right anterior diagonal chain and the left posterior diagonal chain perform rightward trunk rotation.
- The left anterior diagonal chain and the right posterior diagonal chain perform leftward trunk rotation.

- The left anterior and the left posterior diagonal chains perform left translation.
- The two anterior diagonal chains "close the body."
- The two posterior diagonal chains "open the body."

2.5 Paul Chauffour: Mechanical Link in Osteopathy

Paul Chauffour's Biomechanical Chains

In his book *Le Lien Mécanique Ostéopathique*,[45] Paul Chauffour, a French osteopath, provides a very clear description of the topography and functions of fasciae as well as their attachment points on the skeleton. In a chapter about "osteofascial biomechanics" (biomécanique ostéo-faciale), he also illustrates the role of myofascial chains for the four main movements of the body:

- Flexion = curling up.
- Extension = stretching.
- Torsion toward anterior.
- Torsion toward posterior.

He provides detailed descriptions of the biomechanical processes in the areas of the spine, thorax, extremities, and cranium.

Chauffour draws an interesting connection between cranial and parietal biomechanics.

In another part of his book, Chauffour describes his approach to diagnostics and treatment. His method employs very gentle fascial compression and traction tests.

Chauffour's treatment consists of a type of reflective impulse following a complete examination by the osteopath. For this impulse, the therapist detects the greatest resistance in the affected segment in all spatial planes, builds up slight tension and then performs the impulse.

Of interest with this model are the myofascial explanations for the creation of dysfunctions.

In the following section, we will not describe the individual chains. Instead, we will focus on the explanations Chauffour provides for the creation of dysfunctions in the individual segments. Chauffour's myofascial chains are more or less identical to those of Leopold Busquet.

▪ Flexion Patterns

- C1: Tooth of axis (dens axis) prevents flexion of C1.
- C2: Subjected to particular stress, because C1 and lower cervical spine (cervical spinal column) flex less.

- C7: No longer stabilized by ribs and experiences fascial traction from the central tendon of diaphragm.
- T4: Lowest vertebra to experience fascial traction from the central tendon of diaphragm.
- Horizontal part of trapezius ends at T4; ascending part starts at T5.
- T6: Thoracolumbar fascia is securely attached to T7 via latissimus dorsi. This places stress on T6 during flexion.
- T12: Pulled toward posterior by the psoas.
- L1 and L2: Crura of the diaphragm exert traction on L1 and L2.

▪ Extension Patterns

- Region T1–T12 is compressed upward by the traction of the trapezius and downward by the traction of the latissimus dorsi.
- T7 therefore becomes particularly vulnerable.
- T11 is also under special pressure for the above reason.
- L2 is pulled by the diaphragm.

▪ Torsion toward Anterior

- C6: For Chauffour, C7 acts like a thoracic vertebra and C6 like a cervical vertebra. Counter-rotation during torsion causes stress between C6 and C7.
- C7: Has no joint connection with first rib and is therefore less stabilized.
- T4: Central tendon of diaphragm extends to T4 and slows down rotation of the upper thoracic spine (thoracic spinal column) during trunk torsion.
- T6: Aponeurosis of latissimus dorsi is attached to T7. This makes T6 more vulnerable.
- T10: Tenth rib stabilizes T10; this is not the case for T11 and T12.
- Torsion is clearly noticeable between T10 and T11.
- T11: T12 is the center of torsion and barely moves during torsion. This places stress on T11.
- L2: Crura of the diaphragm pull L2 along into the torsion.

■ Torsion toward Posterior

- C1: Subjected to stress because of the opposing lateral inclination between C1 and C2.
- C6: The same applies for C6 and C7.
- T6: Thoracolumbar fascia exerts more traction on the lower spinal column up to and including T7. This can cause conflict between T6 and T7.

- T10: T11 turns further than T10; this creates stress between T10 and T11.
- T12: Trapezius is attached up to T12 and is therefore pulled further into the torsion than L1.

2.6 Summary of Myofascial Chain Models

To our knowledge, Kabat was the first person to emphasize the importance of chains for treating weak muscles. He based his explanation on the fact that the brain knows only motion patterns, not individual muscles. This led Kabat to develop a series of motion patterns without describing continuous chains from hand to foot. His treatment methods are based on neurophysiologic findings, which subsequently formed the basis for other muscle energy techniques.

Godelieve Denys-Struyf was the first person to talk about muscle chains that encompass the whole body. She views psychological factors as the main reason for the development of dominating muscle chains. Inner influences shape the body's outer form—structure follows function. The muscle chains described by Denys-Struyf exhibit continuity in the cranium and influence the shape of the cranium. Since there are genetic causes for the dominance of muscle chains, it is impossible to extinguish a dominant chain. Therapists can only achieve "balance within imbalance."

Thomas Myers presents probably the most complex system of muscle chains. It is difficult to detect motion patterns in his system, but one needs to consider that Rolfing therapists focus on different priorities than osteopaths.

The two French osteopaths Paul Chauffour and Leopold Busquet present interesting models. Paul Chauffour provides detailed descriptions of the biomechanics of the locomotor system and of the cranium with different motion patterns. His holistic motion patterns, which include cranial movements, are interesting. Leopold Busquet deals more directly with the musculature in muscle chains. He also draws connections to the cranial system, without explicitly basing his explanation of the dysfunctions described by Sutherland on muscle chains. Busquet's explanation of visceral causes for parietal posture problems references the fascial connections of the organ suspension system. Depending on the organ dysfunction, the musculature is programmed to create an environment that is most optimal for the organ to function. He provides clear descriptions of myofascial imbalances as the cause of posture problems of the spine, dysfunctions, and pathologies of the joints and periarticular structures.

3 Physiology

In clinical practice, therapists need to be able to diagnose the condition of the tissues to be treated as precisely as possible to provide focused therapy. This requires a good understanding of the tissue components.

3.1 Connective Tissue

Embryologically, connective tissue develops from the mesoderm and forms wide-meshed cell units with intercellular substance.

Cells

Cells consist of fixed cells, connective tissue cells, and wandering (ameboid) cells.

■ Fixed Cells

Fixed cells derive from the mesenchyme and include the following:
- Fibroblasts and fibrocytes.
- Reticular cells.
- Lipocytes (adipocytes).
- Chondroblasts and chondrocytes.
- Osteoblasts and osteocytes.

■ Wandering (Ameboid) Cells

Wandering cells derive from bone marrow cells (hematopoietic stem cells) and include the following:
- Macrophages.
- Monocytes.
- Histiocytes.
- Mast cells.
- Granulocytes.
- Lymphocytes.

Wandering cells play a key role in cellular immune response.

Intercellular Substance

Intercellular substance, also called matrix, consists of all extracellular components of connective tissue. In addition to water, it contains components that are produced by connective tissue cells.

■ Ground Substance

Ground substance consists of proteoglycans and glycosaminoglycans (GAG) (mucopolysaccharides), which connect collagen and elastic fibers and bind with water. Ground substance provides strength and resilience to connective tissues. It stabilizes connective tissue and maintains tissue elasticity. It absorbs some of the forces acting on tissues ("shock absorber") and returns tissues to their original shape following strain. Proteoglycans and GAG linked together create a tension field in the tissue.

Changes in pressure in the tissue cause the cells to absorb or emit water. This creates fluctuations in tissue tension referred to as **piezoelectric activity**. Piezoelectric activity stimulates the cells to synthesize and to orient collagen molecules. This property can be utilized in fascial treatment techniques.[111]

■ Fibers

Fibers can be divided into the following:
- Collagen fibers.
- Elastic and reticular fibers.
- Noncollagenous proteins.

Collagen Fibers or Fibrils

Collagen is derived from the Greek words "kólla" and "-gen," meaning "glue producing." Collagen fibers provide white color to tissue. They are the second largest component of connective tissue besides water. They consist of individual fibers twisted into spirals that can assume certain shapes depending on strain (pressure or traction). Collagen fibers are found in ligaments, capsules, tendons, aponeuroses, intermuscular septa, cartilage, and intervertebral disks.

Functions

- Collagen provides stability to tissue.
- Collagen absorbs tensile (tractive) forces.
- Collagen counteracts compression forces.

Properties

- Collagen exhibits high tensile strength.
- Collagen molecules arrange themselves in the direction of tensile or compressive forces to counteract these forces. Where tensile direction remains constant, collagen fibers align parallel to each other (tendons, ligaments).
- Where tensile directions change, collagen fibers form a crisscross pattern (aponeuroses).
- Thickness and stability of collagen fibers depend on the strain they are exposed to. Targeted exercise or strain increases the thickness and resistance of collagen fibers.
- Turnover for collagen fibers is about 300 to 500 days.

Elastic Fibers

Elastic fibers are found primarily in loose connective tissue (skin, vessels, elastic cartilage), but also in tendons and ligaments. Elastic fibers contain elastin, which is yellow in color. Vessels contain about 50% elastic fibers, skin and tendons about 5%.
Yellow ligaments (ligamenta flava) consist primarily of elastic fibers, which explains their yellow color.

Functions

- Elastic fibers provide elasticity and mobility to tissues.
- In tendons and ligaments, elastic fibers help collagen fibers maintain their wave-shaped arrangement.
- Elastic fibers absorb tensile and compressive forces and then transfer them evenly to collagen fibers.

Properties

- Elastic fibers consist of elastin, a shapeless substance, surrounded by microfibrils. These elastic microfibrils are highly ramified and interconnected, which creates a highly elastic network. Elastic fibers can stretch by more than 150%.
- Elastic fibers exhibit a tensile strength of 300 N/cm².
- The tensile strength of elastic fibers increases with stretching: fiber resistance grows as it is being stretched.

Noncollagen Protein

These networking and interconnection proteins are found throughout the connective tissue. They can be produced by all connective tissue cells.

Functions

Noncollagen proteins:

- Interconnect the extracellular components of connective tissue. This creates a network that enables connective tissue to function.
- Participate in metabolic processes by enabling the transport of substances through connective tissue and by influencing cell polarity.
- Form links between proteoglycans and hyaluronic acid chains to bind water in the tissue, which enables tissues to absorb pressure.

■ Water

About 60% of our body weight consists of water. Seventy percent of this water is intercellular and 30% is extracellular.

In the extracellular space, water is distributed as follows as:

- Interstitial fluid in intercellular tissue.
- A component of blood in blood vessels.
- A component of liquor.
- Axoplasmic fluid in nerves.

Functions

- Acts as transport medium and solvent.
- Provides volume and shape to tissue.
- Absorbs impacts ("shock absorber").
- Plays a role in thermoregulation.
- Facilitates metabolic processes.

Connective Tissue Supply

Capillaries carry nutrients and oxygen into tissues. Veins and lymphatic vessels transport waste out of the interstitial space. Within connective tissue, cells are supplied by diffusion and osmosis.

■ Diffusion

Diffusion involves movement of solutes down concentration gradients. The amount of diffused matter depends on the concentration gradient, particle size, diffusion surface, tissue viscosity, and the distance particles need to travel.

■ Osmosis

Osmosis is a type of diffusion that moves a solute across a semipermeable membrane up a concentration gradient. The particles making up the higher concentration substance are too large to move across the membrane pores. Smaller particles diffuse and join the larger particles until the concentration is in equilibrium.

The autonomic nervous system plays an important role in permeability. Autonomic nerve cells release neurotransmitters that increase the permeability of cell walls. Neuropeptides stimulate adrenaline, noradrenaline, acetylcholine synthesis, and the release of pain substances, immunoglobulins, and histamine.

The development and maintenance of connective tissue requires physiological strain.[12] Muscles, tendons, and ligaments need to be tensed and optimally stretched. Cartilage and disks need to be stimulated by compression and decompression.

Motion improves general circulation in the tissue and promotes piezoelectric activity. Both contribute to cell synthesis. For ligaments and tendons, it is important that they are stretched longitudinally to stimulate the orientation of collagen fibers.

"Creep" Phenomenon

Creep is caused by a distortion of the collagen network and collagen fibrils. It squeezes fluid out of tissues. Since this is a slow process, duration of strain is a key factor. Creep causes tissue to lose its elasticity, because fluid content in the tissue is partly responsible for its malleability.

3.2 Muscles

Myofibrils are the smallest components of muscles and come in two parts, actin and myosin filaments, which provide the stripes that are characteristic of striated muscles. Myofibrils are grouped into bundles of 100 to 200 and form skeletal muscle cells or muscle fibers. Their diameter ranges from 10 to 100 μm.

The cell membranes of muscle fibers are called sarcolemma and enclose not only the myofibrils, but also sarcoplasm, several cell nuclei, mitochondria, lysosomes, glycogen granules, and fat droplets. Muscle fibers join into fiber bundles (100–1,000 μm). These bundles are surrounded by membranes that join the membranes of other fiber bundles to transition into muscle tendons.

We distinguish between two types of muscles:
- Smooth muscles.
- Striated muscles.

Smooth muscles differ from striated muscles as follows:
- Smooth muscles do not contain horizontal striations. They consist of actin and myosin, but lack thick filaments (bipolar myosin filaments) and do not contain sarcomeres.
- Smooth muscles are stimulated autonomously:
  - Either by ion gap junctions as is the case for most organs. These muscles contract largely independent of external nerve impulses. Stretching of smooth muscles causes depolarization and increases muscle tone (myogenic tone).
  - Or by stimuli from autonomic nerves, for example, iris, vas deferens, and blood vessels (which also have a myogenic tone).

3.3 Fasciae

Fasciae are one component of connective tissue. Other components include subcutaneous tissue, skin, muscles, tendons, and ligaments. Connective tissue also contains collagen, elastic and reticular fibers, mucous cells, bone tissue, and cartilage cells. It is made up of fibroblasts, fibroglia, collagen fibers, and elastic fibers.

All body cells are surrounded by fasciae. Fasciae connect all cells. They provide support and shape to the body.

Functions of Fasciae

Fasciae perform several functions, referred to by Kuchera and Kuchera[82] as packaging, protection, posture, and passageway.

▪ Packaging

Fasciae provide investments (covers) for all body structures. They simultaneously separate and connect individual structures. Their resilience keeps them in place and characterizes their mobility.

▪ Protection

Fasciae provide support and protection to structures by enveloping all organs. Varying degrees of tissue density provide resilience to structures, keep them in place, and characterize their mobility.

■ Posture

Posture is determined by the locomotor system. The body's fascial structures contain proprioceptors that provide information about movements and position of the body. Posture tone and necessary adaptations to externally induced posture changes are provided by muscle spindles, Golgi's tendon receptors in the muscles, and Pacini's and Golgi's corpuscles in ligaments and capsules. Muscles play an active role in this process, while fasciae constitute a connecting element.

Fasciae contain large numbers of free nerve endings and pain receptors. Some authors (Becker[8] and Upledger and Vredevoogd[148]) attribute memory functions to tissues. They surmise that certain motion patterns, traumas, and injuries are stored at the fascial level. How this happens remains unresolved. Biochemical, physical, and energetic processes have been proposed as causative factors. Connective tissue stores the energy of an injury in "energy cysts." **Therapists can feel and treat these tissue changes.**

■ Passage

Fascia form vessel passageways for nerves, arteries, veins, and lymphatic vessels. Connective tissue forms secretory and excretory channels. For this reason, fasciae play an important role in all metabolic processes. Fascial tensions can influence organ functions and metabolism because connective tissue shapes organs (liver, pituitary gland, adrenal gland) and forms vesicles that contain enzymes and hormones (gall bladder, lymph nodes).

The condition of connective tissue is a key determinant for homeostasis of the organism.

Manifestations of Fascial Disorders

■ Somatic Dysfunctions

Fascial tensions initiate somatic dysfunctions by impacting receptors, vessels, and nerves.

■ Metabolic Disorders

Tensions impact circulation in the interstitial space and tissue metabolism. This leads to palpable tissue changes (trigger points, swelling, fibrosis).

■ Fascial Disorders

These manifest as swellings. Certain regions are particularly susceptible: supraclavicular triangle, armpit, groin, back of the knee, and epigastrium.

■ Respiratory Changes

Myofascial tensions impact posture and pressure ratios in the abdomen and thorax. This directly influences thoracic pump function.

■ Posture Disorders

Posture is a compromise between stability and mobility. Myofascial chains act like a generator. Unbalanced or excessive strain causes posture problems and malfunctions.

■ Development of Myofascial Patterns

Certain fascial patterns are found in both healthy and ill people. Its causes are unknown (congenital or acquired).

Asymptomatic people exhibit alternating fascial tracks:
- Occipitoatlantoaxial (OAA) complex: right → left.
- Cervicothoracic junction (CTJ): left → right.
- Thoracolumbar junction (TLJ): right → left.
- Lumbosacral junction (LSJ): left → right.

J. Gordon Zink found this pattern in 80% of all cases. In the remaining 20%, fascial tracks presented in the opposite direction.

In cases of dysfunction, we do not find these alternating fascial tracks. Instead, we find the same myofascial track at two consecutive junctions.

■ Systemic Changes

Tissue tension causes changes in tissue circulation. These change structural functions and cause functional and then structural damage.

Evaluation of Fascial Tensions

- Anamnesis: provides clues regarding fascial tensions.
- Observing posture: fascial tensions manifest in posture problems (in the three planes of motion).
- Testing fascial preferences in the junctions: dominant dysfunction is located where rotation is most palpable.
- Palpating the tissue for contractions, fibrosis, and swelling.
- Mobilizing the extremities to identify muscular imbalance by comparison.

> *Important:* The diaphragm is particularly important for myofascial chains as an active factor for muscles and for circulation. It is also the main regulator for pressure ratios in all body cavities.

Causes of Musculoskeletal Dysfunctions

The following factors can cause myofascial changes (listed in random order):
* Posture imbalances.
* Life habits, stress: work, leisure.
* Congenital deformities: differences in leg length, scoliosis.
* Perinatal trauma.
* Emotional stress factors: introverted, extroverted.
* Repetitive stretching, strain during work or leisure activities.
* Hypomobile or hypermobile joints, rheumatic changes.
* Trauma, inflammation.
* Infection.
* Illness.
* Immobilization.
* Metabolic disorders, dietary issues (e.g., lack of vitamin C impacts formation of collagen fibers in tissue).
* Nerve lesions due to changes in trophic nerve function.

Genesis of Myofascial Disorders

Biochemical, biomechanical, and psychological dysfunctions can stress myofascial structures.
Leon Chaitow[40] postulated the following scenario:
* Functional disorders in the organism cause local increases in muscle tone.
* Increase in muscle tone reduces elimination of waste products and causes shortages in local oxygen supply. This leads to ischemia (depends on degree of muscle exertion).
* Increased tone can cause local edemas.
* These factors (waste products, ischemia, swelling) cause tension and pain.
* Tension and pain cause or increase hypertonicity.
* Hypertonicity can cause inflammation or, at a minimum, chronic irritation.
* This causes segmental facilitation at the level of the spinal cord.
* Macrophages and fibroblasts are activated.
* Production of connective tissue increases, creating links. This causes indurations and contractions.
* Because of the continuity of fasciae, tension arises in other areas of the organism and impacts lymph and blood circulation.
* Vascular disturbances cause muscle tissue fibrosis.
* In a chain reaction, this causes contractions of postural muscles and weakens phasic muscles.
* Contracted muscles cause tensions in tendons and pain in the periosteum.

* These muscle imbalances result in movement coordination problems.
* This causes articular dysfunctions and additional fascial changes.
* Segmental facilitation at the spinal cord level continues to progress and trigger points develop in muscles.
* Muscle contractures cause energy loss.
* Other body systems are impacted by hypertonicity, for example, respiratory function and digestion.
* Over time, hypertonicity, muscle contractures, and nerve facilitation cause increased sympathetic tone and negative feedback in the central nervous system (CNS). This results in restlessness and irritability, which further increase tensions.
* In this state, other functional problems can occur.
* This opens the door for acute pathologies. The person is no longer able to extricate themselves from their misery without help.

Pains associated with this process can be explained by the release of tissue hormones. Bradykinin, histamine, serotonin, and prostaglandins irritate alpha, delta, and C-fibers. The limbic system and the frontal lobes of the cerebrum are also involved.

Pain perception varies from one person to the next and differs depending on the situation. Studies[2,40,41,9,113] demonstrated that emotional stress lowers the pain threshold, as do infections.

When stimuli such as microtraumas progressively impact the organism, they are more likely to raise the pain threshold. Acute traumas, on the other hand, lower the pain threshold because the body attempts to minimize the damaging effects of nociceptive stimulation for as long as possible (release of tissue hormones, inflammation, release of macrophages, fibroses, etc.). We should also mention that pain pathways are fast conductors, while the pathways that conduct impulses from the joints are slow.

Pain Patterns

Pain indicated by a person in a certain area of the body can be a manifestation of several phenomena: radicular pain, referred pain syndrome, pseudoradicular pain, myofascial trigger points, tender points, or viscerosomatic reflexes.

■ Radicular Pain

* Pain area matches the regions supplied by the segment.
* Sensory disturbance present in the supplied areas.
* Sometimes loss of strength in the muscles supplied by the segment, to the point of atrophy.
* Weakened tendon reflexes.

Referred Pain Syndrome

Nonradicular projected pain, for example, Head's zones.

Pseudoradicular Pain

Pain caused by a peripheral nerve irritation radiating into certain skin regions: for example, femoral neuralgia due to psoas contracture.

Tender Points

These are pressure-sensitive points (indurations) in certain areas of the locomotor system. These points may originate from strains, stretching, or motor system stress.[40,43,82,145,156] Tender points are not always located in the areas indicated as painful by the patient. They serve as a diagnostic tool and as indicators for treatment progress.

Viscerosomatic Reflexes

Somatic organ dysfunctions send afferent impulses to the posterior horn of the spinal cord, where they communicate with interneurons. Motor and sympathetic fibers then transmit these stimuli to muscles, skin, and vessels.[35,46,79,82,156]

These abnormal stimuli can result in skin hypersensitivity, vasoconstriction, or increased sudomotor activity. Simultaneously, muscular hypertonicity can arise in the muscles motorically supplied by the segment.

Viscerosomatic reflex activity is usually present before an organ consciously manifests symptoms. Skin changes, perspiration changes, and hypertonicity of paravertebral muscles are important diagnostic tools. When the pathology becomes chronic, structural changes in the tissue occur: skin becomes less sensitive (numbness) and muscles tend toward fibrosis.

The intensity of symptoms relates directly to the degree of organ pathology.

Generally, viscerosomatic reflexes indicate that several segments are limited in their mobility.

Trigger Points

Trigger points are a palpable, pressure-sensitive mass found in muscle tissue. The pain experienced when trigger points are palpated is local and radiates out into a predictable region in the same way in every person. Trigger points are "facilitated" musculature areas that can be activated by subliminal stimuli, similar to spinal column segments.[38,40,43,82,145,156]

In general, trigger points are found in tensed fibers of the affected muscle, usually near the insertion of the muscle. These muscle fibers can be "plucked" using a finger, like guitar strings.

> *Important:* Some types of somatization disorders involving impaired vision, respiratory problems, or motoricity disorders and dysesthesia can stem from impulses that originate in trigger points. In fact, people impacted by somatization disorders often exhibit trigger points.

Another phenomenon seen with trigger points is that active trigger points can cause the formation of silent or latent trigger points in muscles located in the region into which the active trigger points radiate. This may explain a snowball effect seen in certain pain syndromes.

Notes:

- Per Melzack and Wall, ± 80% of all acupuncture points are active and inactive trigger points.[38,40]
- Many authors believe that Lawrence Jones' tender points are actually inactive trigger points.[40,145]
- Emotional factors are the strongest stimuli for the formation and activation of trigger points.
- Certain muscles are more frequently impacted by trigger points (e.g., trapezius, pectoralis, piriformis).
- Treatment varies and includes the following:
  - Injections.
  - Acupuncture.
  - Cooling spray.
  - Friction, acupressure.
  - Myofascial release.
  - Muscle energy technique (MET).
  - Strain counterstrain (SCS) technique.
  - Positional release therapy (PRT; relaxation by body positioning).

Some of these treatment methods are covered in detail in later parts of this book.

3.4 Vegetative Innervation of Organs

In this section, we present a brief overview of the segmental supply of organs. Via viscerosomatic reflexes, organ dysfunctions can be starting points for postural imbalances and restricted mobility:

Eyes	T1–T4
Lacrimal and salivary glands	T1–T4
Paranasal sinuses	T1–T4
Carotid sinus, carotid body	T1–T4
Thyroid gland	T1–T4
Trachea	T1–T6
Bronchi	T1–T6
Esophagus	T1–T6
Cardia	T5–T6
Mammary glands	T1–T6
Aorta	T1–T6
Heart	T1–T6
Lung	T1–T6
Stomach	T6–T9
Pylorus	T9
Liver	T5–T9
Gall bladder and cystic duct	T6–T9
Spleen	T6–T9

Pancreas	T6–T10
Duodenum, upper section	T6–T9
Duodenum, lower section	T10–T11
Small intestine	T9–T11
Large intestine overall	T10–L2
Cecum	T11–T12
Ascending colon	T11–L1
Descending colon	L1–L2
Adrenals	T10–T11
Kidneys	T10–T11
Ureter	T11–L1
Bladder (urinary)	T12–L2
Testes	T12–L2
Sigmoid colon	L1–L2
Rectum	L1–L2
Uterus	T12–L2
Ovaries	T10–T11
Prostate	T10–T11
Upper extremities	T2–T8
Lower extremities	T9–L2

3.5 Irvin M. Korr

If osteopathy owes recognition and gratitude to a nonosteopath, it is certainly Irvin M. Korr. In addition to Louisa Burns and John Stedman Denslow, Korr has contributed 50 years of research to provide scientific explanations for the causes and effects of somatic dysfunctions. It is largely due to Korr's work that vertebral blockages are no longer viewed as joint blockages, but rather as neuromusculoarticular dysfunctions.

It is impossible to provide even an overview of Korr's work within the context of this book. We therefore focus on those research results that we view as important for the topics covered in this book and recommend *The Collected Papers of Irvin M. Korr, Vols. I and II*[79] for more information.

Significance of Somatic Dysfunctions of the Spine for the Entire Organism

Somatic dysfunctions of the spine:
- Lead to hypertonicity of the paravertebral muscles surrounding the dysfunctional segment.
- Result in sympathicotonia of the segment.

- Impact nerve conductivity.
- Lower the stimulus threshold of all receptors that depend on this segment.

Korr coined the terms *facilitated segment* and *neurologic lens*.

■ Facilitated Segment

Somatic spine dysfunctions lower the stimulus threshold of all nuclei in the impacted segment.

■ Neurologic Lens

A lowered stimulus threshold makes receptors in the facilitated segment more susceptible to lower stimuli. This has two consequences:
- Cerebral stimuli (emotions, stress, anxiety, anger) reach the stimulus threshold of the segment more easily and cause symptoms there more quickly (e.g., stomach pains in stress situations).
- Stimuli that would normally only reach neighboring segments can impact the facilitated segment.

Role of the Spinal Cord

■ Spinal Cord (Medulla) as Information and Control Center

Spinal cord segments receive information from the brain as well as from the periphery. Likewise, there are pathways from the spinal cord to the brain and to the peripheral structures. At the level of the spine, all nuclei are connected by interneurons. All inputs stimulate or inhibit each other to provide output that is appropriate for the needs of the moment.

The spinal cord is part of the CNS, which receives most afferents. Afferents that arrive in a segment of the spinal cord are in communication with neighboring segments via interneurons. This is important, for example, for the ability to carry out harmonious motions. It enables simultaneous activation of agonists, synergists, and stabilizers, and inhibition of their antagonists.

■ Spinal Cord as Reflex Center

Many vital reflexes are spinal reflexes (flexion reflex, crossed extensor reflex, tendon reflex). They are part of the plastic motion patterns of daily life (running, dancing, swimming, etc.). This prevents overload on the brain.

■ Spinal Cord Segments as Functional Starting Points

To perform a motion, muscles need to be activated and sufficiently vascularized. This is coordinated in a multisegmental plane.

Role of the Autonomic Nervous System

In several experiments, Korr showed how persistent sympathicotonia impacts human health. The sympathetic nervous system:
- Increases muscle strength and reduces muscle fatigue.
- Increases receptor sensitivity and lowers stimuli threshold.
- Impacts neuronal irritability and brain activity.
- Modulates metabolism and stimulates bone growth, lipolysis, and erythropoiesis.
- Influences the entire endocrine system.

These are vital processes that are essential for life. Persistent sympathicotonia has damaging consequences.

Significance of Nerves for Trophism

Nerves are conductors not only for nerve impulses, but also for peptides needed for tissue growth. Korr demonstrated experimentally how denervation leads to atrophy.

In other experiments, Korr's team showed how quickly posture imbalances stimulate the sympathetic nervous system in certain segments of the spine. Initial vegetative manifestations begin to appear as early as 1 hour after the occurence of an imbalance.

Another important discovery is the extreme sensitivity of muscle spindles. Muscle spindles react to a traction of 1 g and a stretch of 1/1,000 mm. This makes muscle spindles one of the most sensitive organs of the human body.

Other researchers have also studied somatic dysfunctions:

J.S. Denslow[2] showed that paravertebral muscles in blocked segments are more irritable and therefore respond to lower stimuli. These muscles respond to stimuli by increasing contraction.

Louisa Burns[2] studied the impact of somatic dysfunction on muscles and organs. She found microscopic tissue changes in as little as 96 hours.

Michael Patterson[112] explained that persistent facilitation leads to somatic dysfunctions.

Akio Sato[82,112] experimentally demonstrated somatovisceral reflex pathways and that somatic dysfunctions lead to organic dysfunctions.

In summary, these researchers showed that somatic dysfunctions of the spine lower the stimulus threshold of segments and stimulate the sympathetic nervous system. This causes visceral dysfunctions, among other things. Persistent facilitated state over a longer period can lead to chronicity of problems. Because of their sensitivity, muscle spindles play a key role in this process.

These findings illustrate the key role of the nervous system as a control and coordination entity. The CNS coordinates all organism functions as well as all adaptations to dysfunctions. For this reason, the spine plays a central role in diagnostics and treatment.

3.6 Sir Charles Sherrington

Sir Charles Sherrington was a neurophysiologist who published a series of interesting research results in 1947[162] Not only his findings contributed toward understanding the development of motion patterns, but we also have him to thank for **neurophysiological explanations** of the effectiveness of certain muscle techniques.

Inhibition of Antagonists or Reciprocal Innervation (or Inhibition)

Stimuli received by agonists lead to simultaneous inhibition of antagonists and activation of synergists.

Postisometric Relaxation

Muscle fibers relax and can be stretched more easily following contraction. This relaxation phase can last up to 15 seconds.

Temporal and Spatial Summation

Temporal (time) or spatial (place) summation (cumulative effect) of several above or below threshold individual stimuli produces impulses or effects that cannot be produced by a single stimulus.

Successive Induction

Antagonistic irritability increases immediately following contraction of the agonist.

These are only a few of the physiologic facts described by Sherrington that need to be kept in mind for the application of muscle techniques.

Another physiologic principle is of importance for posture and motion patterns: the **crossed extensor reflex**.

This reflex is a protective or flight reflex. For example, irritation of the right sole of the foot by a pain impulse causes hip, knee, and foot flexion. At the same time, interneurons stimulate the extensors of the left leg (▶ **Fig. 3.1**).

Certain motion patterns, for example, gait, exhibit the same phenomenon. Mitchell Jr. describes a similar phenomenon in cases of somatic dysfunction.[107]

Example: Right anterior ilium dysfunction is characterized by dominance of the muscles on the right side that cause anterior rotation of the ilium. The crossed extensor reflex activates muscles on the left side that cause a posterior rotation of the ilium. This makes the dysfunction even more obvious.

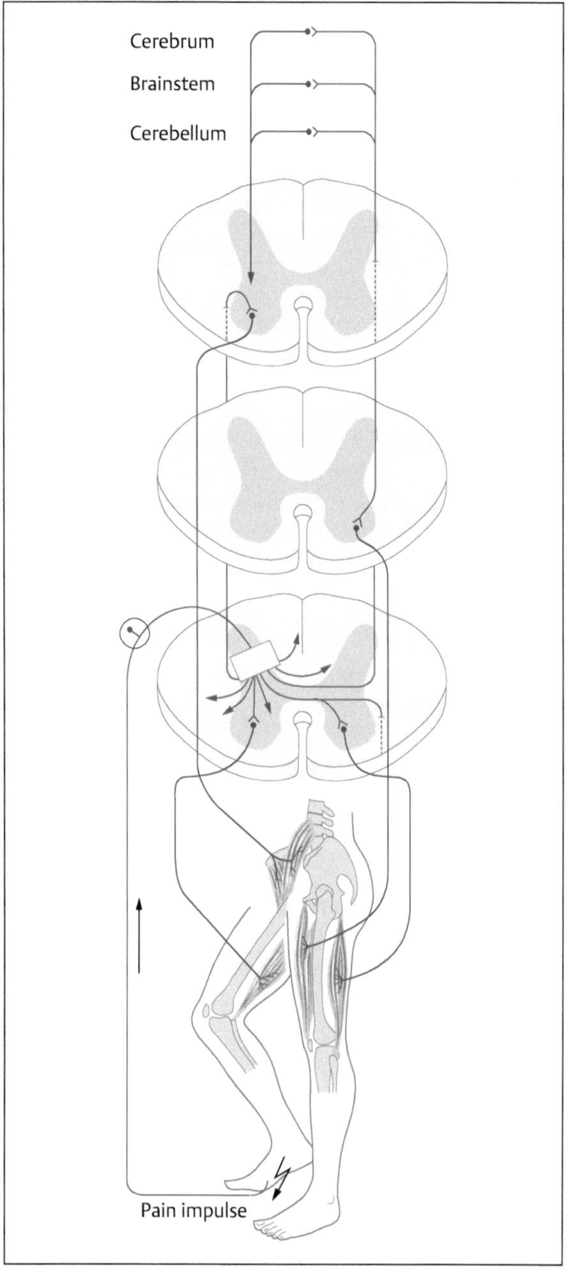

▶ **Fig. 3.1** Reflex communication between muscles. Cerebellum and brainstem participate to control frequently necessary balancing reactions. (From Hüter-Becker A, Hrsg. Das Neue Denkmodell in der Physiotherapie. Bd.1: Bewegungssystem. 2nd ed. Stuttgart: Thieme; 2006:294.)

3.7 Harrison H. Fryette

Harrison H. Fryette, one of Still's most brilliant students, is known in osteopathy for his analysis of the biomechanics of the spine.[56,121,125] Since their publication in the 1920s, "Fryette's laws" have been the primary explanatory model of spine physiology. Even though "Fryette's laws" are being questioned by many experts in manual therapy, his explanatory model nevertheless works well in practice. His discoveries are even more meritorious given that he did not have access to imaging technology for his studies.

Osteopathic dysfunctions are very complex processes that involve not only mechanical factors, but also other important causes. They encompass living tissue with specific characteristics (plasticity, hydrolytic characteristics, piezoelectricity). In addition, all motions are three dimensional and motion amplitudes can differ on each plane. These factors make it difficult to assert "laws." Nevertheless, Fryette's model represents a helpful concept in clinical practice, at least from a purely mechanical point of view.

Examining our patients, we find segmental dysfunctions and group lesions as described by Dr. Fryette. In motion tests, we can palpate the behavior of vertebrae and recognize "Fryette's Laws." It appears normal to us that this is often not possible because of the prevalence of congenital or acquired abnormalities and trauma.

Lovett's Laws

In 1907 another physician, Robert A. Lovett, published a paper in which he described the physiology of the spine. To conduct his studies, Lovett separated vertebral arches from their vertebral bodies, analyzed the behavior of both columns under strain, and derived the following rules:
- **Lumbar spinal column (LSC):** If the lumbar spine is forced into a sidebend, the vertebrae rotate into the concavity.
- **Thoracic spinal column (TSC):** When the thoracic spine performs a sidebend, the thoracic vertebrae always rotate into the convexity.
- **Cervical spinal column (CSC):** With the cervical spine, sidebending causes rotation into the concavity.

Since these findings were not borne out in practice, Fryette used a different method to examine the mechanics of the spine. He discovered that the behavior of the vertebrae differed, depending on whether the facets of the zygapophyseal (facet) joints were in contact or not. He found concordant rotation and sidebending of all vertebrae below C2 when the joint facets are in contact. If the facets are not in contact, the vertebrae sidebend and rotate in the opposite direction.

The starting point for a motion is essential for determining whether the joint surfaces of the zygapophyseal (facet) joints touch each other or not. Curvature of the spine and orientation of joint surfaces are other factors.

■ Lumbar Spinal Column

- The LSC is concave posteriorly.
- The facets are almost vertical in the sagittal plane.
- This isolates and limits rotation and sidebending, and facet contact occurs very quickly.

- Flexion of the LSC quickly causes contact of joint surfaces. During extension, on the other hand, contact occurs relatively late.

■ Thoracic Spinal Column

- The TSC is convex toward the back.
- The facets are oriented toward the back and outward and are located almost in the frontal plane.
- Due to the facets' position and kyphosis of the thoracic spine, extension is the parameter that first leads to facet contact.

■ Cervical Spinal Column

- The CSC is lordotic.
- The facets are oriented outward posteriorly and their position is impacted by lordosis. In the lower CSC (C5–C7), their vertical position is very pronounced; in the central and upper CSC distinctly less so.
- The uncinate processes of cervical vertebra and the saddle shape of the cervical plateau, however, only allow for concordant rotation and sidebending of the cervical vertebrae.
- The OAA complex exhibits its own physiology (atypical vertebra).

Fryette's Laws

■ First Law: Neutral Position– Sidebending–Rotation

Fryette called the neutral position "easy flexion." This refers to the range of motion in the sagittal plane between the points where facet contact occurs in flexion and extension.

When the spine sidebends from a neutral position, the vertebrae rotate into the newly formed convexity. This involves several vertebrae (▶ **Fig. 3.2**).

■ Second Law: Flexion (or Extension)– Rotation–Sidebending

When the spine sidebends from a flexion or extension position in which the facets are in contact, the vertebrae are forced to rotate to the same side (▶ **Fig. 3.3**). This is due to the orientation of the joint plane. This movement can be performed by a group of vertebrae, but also in isolation.

These are everyday physiological movements of the spine:
- With each step, the LSC and TSC perform neutral position–sidebending–rotation (NSR) movements and the CSC performs extension–rotation–sidebending (ERS) movements.

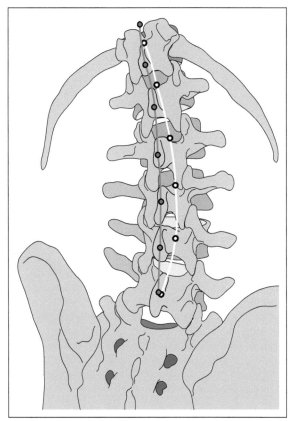

▶ **Fig. 3.2** Lumbar vertebrae adaptation to sidebending from neutral position (neutral position–sidebending–rotation). Adaptive lumbar curvature.

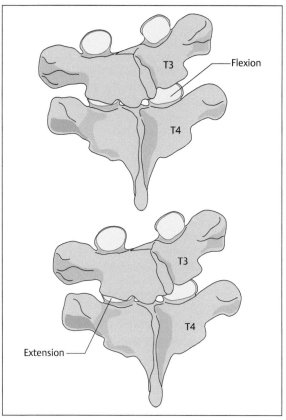

▶ **Fig. 3.3** Facet positions in flexion and extension.

- Each time we bend sideways while in a forward bend, at least one vertebra performs a flexion–rotation–sidebending (FRS) movement.

Similarly, during trunk extension with sidebending or rotation, at least one vertebra performs an ERS movement.

Gait as a Global Functional Motion Pattern

Gait is perhaps the most impressive example of an activity that involves the entire body. It illustrates how the entire locomotor system follows a certain motion pattern.[10,19,63,107]

All myofascial structures and all joints act as both propulsion organ and shock absorber.

The physiological processes of winding and unwinding (torque) that occur in the legs and trunk follow a specific pattern. The forward impulse during walking converts chemical energy created by muscle activity into kinetic energy that propels the body forward.[155] We can compare this motion pattern to a spring that unwinds when the leg swings and winds back up when

the weight lands on the heel again. The gait impulse starts when the heel touches the floor, the weight shifts forward, and the leg muscles transmit the movement through the pelvis toward the spine.

Harmonious and economical locomotion is made possible by (1) the fact that almost all joints support three-dimensional movement, (2) the sequence of lordosis and kyphosis from the sole of the foot up to the root of the nose, and (3) the arrangement of muscles into lemniscates. **This illustrates how function depends on structure.**

Note: In an interesting article, Gracovetsky (in[155]) sets forth the hypothesis that the anteroposterior curves of the spine not only are an adaptation to gravity, but also make forward movement more economical. Kypholordoses act like an anteroposterior leaf spring that is pressed together when the foot is set down and stretches out when the leg swings.

Howard J. Dananberg, a podiatrist and director of the Walking Clinic in New Hampshire, United States, impressively describes in an article titled "Lower Back Pain as a Gait-related Repetitive Motion Injury" (in[155]) how an extension deficit in the metatarsophalangeal (MTP) joint of the great toe can be the starting point for lumbar pain.

A stretch deficit of the great toe prevents the foot from rolling off completely while walking. The body compensates by increasing the posterior extension of the foot, flexing the knee, and flexing the hip. This creates imbalance between hip flexors and hip extensors, which shortens the length of the stride. The iliopsoas and quadratus lumborum respond with increased pelvis rotation to reestablish balance.

This example shows how a foot lesion is compensated by a specific muscle chain, which can lead to predictable dysfunction.

Gait Analysis

The following describes the gait cycle as viewed by most experts. The gait cycle can be divided into several phases. We focus on two phases:
- Swing phase.
- Stance phase.

Both phases occur simultaneously, with one leg being the stance leg and the other the swing leg. Body weight is balanced on the stance leg so that the other leg can be propelled forward (▶ **Fig. 3.5a-c**).

Swinging one leg forward rotates the pelvis toward the stance leg. This causes a counter-rotation toward the swing leg at the TLJ. This is illustrated by the movements of the arms, which oppose the leg movements.

During the swing phase, the hip is bent and the foot is extended posteriorly. The knee is bent during the first half and stretched during the second half, before the heel touches the ground.

In the stance phase (▶ **Fig. 3.5d-f**), the hip is stretched. The knee is initially slightly bent and then stretched completely. The stance phase begins the moment the heel touches the ground. Then the foot rolls off from the heel to the great toe (▶ **Fig. 3.5g-i**).

In this context, the lower ankle joint takes on a special role. Dysfunction here will change the entire gait cycle. The opposing movements between pelvic girdle and shoulder girdle enable minimal movement of the head and the ability to look straight ahead.

While walking, the spine performs a snaking or "scoliotic" motion. The lumbar spine (LSC) becomes convex and turns into the swing side. The thoracic spine (TSC) becomes convex and turns into the stance side.

The pelvis performs a global rotation toward the stance side and a slight tilt to the swing side. During the gait cycle, changes also occur in the pelvis between sacrum and ilia. In this context, the pubic symphysis plays the role of a half-mobile rotational pivot. In the symphysis, rotations take place in accordance with the ilia rotations.

We can use the swing phase of the right leg as an example (▶ **Fig. 3.4**). This cycle begins when the left heel touches the ground and the right great toe loses contact with the ground. This orients the left ilium posteriorly and the right ilium anteriorly. The sacrum is in a neutral position between the two ilia. As soon as the right foot leaves the ground, weight is placed on the left leg. This causes ligamentous (and muscular) locking of the left sacroiliac joint (SIJ), which contributes to stabilizing the body.

To shift the weight to the left leg, the LSC makes a left sidebend, which shifts pressure to the short shank of the left SIJ. Concurrently, the pelvis tips to the right (by 5°, as per Di Giovanna and Schiowitz.[49]) The lower pole of the right SIJ is compressed by the weight of the right leg and the resulting muscle tension. This creates a left diagonal axis. The lumbar spine is in a neutral position, with a left sidebend and right rotation (NSR, as per Fryette). The sacrum below it rotates left, around a left diagonal axis (as per Mitchell.[107]) The ilia rotate together with the spine, which maintains constant tension in the ligaments.

During the swing phase of the right leg and the propelling phase of the left leg, the ilia rotate in the opposite direction. The right ilium rotates backward and the left ilium rotates forward. This motion is initiated by muscles and completed by the momentum of the motion (the law of economy is observed).

Note: The sacrum moves with the ilia and performs the same rotation and sidebend, only more slowly. It takes on the role of a ball bearing, whose task it is to maintain the force lines between the spine and the two ilia.

Muscle Activity while Walking

A detailed description of muscle activity would exceed the scope of this book. First, statements in the literature regarding the activity of individual muscles vary widely. Second, muscle chains are, in our opinion, more important than isolated muscles. Furthermore, analysis is made more difficult by the fact that some joints must be stabilized in several planes and motions happen three-dimensionally. Nevertheless, in Part B of this book, we describe the functions of individual muscles in the discussion about trigger points.

A classic example of muscle activity is the knee joint at the beginning of the stance phase. The hamstring muscles and the quadriceps muscle stabilize the knee in the sagittal plane. The muscles of the pes anserinus prevent valgus of the knee. The iliotibial tract is tensed because the tensor fasciae latae helps prevent adduction of the hip.

■ Swing Phase

At the onset of the swing phase, when the great toe leaves the ground, the iliopsoas and rectus femoris bend the hip, while the hamstring (ischiocrural) muscle group bends the knee. The anterior tibial muscle together with the toe extensors lifts the foot. At the conclusion of the swing phase, the quadriceps extends the knee. Shortly before and during the moment the heel

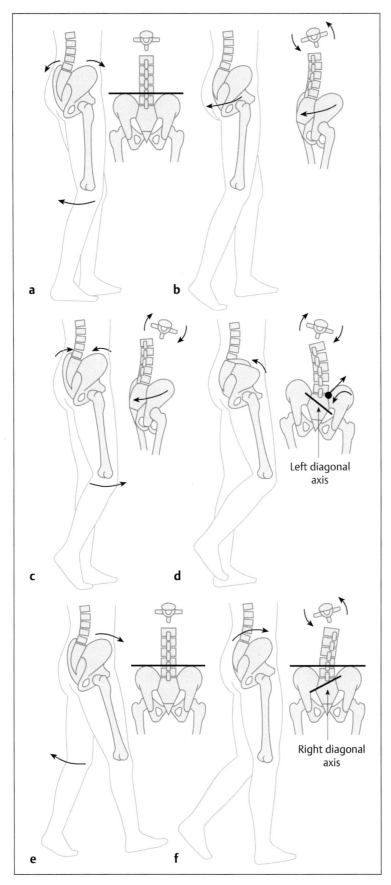

▶ **Fig. 3.4 (a–f)** Biomechanics and pelvic motion during each phase of the gait cycle. (From Brokmeier AA. Kursbuch Manuelle Therapie. Biomechanik, Neurologie, Funktionen. 3rd ed. Stuttgart: Hippokrates; 2001:86.)

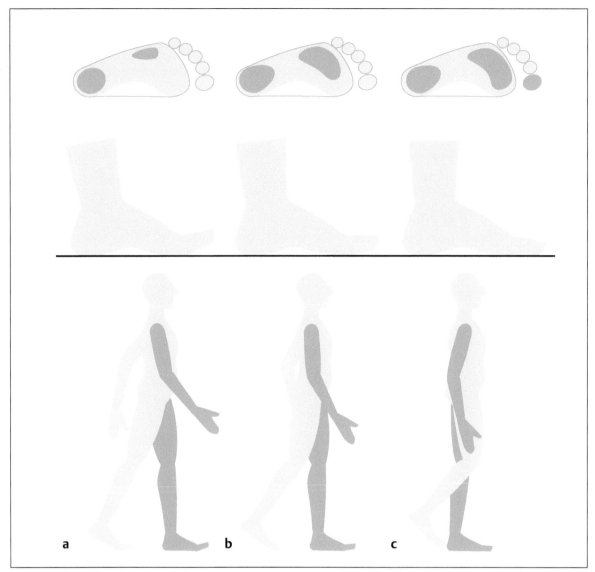

▶ **Fig. 3.5 (a–c)** Weight distribution during gait cycle phases.

touches the ground, the knee stabilizers are activated (see above). The leg swing phase therefore encompasses activation of the leg flexors.

■ Stance Phase

The stance phase begins when the heel touches the ground. The hip is flexed, the knee is extended, and the foot and toes are extended posteriorly.

The stance leg has two tasks:

- Maintaining leg and pelvis stability (abductors).
- Propelling the upper body forward (extensors).

Pelvis stability is maintained by the gluteal muscles, the tensor fasciae latae, and the iliotibial tract. Valgus of the knee is maintained by the pes anserine muscles and by the muscle chain of gluteus maximus–vastus lateralis–lateral patellar ligament. The varus of the foot is limited by the peroneal muscles. This chain is continued cranially via the gluteal muscles to the latissimus dorsi of the opposite side.

The upper body is propelled forward by extending the hip, knee, and foot. The main muscles responsible for this action are the gluteus maximus, quadriceps, triceps muscle of calf (triceps surae), posterior tibial muscle, peroneal muscles, and the toe flexors.

Of interest is that muscles that are activated in one motion phase are optimally positioned in the preceding phase, that is, they are placed into a stretched position. This is well illustrated by the counter-rotation of pelvis and shoulder girdles and the opposing movement of the arms and legs.

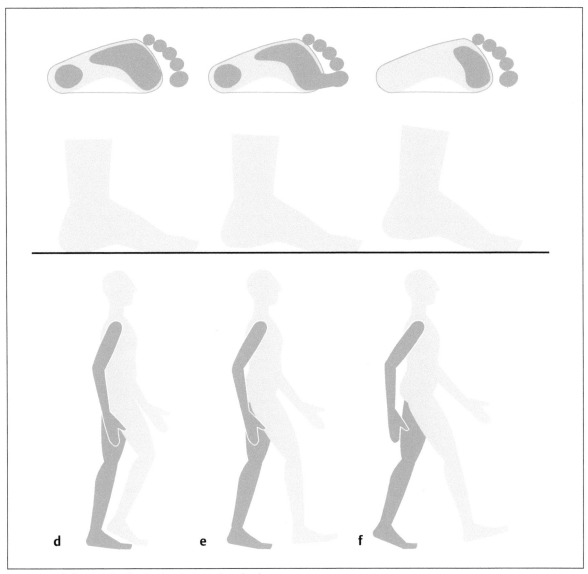

▶ **Fig. 3.5 (d–f)** Weight distribution during gait cycle phases.

When the right iliopsoas needs to pull the right hip forward, the left latissimus dorsi pulls the left arm backward and stabilizes the spine. This provides a stable basis for the psoas.

In their book *Les Pivots Ostéopathiques*, Ceccaldi and Favre[36] present gait as a harmonious interplay of muscle chains. The entire locomotor system follows the same pattern, which repeats itself with every step. The pelvis and spine perform specific movements around the pivots described by J.M. Littlejohn. These two authors extend Littlejohn's model to the extremities and describe additional pivot points in the sternocostoclavicular joint, knee joint, and lower ankle joint.

As mentioned earlier, the spine performs a scoliotic motion when the pelvis bends sideways during the swing phase. In this process, the lumbar vertebrae rotate to the side of the swing leg and the thoracic vertebrae rotate to the side of the stance leg, with L3 and T6 as the respective apex of the curvatures. The cervical spine performs a translation to the swing leg side while rotating to the other side (Fryette's second law).

This behavior can be illustrated by the hip drop test. This test imitates the gait cycle. We describe the behavior of the extremities in the section on muscle chains.

By recalling W.G. Sutherland's craniosacral model, we can deduce the movements of the sphenobasilar synchondrosis (SBS) and the entire cranium with every step.

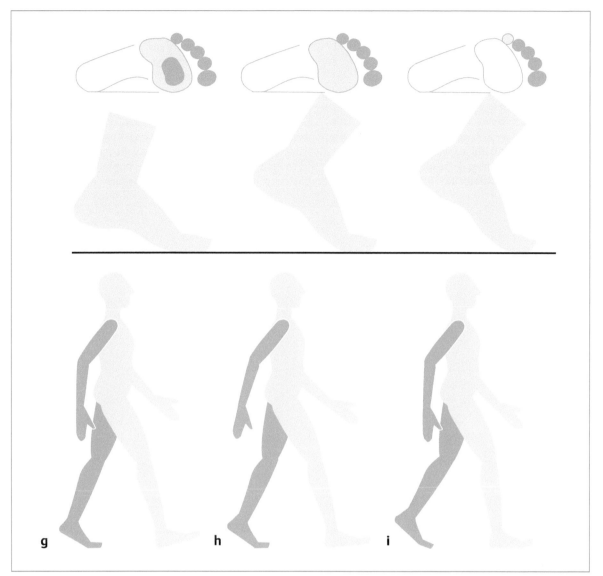

▶ **Fig. 3.5 (g–i)** Weight distribution during gait cycle phases. (From Brokmeier AA. Kursbuch Manuelle Therapie. Biomechanik, Neurologie, Funktionen. 3rd ed. Stuttgart: Hippokrates; 2001:114–116.)

Conclusion

Gait is a physiologic function of the entire locomotor system in which the organism acts like a spring. Opposing arrangements of lordosis and kyphosis from the sole of the foot to the head and the elasticity of ligaments, tendons, and fasciae make it possible to release the energy gained during the stance phase for the swing phase. This process maintains the law of economy.

The gait cycle illustrates two motion patterns. Flexion and extension alternate rhythmically.

While the extensor chain is active on one side, the flexor chain dominates on the other side (Sherrington's second law). This causes a torsion pattern of the spine (opposing rotation of pelvic and shoulder girdle). From a craniosacral perspective, this results in torsion of the SBS.

Harmonious locomotion requires structures that function normally. Hypomobility as well as hypermobility impact the motion pattern and result in postural and motoric dysfunctions.

Example: Dysfunctions of the first metatarsal bone toward posterior or of the talus toward anterior prevent the foot from rolling off. Over time, this causes a flexed position of the lower extremities and subsequent shortening of the psoas. This impacts the entire spine.

The motion pattern a therapist finds in a patient reflects the adaptive pattern of the entire organism to its dysfunction.

This phenomenon accords with the laws of economy, comfort (freedom from pain), and globality.

Note:

- Vleeming et al[155] postulate that the reason for premature fatigue while walking slowly, for example, during window shopping, is that walking slowly does not engage the spring principle. This means that muscles must work harder, especially muscles that are already overburdened by posture dysfunctions and imbalance.
- H.J. Dananberg makes some interesting statements about walking in his article [in[155]]. He puts forward that walking is a daily activity. Considering that a person walks an average of 80 minutes every day, this translates into around 2,500 steps a day and about 1 million steps a year.
- Certain occupations or sports activities can double or triple this number. Even minor imbalances can cause pain symptoms.
- In another article (in[155]), Gracovetsky hypothesizes that the reason for the special biomechanics of the cervical spine (CSC; Fryette's second law) could be that the CSC neutralizes the rotation of the shoulder girdle to maintain forward vision.

4 The Craniosacral Model

4.1 William G. Sutherland

Osteopaths need no introduction to William G. Sutherland. Therapists who utilize cranial osteopathy in their treatments have most likely heard of him. We do not want to present Sutherland's life and work here, but highlight those aspects that fit within the framework of this book.[54,89,101,102 136,142,143,144]

Among Still's students, Sutherland was probably the one who came closest to the master in his work. He recognized the significance of anatomy and biomechanics in the development and treatment of dysfunctions. At the same time, he was also aware of other factors that influence a person's health. Like Still, Sutherland was a religious person and this aspect influenced his treatments. The "breath of life," as he called it, flows through the entire body via the liquor and interstitial fluid. This was an important aspect of Sutherland's treatment method.

Sutherland underwent a remarkable development in his osteopathic work. Originally, mechanical aspects clearly dominated in his treatments. This is illustrated by the fact that in his beginning years, he considered cranial lesions to be mechanical malpositions and treated them accordingly. He developed a kind of turban or helmet to target specific cranial regions for treatment. He also compared the bones of the cranial base to vertebrae and the cranial dome (calvaria) to the transverse and spinous processes of vertebrae.

In the same way that we can deduce the position of vertebral bodies from the position of the spinous and transverse processes, the cranial dome can inform us about the position of the sphenoid and occiput.

From an embryological point of view, we can view the cranium as consisting of three modified vertebrae, with the occiput, sphenoid, and presphenoid (ethmoid) bones extending the spine toward the cranium (▶ **Fig. 4.1a**). Occiput and sphenoid form a concave forward curve that can be compared to the kyphosis of the thoracic spine (thoracic spinal column).

Sutherland used the same terms to describe the motions of the spine and the cranium (flexion, extension, torsion, and sidebending rotation). Sidebending rotation corresponds to extension–rotation–sidebending (ERS) or flexion–rotation–sidebending (FRS).

The embryonic development of the brain and head is responsible for the fact that the planes of movement in rotation and sidebending differ for the sphenobasilar synchondrosis (SBS). During the process of phylogenesis, the head bent forward to direct vision forward in the upright position.

While the sphenoidal and occipital bones rotate in a frontal plane, in sidebending rotation they bend around a vertical axis in a transversal plane (▶ **Fig. 4.1b, c**). Flexion and extension take place in a sagittal plane.

Years of clinical experience and experimentation led Dr. Sutherland to evolve his treatment methods over time toward increasingly gentle methods. For example, he realized that dysfunctions can also be treated indirectly by placing the joint or bone to be treated into a position that is as relaxed as possible and then allowing the body to do the work of correcting itself.

At the end of his career, Sutherland used liquor—or tide—for therapeutic purposes by directing liquor flow and utilizing respiration and motions of the extremities for support.

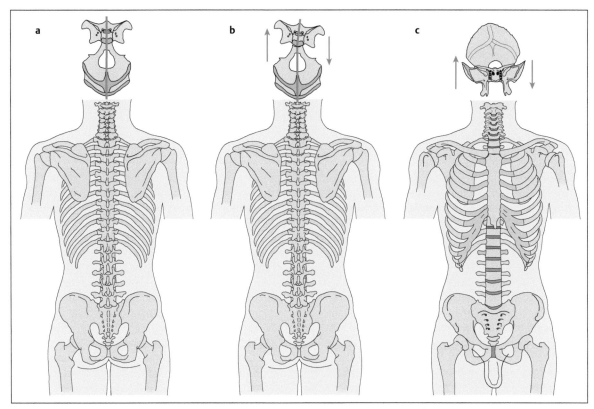

▶ **Fig. 4.1 (a)** Cranial "vertebrae." **(b)** Right bend of sphenoid bone. **(c)** Right rotation of sphenoid bone.

4.2 Biomechanics of the Craniosacral System

Craniosacral mechanism theory is based on five elements:

- Motility of the nervous system.
- Fluctuation of the cerebrospinal fluid (CSF).
- Reciprocal tension membranes (RTM): cerebral and cerebellar falx, cerebellar tentorium, and spinal dura mater (▶ **Fig. 4.2**).
- Mobility of the cranial bones.
- Involuntary mobility of the sacrum between the ilia.

We do not intend to present these five components of craniosacral therapy in detail and refer the reader to the relevant literature.[37,54,57,67,89,90,91,101,102,117,142,143,144,148,150] Nevertheless, a good understanding of this theory requires that we describe a few aspects in more detail.

Nervous system motility and liquor fluctuation are most likely at least partly responsible for the motions of the craniosacral system, that is, they serve as a kind of motor. However, harmonious motion patterns are primarily determined by interconnected membranes and bones.

The cranial dura mater adheres to the inside of the cranial bones with its parietal layer and connects to the periost via the sutures. The visceral layer is partly detached from the parietal layer and constitutes the cerebral membranes. These are arranged in such a way that they force the cranial bones to perform very specific motions during a cranial impulse.

The cerebral and cerebellar falx form a vertical sickle in the sagittal plane that runs from the crista galli of the ethmoid bone along the metopic suture and the sagittal suture to the internal occipital protuberance and from there to the foramen magnum. They form a dividing wall between the cerebral hemispheres and between the cerebellar hemispheres (▶ **Fig. 4.2**). The cerebral and cerebellar falx also connects the ethmoid bone, frontal bone, both parietal bones, and the occipital bone.

The cerebellar tentorium runs from the clinoid processes along the upper edge of the petrous part of temporal bone, the inside of the asterion, and then along the occiput up to the internal occipital protuberance. As such, the cerebellar tentorium separates the cerebrum from the cerebellum. The free edge of both sickles is in contact with the corpus callosum for the falx and with the midbrain (mesencephalon) for the tentorium. The tentorium connects the sphenoid, temporal, parietal, and occipital bones.

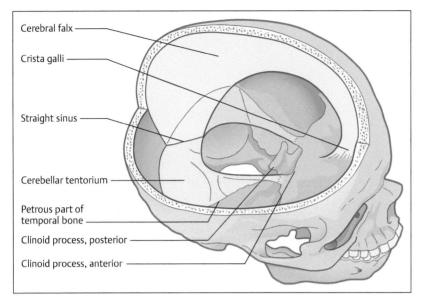

Cerebral falx

Crista galli

Straight sinus

Cerebellar tentorium

Petrous part of
temporal bone

Clinoid process, posterior

Clinoid process, anterior

▶ **Fig. 4.2** Intracranial membranes:
falx and tentorium. (From Liem T.
Kraniosakrale Osteopathie. Ein praktisches Lehrbuch. 5th ed. Stuttgart:
Hippokrates; 2010:233.)

It is significant that the intracranial membranes form the venous sinuses, the venous blood channels of the brain. Tensions in these membranes can impact venous drainage from the head. The two sickles, falx and tentorium, meet in the straight sinus, also called the "Sutherland fulcrum."

Another notable fact is that on the outside of the occiput the external occipital protuberance, which corresponds to the internal occipital protuberance inside the skull, serves as attachment point for the nuchal ligament.

Likewise, the transverse sinus, which is formed by the cerebellar tentorium on the inside of the occiput, is located on a line with the superior nuchal line, which serves as attachment point for the trapezius muscles.

Therefore, the nuchal ligament is the extension of the falx on the outside of the cranium (▶ **Fig. 4.3**), and the fascia of the trapezius muscles is the extension of the tentorium (▶ **Fig. 4.4**).

The cerebellar falx is solidly attached to the foramen magnum and transitions from there into the spinal dura mater. The spinal dura mater is formed only by the visceral layer, like the falx and tentorium, while the parietal layer passes into (or forms) the periost. The spinal dura mater hangs loosely in the entire spinal canal and is only solidly attached to the vertebrae at certain points.

In the cranial section, the spinal dura mater is connected to the foramen magnum and the second cervical vertebra and is solidly attached at the level of S1/S2 in the sacral area.

The spinal dura mater encloses the spinal cord and follows the peripheral nerves up to the intervertebral foramen, where it transitions into the outer nerve sheath. It is also attached to the bone in the intervertebral foramen.

There are also relatively loose attachments at the vertebrae bodies via the denticulate ligaments.

The dura mater is the outer envelope of the three meninges that envelop the central nervous system. The pia mater rests on top of the nerve mass. The arachnoid mater fills the space between the pia and dura mater, called subarachnoid space. This space is filled with liquor and serves as a kind of water bed for the brain and spinal cord.

The subarachnoid space is connected to the cerebral ventricles in which the liquor is produced (choroid plexus). Ninety-five percent of liquor reabsorption takes place in the arachnoid villi of the cranial venous sinuses. The remaining 5% is reabsorbed via the lymphatic system.

The dural system is a very resistant membrane that attaches to specific locations and forms a hoselike structure filled with CSF and nerve mass. It stands to reason that pressure or tension at one location spreads to the entire system. We can compare this to an air-filled balloon that is compressed in one spot. This pressure can be felt everywhere on the balloon. The entire dural system has five points of attachment. Their common anchor is the "Sutherland fulcrum" (▶ **Fig. 4.5**):

- In front, crista galli and clinoid processes.
- Laterally, two temporal bones.
- In back, occipital bone.
- Below, sacrum.

Of clinical significance is the fact that traction on one of these points affects all others via the Sutherland fulcrum. In other words: sacral malpositions impact the occipitoatlantoaxial (OAA) complex just as much as the temporal bone or sphenoid bone. The impact is even greater for the spine because sensitive muscle spindles here potentiate the impact.

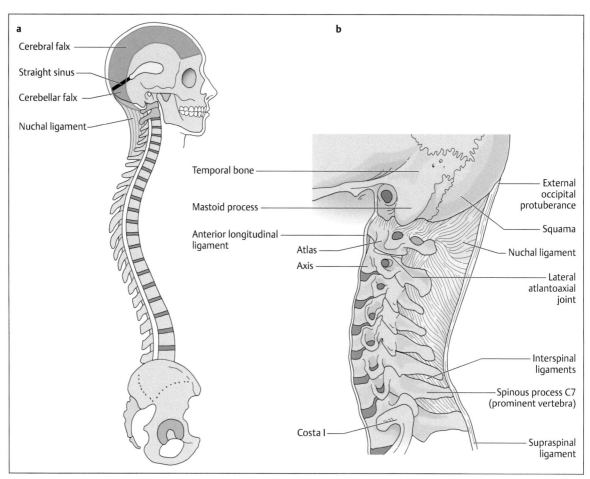

Cerebral falx

Straight sinus

Cerebellar falx

Nuchal ligament

Temporal bone

Mastoid process

Anterior longitudinal ligament

Atlas

Axis

Costa I

External occipital protuberance

Squama

Nuchal ligament

Lateral atlantoaxial joint

Interspinal ligaments

Spinous process C7 (prominent vertebra)

Supraspinal ligament

▶ **Fig. 4.3 (a, b)** Nuchal ligament as extension of falx.

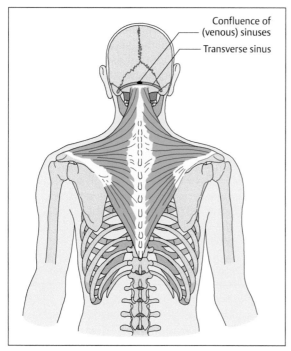

Confluence of (venous) sinuses

Transverse sinus

▶ **Fig. 4.4** Fascia of trapezius muscles as extension of the tentorium.

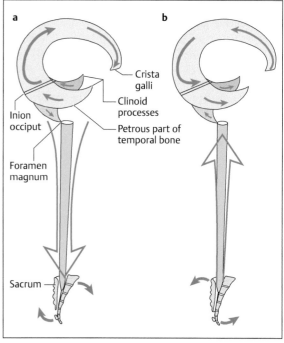

Crista galli

Clinoid processes

Petrous part of temporal bone

Inion occiput

Foramen magnum

Sacrum

▶ **Fig. 4.5 (a, b)** "Reciprocal tension membranes" with attachments.

While cranial sutures do not permit motion like the extremities or the spine, they do allow for plasticity. Motions related to craniosacral impulses do not cause volume changes in the cranium, but they do result in deformation of the entire hydraulic system, including the spine and pelvis. Since these motions proceed harmoniously, restrictions at one point of the system manifest everywhere.

If the dysfunction is significant enough, the whole system adapts to maintain function. This leads to structural adjustments, which ultimately cause structural or positional changes. This is the meaning of the term **reciprocal tension membranes.**

Note: Opinions differ about what triggers craniosacral motions. In general, it is assumed that fluctuations in the liquor cause tensions in the dural system, which in turn impacts the bones. The special anatomy of cranial sutures and the attachments of the dura are responsible for the specific motion patterns.

4.3 Motions and Dysfunctions of the Craniosacral Mechanism

For a detailed description of this topic, we refer the reader to the relevant literature. In this section, we focus on the information needed to understand the content that follows.

Flexion–Extension

When Sutherland defined the two stages of the craniosacral rhythm, he called them flexion and extension because he considered the SBS to be the center of motion. In this nomenclature, flexion of the SBS corresponds to a reduction in the angle between the basilar part of the occiput and the body of sphenoid bone. Extension corresponds to an increase of this angle.

■ Flexion

The occipital bone rotates posteriorly, and the sphenoid bone rotates anteriorly, while the SBS rises. Globally, both bones move anteriorly. This is important for the relationship between occiput and atlas. **In cranial flexion, the occipital bone slides forward over the atlas** (▶**Fig. 4.6a**). This corresponds to a mechanical extension of the occiput. The ethmoid bone, which is in front of the sphenoid bone, performs the same rotation as the occipital bone. The paired or peripheral bones rotate externally during flexion.

The forward motion of the occipital bone and upward motion of the basilar part shift the foramen magnum forward. This results in traction on the spinal dura mater toward cranial, which causes the base of the sacrum to be pulled upward. The sacrum then performs an extension motion and stretches the spine.

■ Extension

Extension of the craniosacral mechanism (▶**Fig. 4.6b**) causes motion in the opposite direction. The SBS drops, the occiput rotates forward, and the sphenoid bone rotates backward. **The basilar part and the foramen magnum move backward.** From a mechanical standpoint, this corresponds to a flexion of the occiput.

The dural tube drops and the sacrum moves forward into nutation. The ethmoid bone rotates forward, like the occiput. The peripheral bones rotate internally.

In addition to the physiological movements of flexion–extension, which are induced by the organism's inherent powers, the primary respiratory mechanism (PRM), Sutherland described other movements (torsion, sidebending rotation, vertical strain, and lateral strain), which are explained in the following sections.

Torsion

Like flexion and extension, torsion is a physiological motion. The occiput and sphenoid bone rotate around an anteroposterior axis in the opposite direction (▶**Fig. 4.7**). The motion derives its name from the rotation of the sphenoid bone (like the motion in the spine derives its name from the rotation of the cranial vertebra).

Let us take right torsion as an example (▶**Fig. 4.8b, c**). During this motion, the sphenoid bone rotates to the right, and the right greater wing of sphenoid (ala major) moves upward. Since the joint face of the SBS is not in a vertical but in a diagonal plane that stretches, more or less, through the vertex and the gnathion, both joint partners move in this diagonal plane. With right torsion, this causes the basilar part of the occiput to move forward and downward on the right, while the sphenoid body moves upward and backward and in the opposite direction on the left side.

This has consequences for the occipitoatlantal (OA) joint. **On the right side, the occiput moves forward. On the left side, it moves backward. This means that in a left rotation and right sidebend, the occiput is located above the atlas.**

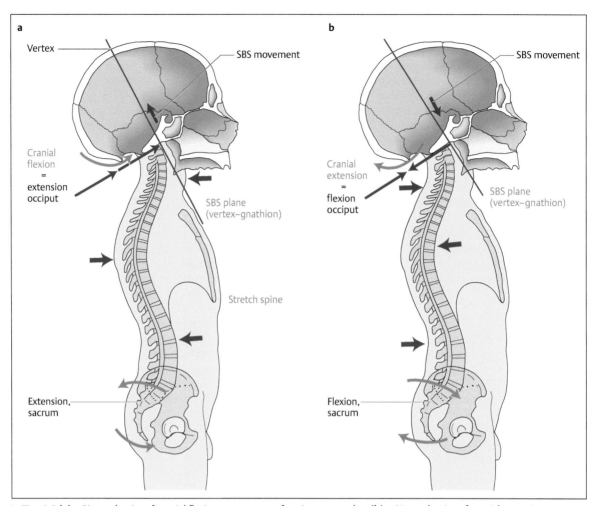

▶ **Fig. 4.6 (a)** Biomechanics of cranial flexion: movement of occiput over atlas. **(b)** Biomechanics of cranial extension: movement of occiput over atlas.

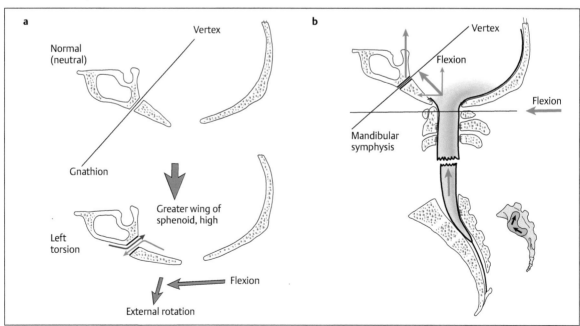

▶ **Fig. 4.7 (a)** Cranial extension. **(b)** Cranial flexion.

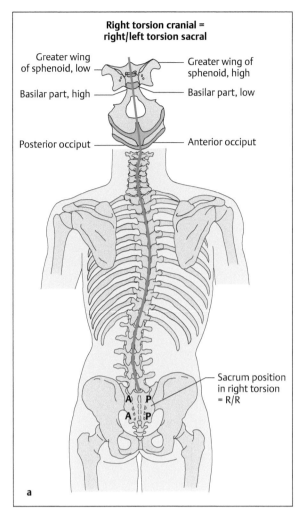

Right torsion cranial = right/left torsion sacral

Greater wing of sphenoid, low — Greater wing of sphenoid, high

Basilar part, high — Basilar part, low

Posterior occiput — Anterior occiput

Sacrum position in right torsion = R/R

a

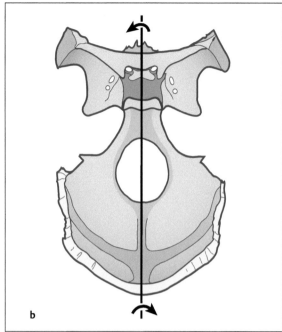

b

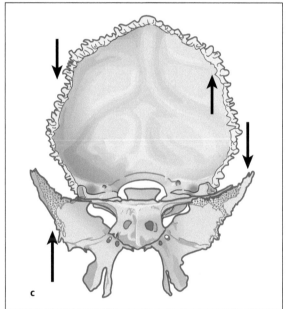

c

▶ **Fig. 4.8 (a, b)**   Right torsion and impact on spine and sacrum. (From Liem T. Kraniosakrale Osteopathie. Ein praktisches Lehrbuch. 5th ed. Stuttgart: Hippokrates; 2010: 576). **(c)** Right torsion. (From Liem T. Kraniosakrale Osteopathie. Ein praktisches Lehrbuch. 5th ed. Stuttgart: Hippokrates; 2010:578.)

Since the peripheral bones follow the movement of the central bones, we find the following in the case of right torsion:

- Right basilar part anterior and low: right temporal bone in external rotation (= back right quadrant in external rotation).
- Left basilar part posterior and high: left temporal bone in internal rotation (= back left quadrant in internal rotation).
- Body of sphenoid bone and right greater wing of sphenoid bone high: front right quadrant in external rotation.

- Body of sphenoid bone and left greater wing of sphenoid bone low: front left quadrant in internal rotation.

■ Impact on the Pelvis

During right torsion of the cranium, the basilar part of the occipital bone is in flexion on the right, that is, anterior and left posterior. From a craniosacral perspective, it is in extension. This places traction on the dura mater on the right, while it becomes relatively relaxed on the left. This lowers the base of the sacrum on the left and raises

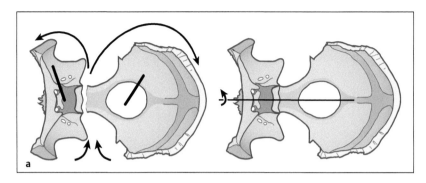

▶ **Fig. 4.9 (a, b)** Sidebending–rotation right. (From Liem T. Kraniosakrale Osteopathie. Ein praktisches Lehrbuch. 5th ed. Stuttgart: Hippokrates; 2010:579.)

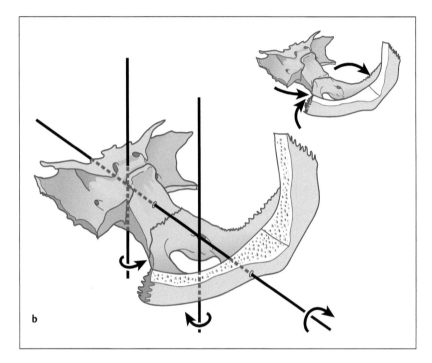

it on the right. In Mitchell's model, this position corresponds to a right torsion around a right axis (▶ **Fig. 4.8a**).

Note: In Sutherland's time, sacrum dysfunctions were not named in keeping with Mitchell's model.[107,156] The following terminology was used instead:

- Sacrum in flexion:
  – Base anterior–inferolateral angle (ILA) posterior.
- Sacrum in extension:
  – Base posterior–ILA anterior.
- Torsion:
  – Base and ILA on the same side or anterior or posterior.
- Sidebending rotation:
  – Base anterior and ILA posterior on one side, and the other way around on the other side. This corresponds to the sacrum anterior or posterior unilaterally.

The posterior base of the sacrum determines the rotation, while the lower ILA determines the sidebending.

Sidebending–Rotation

Sutherland maintained that sidebending rotation is also a physiological motion of the SBS. During this motion, the sphenoid bone bends sideways toward the occiput on one side, and both bones rotate together to the same side (▶ **Fig. 4.9**). This motion is named for the side where the greater wing of sphenoid (ala major) is low.

Example: Sidebending-rotation left.

Sidebending moves the sphenoid and occiput closer together on the right side. The left rotation causes the body of sphenoid bone and the basilar part of occipital bone on the left to incline. This imparts a characteristic shape to the cranial dome. While cranial girth is shorter and straighter on the right side, the left side becomes longer and rounder.

Right sidebending of the SBS causes "the joint to open up on the left," which impacts the position of the occiput over the atlas. On the left side, the occiput slides backward. On the right side, it is pulled forward by the sidebend.

In left rotation and right sidebending, the occiput is located over the atlas (which restores horizontality).

The descent of the SBS on the left side is compensated by right sidebending of the occiput.

The peripheral cranial bones adapt as follows:
- Left basilar part low: left temporal bone in external rotation = back left cranial quadrant in external rotation.
- Right basilar part high: right temporal bone in internal rotation = back right quadrant in internal rotation.
- Left greater wing of sphenoid low = left front quadrant in internal rotation.
- Right greater wing of sphenoid high = right front quadrant in external rotation.

In the same way that cranial bones are forced to adapt to restore harmony, the spine and the rest of the organism are forced to adapt as well. The left rotation–right sidebending of the occiput over the atlas impacts the OAA complex and the spinal dura mater as much as the lumbosacral junction.

The occiput in posterior on the left corresponds to occiput in extension on a craniosacral level.

■ Impact on the Pelvis

The dural tube is relaxed on the left side, which allows the base of the sacrum to drop forward and down on the left. On the right, the occiput is anterior, that is, in flexion from a craniosacral point of view. The dural tube is tensed and the base of the sacrum is maintained cranial–posterior. The sacrum rotates to the right. This corresponds to right rotation of the occiput and sphenoid in a sidebending rotation to the left (▶ **Fig. 4.10**).

Note: The vestibular organs (comparable to a spirit level) and the eyes need to be horizontal to perform their balancing task. The eyes also must be in the same frontal plane to avoid excessive strain on the eye muscles. The ideal adjustment zone for this purpose is in the OAA joints.

Vertical and Lateral Strain

In addition to the four physiological movements described earlier, the SBS also exhibits so-called unphysiologic movements.

Vertical strain causes a cranial inferior shift in the SBS. The body of sphenoid bone shifts upward or downward in relation to the basilar part of the occipital bone. This impacts the visceral cranium, spine, and pelvis (flexion–external rotation or extension–internal rotation position).

Lateral strain causes the occiput and sphenoid to shift in the horizontal plane. This does not lead to obvious impacts on the spine.

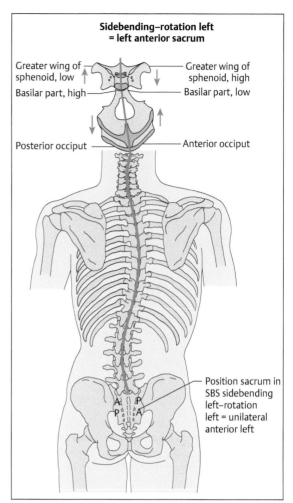

▶ **Fig. 4.10** Sidebending—rotation left and impact on spine and pelvis.

Lateral strain is most commonly found in combination with other cranial dysfunctions, such as flexion, extension, torsion, or sidebending rotation. Frequently, this type of strain is traumatic in nature or results from persistent tensions in the areas influenced by the sphenoid or occiput:
- Falling on the buttocks, blows to the back of the head, or tensions on the spinal dural mater all put strain on the occiput.
- Facial traumas or persistent anterior fascial traction, on the other hand, impact and cause strain for the sphenoid bone.

Compression Dysfunction in the Sphenobasilar Synchondrosis

Compression dysfunctions do not create malposition and, therefore, do not significantly impact the spine or other cranial bones. They do, however, produce extremely negative outcomes for the mechanics of the PRM and must receive primary treatment when they occur. They involve traumatic lesions that significantly limit the motion of the occiput and sphenoid.

Compressions can be caused by a fall on the buttocks or blows to the occiput, glabella, or nasion.

Compressions often arise during birth when the head becomes stuck in the birth canal and the baby is exposed to pressure during contractions.

Intraossal Dysfunctions

■ Lesions of the Cranial Vault

Because bones grow from ossification points out into the periphery, compression of the cranial sutures is the most likely cause of intraossal lesions of the cranial dome. Tensions in the cranial membranes can also be a cause of dysfunctions.

Intrauterine and perinatal factors are mainly responsible for the compressions of sutures. It is obvious that these lesions, as they are viewed from an osteopathic perspective, only arise during the growth phase.

■ Intraossal Lesions of the Cranial Base

Trauma, compression, or persistent tension that impacts the growth sutures can also lead to cranial bone deformities, as is the case for bones in the extremities. This can be particularly dramatic when it impacts the sphenoid, temporal, or occipital bones or the sacrum.

At birth, these bones consist of several parts that do not fuse together completely until the age of 8 to 12 years. Deformities in these bones can result in malpositions of the SBS and craniocervical junction, which impacts the locomotor system.

Intraossal lesions in these bones can cause specific damage in specific areas of the body:
* Lesions between the presphenoid and postsphenoid parts of the sphenoid bone impact the visceral cranium (especially the eyes).
* Lesions in the temporal bone can negatively impact the auditory system, the vestibular system, and the temporomandibular joint (TMJ).
* Intraossal lesions in the sacrum negatively impact posture and motor functions of the spine and lower extremities.
* Lesions in the OA region likely have the most far-reaching impact, not only on posture.
* Sutherland viewed deformities of the basilar and condylar part as partly responsible for several problems:[101,102]
  – Disorders in cranial nerves VI to XII due to compression in the area of the foramina or tension of the membranes. It is important to remember that the dura mater accompanies the cranial nerves up to the foramina and is securely attached there.
  – Impaired circulation: 95% of venous blood leaves the head via the jugular foramen. Shifts in the condylar or basilar parts can change these openings.
  – On the other hand, malpositions of the cranial base can cause SBS lesions and create tension in the membranes. This can impact the dural venous sinuses and, in turn, influence circulation in the brain.
  – A change in the lumina of the foramen magnum can exert pressure on the brain stem, which can have far-reaching impacts.

The medulla and pons rest on top of the basilar part of the occipital bone and the SBS. Damage to the pyramidal tracts is a common cause of spastic states in cerebral palsy.

Malpositions in the basilar part region could be implicated as well.

Note: Nerve dysfunctions do not necessarily require nerve tissue compression. Vascular supply impairment may suffice. Pressure or membrane tensions can irritate the vessels that supply the nerves.

As mentioned earlier, tensions in one part of the cerebral membranes transmit to the entire dural system. The dura mater is solidly attached to the foramen magnum and S2, and deformities in these areas impact the entire postural system. For this reason, we are going to take a closer look at intraossal lesions of the occiput.

■ Intraossal Lesions of the Occiput

It is important to point out again that the cranial base originates from cartilage, while the cranial vault is made from membranes. This makes the cranial dome (calvaria) more adaptable than the base.

During birth and early childhood, membranes are more resilient than bones. Membranes hold together the bones, which consist of several parts.

Perinatal trauma or tensions as well as accidents in infancy can impact the growth sutures of these bones and, either immediately or frequently later, manifest during growth spurts (scoliosis, kypholordosis, cross-bite, etc.).

At birth, the occiput consists of four parts that are held together by the dura mater and the pericranium (▶ **Fig. 4.11**):
* Squamous part of occipital bone.
* Two lateral masses or condylar parts.
* Basilar part.

These four parts frame the foramen magnum.

The two occipital condyles are not fully developed at birth and consist two-thirds of the condylar part and one-third of the basilar part. The atlas also consists of several parts.

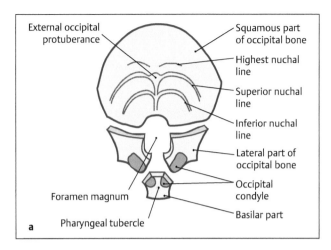

External occipital protuberance

Squamous part of occipital bone

Highest nuchal line

Superior nuchal line

Inferior nuchal line

Lateral part of occipital bone

Occipital condyle

Basilar part

Foramen magnum

Pharyngeal tubercle

a

▶ **Fig. 4.11 (a)** Occipital bone. (From Liem T. Kraniosakrale Osteopathie. Ein praktisches Lehrbuch. 5th ed. Stuttgart: Hippokrates; 2010:92.) **(b)** Atlas and Axis in newborn.

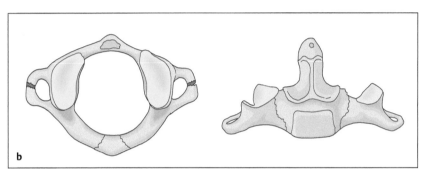

b

In contrast to the occiput, the facets in this area are formed earlier. In addition, the atlas arches are stabilized by the strong transverse ligament of the atlas. For this reason, deformities of the occiput condyles and the foramen magnum are more likely than changes to the atlas. It is also significant that the occiput condyles and atlas facets are oriented medially forward.

The longitudinal axes of both joints converge in front in a point below the SBS. They form an angle of ± 30°. Forced flexion and extension motions can result in compression of the growth sutures because the condyles "threaten to derail."

The most common deformations of the cranial base likely occur during childbirth.

In a normal, natural birth, the head of the newborn is compressed according to a certain pattern during passage through the birth canal. In addition, the cervical spine performs a rotation and flexion–extension motion. If for any reason the birth canal is too narrow for the child's head, the mother's contractions can exert such pressure on the child's cervico-occipital junction that the weakest structures must yield. These forces focus on a specific point determined by the position of the head at the time and cause characteristic lesions to develop at that location.

Compression in the sagittal plane (symmetrical pressure on the supraoccipital bone) can push the condyles forward too strongly. This can change the position of the condylar parts.

The lumen of the foramen magnum and of the jugular foramina may become reduced. This can result in compression of the sutures between the occiput and the temporal bone. The pressure can also shift the basilar part, which may cause vertical strains (an inferior shift of the basilar part).

Therapists can palpate this position by examining the shape of the supraoccipital bone and the position of the inion, among other things. When diagonal pressure is exerted on the occiput while the baby's head is in a rotated position above the atlas, a condyle may be pushed forward. This condyle is then shifted forward medially and the condyle on the other side is shifted laterally. This can cause torsions, sidebending rotation, or lateral strains (a lateral shift of the basilar part) in the SBS.

The foramen magnum and jugular foramina may also change. The sutures between the occiput and the temporal bone may become compressed. Therapists can recognize this malposition by examining the relation between the occiput and the lateral mass of atlas, and by comparing the nuchal line (or supraoccipital bone) on the left and right sides. Both cases impact spinal posture and muscle tone:

- Condyle position impacts dural tube tension down to the sacrum as well as forward to the crista galli.

- Symmetrical malpositions manifest as increases in posture flexion or extension.
- Asymmetrical positions of the occiput condyles lead to dural torque that results in pelvic torque.
- The suboccipital muscles are particularly important for muscle tone.
- Muscle spindles are highly sensitive and the short neck muscles in the suboccipital region are richly supplied with muscle spindles. That makes this area very important for regulating muscle tension in general and especially for posture.

Notes:
- Posturologists demonstrated experimentally—by measuring the weight distribution on both feet—that manipulation of C2, relaxation of the falx, and treatment of the TMJ result in obvious improvement in the distribution of weight.[153,154] All osteopaths are likely familiar with the connections between these three structures and the short neck muscles.
- Microscopic examinations of the short neck muscles showed that they contain ± 6 times as many muscle spindles than the gluteal muscles (per cubic centimeter of muscle mass).
- Viola Frymann assembled an impressive collection of skulls and concluded that deformities of the cranial base are common. She also showed that malpositions and deformities of the condyles and changes in the foramen magnum, jugular foramen, and hypoglossal canal (anterior condyloid canal) frequently occur together.[57] In most cases, these are accompanied by asymmetries in the cranial vault.
- When cranial scoliosis is visible, parietal scoliosis is also present. How pronounced it is depends on the adaptive capabilities of the organism.
- The research results of Korr[79] and Patterson[112] provide sufficient evidence to postulate that persistent myofascial tensions and imbalances cause structural changes.
- One interesting observation in this context is that the clivus and the SBS plane exhibit the same

inclination toward vertical as the longitudinal axis and the promontory of the sacrum.

Sacrum Dysfunctions

Sacrum dysfunctions are impacted by the spinal dura mater, which acts as a "core link" for the craniosacral mechanism:
- Sacrum nutation → cranial extension.
- Sacrum counternutation → cranial flexion.
- Sacrum torsion → SBS torsion.
- Unilateral sacrum flexion → sidebending–rotation.

Causes of sacrum dysfunctions include trauma, persistent malpositions, lumbar spine (LSC) dysfunctions, and visceral disorders. Not to be forgotten is that infants frequently fall on their buttocks.

If one develops the idea of asymmetry of membranous tensions and corresponding muscular imbalance further, one could conclude that these problems, if left untreated, can easily explain scoliosis and other asymmetries.

Some authors, including Harold Magoun, hypothesized that asymmetric dural tensions can negatively impact growth. It seems that leg length differences present in children and youth do not completely disappear in adults (Travell and Simons.[145]) Nerves, in addition to conducting nerve impulses, also transport molecules that are vital for the trophicity of the supplied structures. This means that fascial or membranous tensions can easily impact tissue trophicity during growth spurts in a manner that results in the development of asymmetries.

> We can only conclude from the above that newborns should be examined and, if necessary, treated osteopathically to facilitate optimal, harmonious development.

4.4 Impact of Cranial Dysfunctions and Malpositions on the Periphery

Cranial dysfunctions impact not only the axial skeleton, but also the extremities and even the organ system.

Sutherland was an outstanding osteopath in all respects. He integrated Still's mindset like no other and was also an excellent observer. His keen sense of observation and palpation and his passion for experimentation enabled him to "decode" the craniosacral mechanism. He also recognized how the craniosacral

mechanism impacts the entire body. He determined that the entire organism acts analogous to the craniosacral mechanism.

During thoracic inspiration, the cranium expands like in the cranial flexion phase. Expiration results in a motion that corresponds to the extension phase. Sutherland also discovered that during thoracic inspiration, as during the cranial flexion phase, the entire body rotates externally. It rotates internally during the opposite phase. This discovery led him to conclude that there are two motion patterns:

- A flexion pattern associated with external rotation and abduction.
- An extension pattern associated with internal rotation and adduction.

A simple experiment can demonstrate these conclusions. Compare inspiration with completely internally rotated arms and legs and with completely externally rotated arms and legs. Inspiration is much deeper with externally rotated extremities.

Our description of muscle chains (see Chapter 8) is consistent with Sutherland's model. We are convinced that there are two myofascial chains in each half of the body:

- One flexion chain.
- One extension chain.

Bilateral dominance of the extension chain stretches the spine and places the head and the extremities into flexion and external rotation (and abduction for the extremities).

Dominance of the flexion chain amplifies spinal curves and places the extremities and the cranium in extension and internal rotation (and adduction for the extremities).

Asymmetrical dominance causes one half of the body to act in a flexion pattern and the other half in an extension pattern.

Chapter 8.1 provides a detailed description of how bones and joints respond if one chain is dominant. This explains the possible dysfunctions that may ensue.

Muscle chain dominance may be triggered by the extremities, organs, or the cranial base. In all cases, however, we find a specific SBS position along with a corresponding position of the OAA complex and a specific position of the lumbosacral junction.

5 The Biomechanical Model of John Martin Littlejohn: Mechanics of the Spine

5.1 History

John Martin Littlejohn emigrated from Great Britain to the United States in 1892 for health reasons. He suffered from what was thought to be an incurable throat disorder. After he arrived in the United States, he heard about Dr. Still's unbelievably successful cures and decided to go see him in Kirksville, Missouri.

Still was not only able to cure Littlejohn, he also instilled such excitement about osteopathy in him that Littlejohn decided to stay in Kirksville and train with Still. Littlejohn remained with Still for several years. He also taught and served as deacon of the American School of Osteopathy (now A.T. Still University) founded in Kirksville by Still in 1892. In 1900, Littlejohn founded the American College of Osteopathy and Surgery in Chicago together with his two brothers.

After obtaining his doctorate in osteopathy, Littlejohn stayed at the American College of Osteopathy and Surgery in Chicago until 1913, when he moved to London. In 1917, he founded the British School of Osteopathy. Littlejohn was not the first osteopath to move from the United States to Europe. Others, such as Drs. Jay Dunham, L. Willard Walker, and F.J. Horn had gone to Great Britain and founded the British Osteopathy Association in 1911. Nevertheless, it can be said that Littlejohn brought osteopathy to Europe. After all, it was his theories about spine biomechanics that shaped American (and English) osteopathy for decades.

Littlejohn is known as the mechanic in osteopathy. His views on spine functions are indeed very mechanical, but they are nevertheless dominated by functionality and globality. For Littlejohn, the spine (and its locomotor system) is a unit that is governed by certain mechanical laws. For example, the spine is always subject to gravity. Individual segments of the spinal column do not act in isolation. The entire trunk responds to external and internal forces as a unit.

Littlejohn, like all osteopaths, observed that patients presented with the same, repeating patterns, the same regions of dysfunction, and often also the same symptoms. This motivated him to search for a mechanical explanation of these patterns. It should be noted that in the beginning years of osteopathy, cranial osteopathy and visceral osteopathy as we know them in Europe and in the United States today were not known then.

Still and Littlejohn were both convinced that the spine plays a decisive role in the development and treatment of disease. As a passionate physiologist, Littlejohn applied physical laws to explain the biomechanics of the spine.

In his book *Mechanics of the spine and pelvis,* John Wernham[157] describes in detail the mechanical model of the spine as elaborated by John Martin Littlejohn.

5.2 "Mechanics of the Spine" and the Body's Lines of Force

In physics, compressive and traction forces play an important role and this is no different in human physiology. Cellular metabolism depends on stress ratios (see the development of arthrosis or the supply of intervertebral disk, cartilage, etc.).

Kapandji[74] writes about the significance of spinal curves for spine stability ($R = N^2 + 1$; R = resistance; N = number of curves).

Another law of physics posits that when an arch is bent to one side, it tends to rotate its convex side into a newly formed convexity (see Neutral position–Sidebending–Rotation [NSR] in Chapter 3).

Note: An interesting fact to note is that our trunk consists of two cavities that both exhibit expanding force. Lungs as well as intestines contain air and tend toward expansion. The thorax and the abdominal cavity are encircled by muscles that exert inward directed force.

One characteristic of muscles is that they maintain the same base tension in all positions. Normally, these forces neutralize each other.

This phenomenon can be compared to the dural sac, which is turned into a water column by liquor and functions as a unit. The entire trunk acts as a unit.

Littlejohn described six lines of force to explain the impact of gravity on the behavior of the spine and the development of repetitive patterns of dysfunction.[94,97,126]

Central Gravity Line

This line actually encompasses two lines: one on the right and one on the left. Its course is as follows (▶ **Fig. 5.1**):

- ±1 cm behind the sella turcica.
- ±1 cm in front of the atlas facets.
- Through the center of the transverse processes of C3–C6.
- In front of the vertebral body of T4.

- Through the costovertebral (CV) joints of T2–T10.
- Through the vertebral body of L3.
- At the level of L3, the two lines separate and travel through the legs to the midfoot.

These lines are mobile and can change their course to adapt to posture.

Anterior Body Line

This line runs parallel to the central gravity line from the mandibular symphysis to the pubic symphysis (▶ **Fig. 5.2**). Its course depends on the pressure ratios in the thorax and abdomen. This line is an indicator of the correlation between posture and pressure ratios in the cavities. If posture changes, the pressure ratios

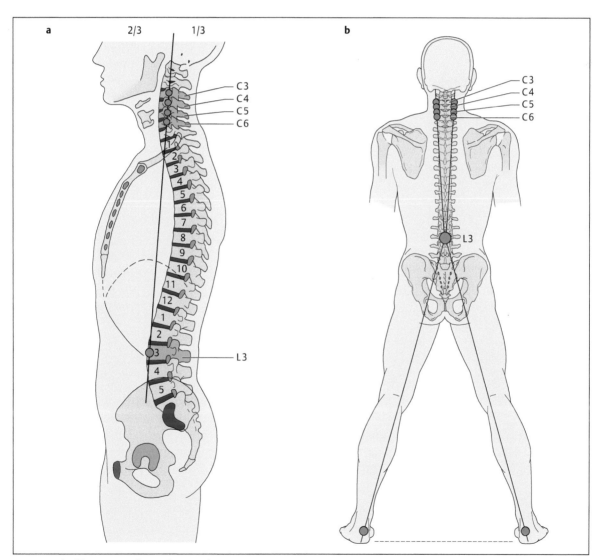

▶ **Fig. 5.1 (a, b)** Course of central gravity line.

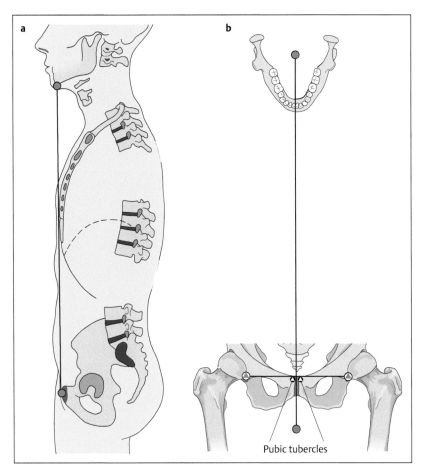

► **Fig. 5.2 (a, b)**   Course of anterior body line.

Pubic tubercles

in the abdominal and thoracic cavities adapt. For example, increased abdominal pressure changes the course of the anterior body line, and this changes the course of the central gravity line (► **Fig. 5.3**).

Diaphragms are important for balancing the pressure ratios in the cavities. That is why there is a close connection between the diaphragms and the anterior body line. Abdominal wall tension is related to diaphragm tension. The following two scenarios can be found:

■ Anterior Body Line Runs in Front of the Pubic Symphysis

- Abdominal wall pressure increases.
- Inguinal ligament tension increases, which can lead to inguinal hernias.
- Cervical spine (cervical spinal column [CSC]) lordosis increases.
- Chin is extended forward and upward.
- Tension in the cervicothoracic junction (CTJ), thoracolumbar junction (TLJ), and lumbosacral junction (LSJ).

- Recurvation of the knee.
- Susceptibility to otolaryngology (ear, nose, and throat [ENT]) problems.

■ Anterior Body Line Runs behind the Pubic Symphysis

- Abdominal pressure shifts backward onto the lower abdominal organs, aorta, and iliac vessels.
- CSC stretches and chin pulls backward.
- Thoracic spine (thoracic spinal column [TSC]) kyphosis and tension between shoulder blades.
- Drooping shoulders.
- Tendency toward lumbar hyperlordosis.
- Flat thorax.
- Tendency toward organ prolapse.
- Tension in the sacroiliac joint (SIJ) area.
- Knee flexion.
- Traction on hamstring (ischiocrural) muscles.
- Weight shifts to the heels.

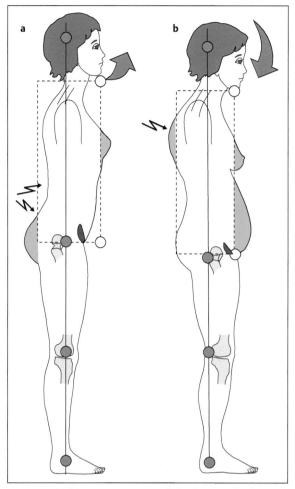

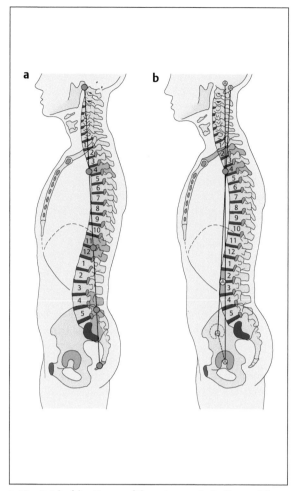

Anteroposterior Line

This line begins in the opisthion and runs through the anterior tubercle of atlas, through the vertebral bodies T11 and T12, through the zygapophyseal (facet) joints of L4–L5, through S1, and ends at the tip of the coccygeal bone (▶ **Fig. 5.4**).

The anteroposterior line turns the entire spine into one unit, and turns T11 and T12 into key vertebrae for anteroposterior balance and trunk torsion. Asymmetric strain on arms and legs, trunk torsions, or straightening of the spine place strain on T11 and T12. These vertebrae also have a role in abdominal blood circulation.

Two Posteroanterior Lines

These two lines run from the posterior margin of the foramen magnum through the second ribs, through the vertebral bodies of L2 and L3, and end in the hip joints (▶ **Fig. 5.4**). Like the anteroposterior line, the posteroanterior lines run in front of T4.

Both lines connect the occipitoatlantal (OA) joints with the second ribs and T2. This assures balanced tension in the CSC. These lines direct the pressure ratios to the hip joints when standing and to the tuberosities when sitting. The main function of these lines is to maintain optimal tension ratios between neck, torso, and legs and between abdomen and thorax.

The anteroposterior line and the two posteroanterior lines form the so-called "polygon of forces."

5.3 Polygon of Forces

Littlejohn's polygon of forces consists of two pyramids. The tips of the pyramids attach in front of the vertebral bodies of T4 (▸**Fig. 5.5**). The two posteroanterior lines and the anteroposterior line balance each other and cross in front of T4. The resultant of these three lines is the central gravity line, which runs through L3.[51,52,53,88]

The lower pyramid has a solid base provided by the hip joints and the coccyx. The foramen magnum provides the base for the upper pyramid. The upper pyramid is stabilized by myofascial structures. Pelvic dysfunctions as well as occipitoatlantoaxial (OAA) lesions impact T3 and T4.

When walking, both pyramids rotate in opposite directions, as is evidenced by opposing arm and leg motions.

When the left leg is the stance leg and the right leg is the swing leg, the lower pyramid forms a convexity and rotates right. The upper pyramid forms a convexity and rotates left. The central gravity line connects L3 with the hip joints.

The anteroposterior line connects the atlas and the coccygeal bone and runs through L3. This creates a third pyramid. It also has a solid base provided by the pelvis and the tip of L3.

All three pyramids depend on the pressure ratios in the cavities: the two lower pyramids directly and the upper pyramid indirectly via myofascial tensions.

Inspiration and expiration not only change the pressure in the thorax and abdomen, but also stretch the spine during inspiration.

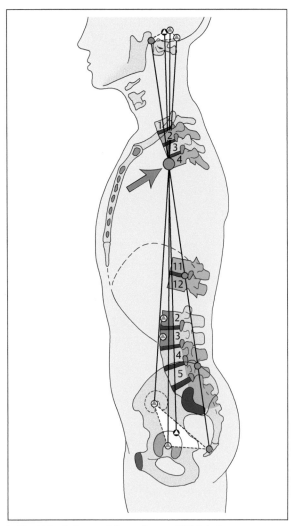

▸ **Fig. 5.5** Polygon of forces (as per Littlejohn).

5.4 Arches, Pivots, and Double Arches

Arches

Anatomically, the spine consists of four arches:
- Cervical: atlas to T1.
- Thoracic: T2–T12.
- Lumbar: L1–L5.
- Sacral: sacrum to coccyx.

Littlejohn[94,96] also divided the spine into four arches, but from a functional perspective. He defined the arches as areas of the spine between pivots. The arches move as a unit.

The following are the functional arches (▸**Fig. 5.6**):
- Upper arch: C1–C4.
- Middle arch: C6–T8.
- Lower arch: T10–L4.
- Sacrum.

This classification of functional arches allows us to illustrate how the individual segments of the spine relate to each other. By accepting Littlejohn's model of lines of force and by understanding the functions of individual muscle groups and the anatomical peculiarities of individual vertebra, we can accept certain vertebrae as pivots.

Pivots

There are anatomical, physiologic, and functional pivots (▶**Fig. 5.6**).[36,53,126]

Anatomical pivots are the atypical vertebrae. Their special anatomical shape forces spine segments to behave in certain ways. Anatomical pivots are C2–L5–sacrum.

Littlejohn viewed the atlas as part of the head and did not consider it a pivot.

Physiologic pivots are located between the curves, where a lordosis transitions to kyphosis: C5–T9–L5.

Functional pivots are vertebrae that have special significance because of their mechanical function: C2–T4–L3.

- C2 is a pivot for the head. The extremely sensitive suboccipital muscles connect the OAA complex.
- T4 is a pivot because head rotation extends to T4–T5. T4 is also an important crossing point for Littlejohn's lines of force.
- L3 is the lowest lumbar vertebra that is not directly connected to the pelvis by ligaments.

L4 and L5 belong to the pelvis because they are connected by the iliolumbar ligaments (like C1 and C2 for the head). Littlejohn also viewed L3 as the center of gravity for the entire body. Dysfunctions of these vertebral pivots are very common. They are rarely manipulated in isolation. Treatment should always include the associated arches.

Double Arches

Littlejohn described two double arches (▶**Fig. 5.6**):[94, 95]
- Upper posterior arch: C7–T8.
- Lower anterior arch: T10–sacrum.

From a mechanical perspective, it is interesting to observe that the upper posterior arch carries the weight of the head, thorax, and upper extremities, and shifts it posteriorly. This allows the anterior arch to balance and direct the weight toward the hips.

The apex of the upper arch is located at the level of T4–T5. The apex of the lower arch is located at the level of L2–L4. Both segments are very susceptible to dysfunctions. Littlejohn described the following weak points in this system: C7, fifth rib, T9, T11, T12, L2, and L3 (▶**Fig. 5.7**):
- C7 is located at the transition between a mobile and a rigid spinal segment.
- T9 is a functional pivot between two arches and between an anterior and a posterior double arch.
- T11 and T12 are the torsion center of the spine.
- The fifth rib is in a transition zone between the upper thorax and CSC and between the lower thorax and lumbar spine (LSC).

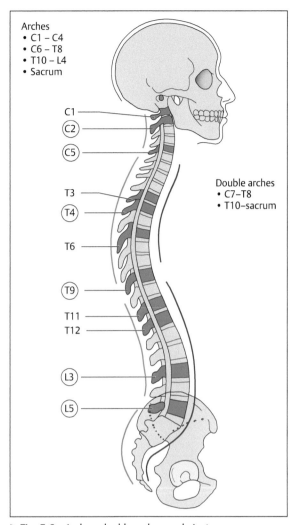

Arches
- C1 – C4
- C6 – T8
- T10 – L4
- Sacrum

C1
C2
C5
T3
T4
T6
T9
T11
T12
L3
L5

Double arches
- C7–T8
- T10–sacrum

▶ **Fig. 5.6** Arches, double arches, and pivots.

- L2 and L3 are the weakest point of the entire spine, because the weight of the entire body manifests here: The weight of the trunk pushes down from above and the lower extremities pull downward while walking.

Posture imbalances are often compensated in these weak points of the spine.

Littlejohn and later also his students John Wernham and T.E. Hall describe the connections to the organs, the neurovegetative system, and the endocrine system. Littlejohn also explains and justifies his treatment approach. We focus on presenting the information that fits within the context of this book.

Further development of this model led to an interesting osteopathic treatment method: specific adjusting technique (SAT). We will introduce this method in the next section.

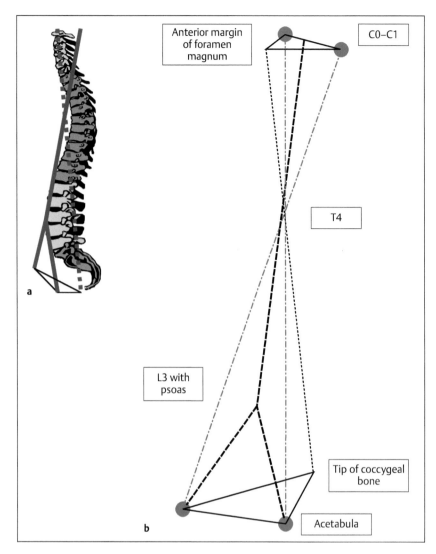

Fig. 5.7 (a) Littlejohn's model. Intercurve pivots C5, T9, and L5, atypical vertebrae C1, C2, C3, and L5/S1. (From Hermanns W. GOT: Ganzheitliche Osteopathische Therapie. 2nd ed. Stuttgart: Hippokrates; 2009:53.) **(b)** Polygon of forces (as per Littlejohn) exhibiting mechanical connections and functions of spine. Anteroposterior line (......) and posteroanterior line (_ _ _ _) form two pyramids. PA line is split into two lines: one line running from the left occipitoatlantal joint to the right acetabulum and the other line running from the right occipitoatlantoaxial joint to the left acetabulum. All lines cross in T4. (From Hermanns W. GOT: Ganzheitliche Osteopathische Therapie. 2nd ed. Stuttgart: Hippokrates; 2009:52.)

Labels in figure: Anterior margin of foramen magnum; C0–C1; T4; L3 with psoas; Tip of coccygeal bone; Acetabula

5.5 Specific Adjusting Technique as per Dummer

History

It appears that the invention of SAT was serendipitous. During a flu epidemic in the 1950s, the osteopath and chiropractor Parnall Bradbury was the only therapist on duty in his clinic. Bradbury was faced with an immense number of patients and had very little time for each treatment. Therefore, he decided to manipulate only the most conspicuous segment in each patient.

His approach was so successful that he analyzed this method further. The most successful treatments involved manipulation of the atypical vertebrae. Parnall Bradbury was a student of Littlejohn and was familiar with his model of lines of force. During his chiropractic

training, he learned the H.I.O. (hole-in-one) manipulation of the upper CSC. Treating only the one key segment also conformed to Still's principle of "find it, fix it, and leave it alone."

Bradbury conducted several studies together with the physician Dudley Tee to analyze the effectiveness of treating key lesions. He introduced a specific methodology and coined the term "positional lesions," which refers to mostly traumatic blockages of atypical vertebrae that happen, for example, in whiplash injuries. Bradbury posits that this vertebra must be repositioned using impulse techniques. The impulse vector must be exactly opposite to the force vector that caused the blockage. After Bradbury's death, this method was further developed and refined by his student Tom Dummer. It is not only used for traumatic lesions.

The location of the "primary lesion" (cervical or sacral) determines the sequence in which the key segments are manipulated. Only one segment is manipulated during each treatment.[53]

Procedure

The therapist locates the key segment to be treated by dividing the locomotor system into three units. There are a series of specific tests for each unit. The goal is to identify the dominant unit.

Each unit contains certain vertebrae of special significance. These are the pivots in Littlejohn's model: C1, C2, C3, C5, T3, T4, T9, T11, T12, L3, L5, and sacrum.

Note:
- Traumatic and adaptive cases involve different pivots.
- Opinions vary as to whether the pivot vertebrae should be manipulated.

Pivots always involve groups of vertebrae. Therefore, it is always recommended to include this group of vertebrae into treatment. Gentle techniques are more suitable in these cases.

Three Units

Dividing the organism into three units fits within Littlejohn's model and makes sense in clinical practice, because it makes sense neurologically as well as mechanically. The three units derive from the three pyramids of the polygon of forces.

Unit 1

Lower extremities, pelvis, and lower LSC starting at L3. This unit represents locomotion.

Unit 2

Cranium, CSC, TSC to T4, shoulders and arms, and upper thorax.

Autonomic functions of the head, throat, and thorax.

Unit 3

Lower thorax and vertebrae T4–L3.

Autonomic functions of the abdomen.

Note: It is interesting to see that these three units correspond, more or less, with the three lower hinge areas in Zink's model. Littlejohn's model is missing the cervico-occipital junction (COJ) as a separate unit. It is included in Unit 2 along with the CTJ.

In our opinion, the COJ, because of its special characteristics (atypical vertebrae, parasympathetic zone), can be viewed as a separate unit with special significance for the craniosacral system.

6 Postural Muscles, Phasic Muscles, and Crossed Syndrome

Vladimir Janda's Contributions to Myofascial Treatment Methods

The locomotor system has two important tasks, in addition to other functions:
- Stability = posture.
- Mobility = motor function, motion.

6.1 Posture

Maintaining balance is one of the most impressive tasks of the locomotor system. To perform this task, the organism compiles large amounts of information from receptors in the entire organism.

The vestibular system, as well as muscles, tendons, fasciae, and joints, play an important role in maintaining balance. Eyes and ears are also very important. The fact that the temporomandibular joints and the organs indirectly impact posture and motor function by influencing muscles is less known.

6.2 Motor Function

Motor function serves to satisfy human requirements and is carried out by muscles. Muscles need good balance and coordination between individual muscle groups to function optimally. Coordination between muscles includes inhibition of antagonists and coactivation of synergists. Balance and coordination are both controlled by the central nervous system (CNS). Postural and motion patterns acquired during ontogeny play an important role in this process.

A person's characteristic gait or typical posture is an example of motion patterns. Imbalances between individual muscle groups represent deviations from optimal motion patterns that often develop in early childhood. Many deviations likely develop prenatally.

Microtraumas and macrotraumas as well as lifestyle habits contribute to the development of motion patterns. Posture imbalance patterns as well as uncoordinated patterns cause muscle imbalances and excessive strain. Every functional joint problem initiates reflexive muscle tension, which impairs posture and motion patterns.

Pain plays an important role in this process. Pain thresholds determine if a joint malfunction manifests as illness. As soon as this is the case, the entire locomotor system strives to adapt and compensate to make the condition more bearable and to maintain organism functionality.

It has been demonstrated in cases of spastic paralysis that muscles were inhibited even though they were not paralyzed. The same phenomenon occurs with trigger points. Pain causes muscle weakness and this promotes posture imbalances.

Vladimir Janda,[40,41,86,87] a Czech physician, conducted interesting research in manual medicine and especially about muscle function. Some of his observations are of great interest for the treatment of locomotor dysfunctions. For example, he discovered that **patients with poor motion stereotypes and muscle imbalances also exhibited neurologic deficits**. Their motions were poorly coordinated and awkward. Sensibility impairments, especially of the proprioceptors, as well as poor adaptation to stress situations led to uncontrolled behavior. Janda discovered these signs both in children and in adults. Adults also exhibited vertebral dysfunctions and pain.

Understanding motor stereotypes and the function of individual muscles as they interact with muscle groups enables therapists to more effectively target their treatment to pathologic patterns.

Example: The quadriceps muscle of thigh and the hamstring (ischiocrural) muscles are antagonists for knee flexion and extension. However, while walking, these muscles are synergists for stabilizing the knee. While walking, the foot, knee, and hip flexors work together synergistically.

Muscle activity synergies are even more evident in pathologic states. It is more important to view a muscle in the context of the entire motion pattern than to view it in isolation.

Another important observation described by Janda is that the ratio between weakened and contracted muscle groups is not random, but is subject to certain regularities.

Microscopic and electrophysiological research has shown that, from a functional point of view, there are two different types of striated muscle fibers: red and white. All muscles contain both fibers, but in varying numbers. How a muscle behaves is determined by the number of certain types of muscle fiber it contains.

The following sections describe the characteristics of both muscle fiber types.[40,41,86,87,107]

6.3 Postural Muscle Fibers (Red Fibers)

■ Type I Fibers (Slow Twitch Fibers)

- Diameter of ± 50 nm.
- High myoglobin content (red color).
- Thick Z-disks.
- High number of mitochondria.
- High amount of neutral fats.
- Oxidative metabolism processes predominate.
- Low glycogenolytic and glycolytic activity.
- High mitochondrial enzyme activity.
- Slow contraction speed.
- Suited to endurance and support functions.
- Tendency toward contraction.
- Treatment: stretching.

6.4 Phasic Muscle Fibers (White Fibers)

■ Type II Fibers (Fast Twitch Fibers)

- Diameter of ±80 to 100 nm.
- Strongly developed sarcoplasmic reticulum.
- Thin Z-disks.
- Contain few mitochondria, lipids, and glycogen.
- High myosin and actomyosin ATPase activity.
- Anaerobic metabolism dominates.
- High glycogen consumption.
- Used for quick, brief activity.
- Strengthened by increased impulse frequency.
- Tendency toward weakening.
- Treatment: strengthening.

Muscles that contain predominantly red muscle fibers tend toward hyperactivity, tension, contraction, and hypertonicity. Muscles that contain predominantly white muscle fibers tend toward weakening and atony.

There are contending naming conventions in use for these two muscle types. We use Janda's terminology: he refers to muscles that contain predominately red fibers as **postural muscles** and muscles that contain predominately white fibers as **phasic muscles** (▶ **Fig. 6.1**).

In his research, Janda found that with most people, certain muscles always exhibit a tendency toward contraction and others toward weakening.

6.5 Muscles that Tend toward Contraction

- Short extensors of the occipitoatlantoaxial (OAA) joints.
- Levator muscle of scapula.
- Middle and upper part of trapezius.
- Lumbar part of erector muscle of spine.
- Quadratus lumborum.
- Muscles of mastication.
- Sternocleidomastoid (SCM).
- Scalene muscles.
- Subscapular muscle.
- Smaller and greater pectoral muscles.
- Oblique abdominal muscles.
- Hamstrings (ischiocrural muscles).
- Rectus femoris.
- Tensor fasciae latae (TFL).
- Iliopsoas.
- Short hip adductors.
- Triceps muscle of calf (triceps surae).
- Flexors of the upper extremities.

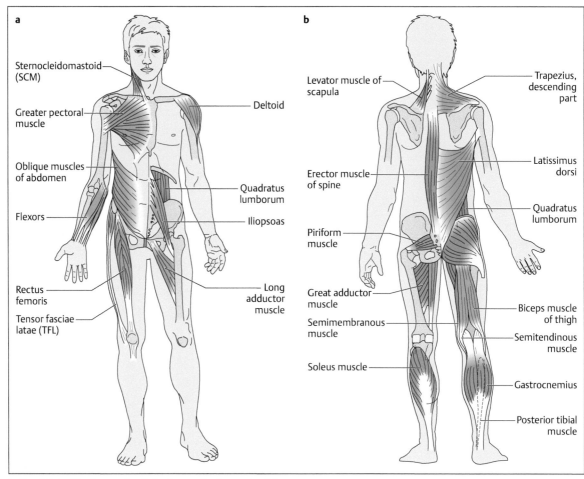

a

Sternocleidomastoid (SCM)

Greater pectoral muscle

Oblique muscles of abdomen

Flexors

Rectus femoris

Tensor fasciae latae (TFL)

Deltoid

Quadratus lumborum

Iliopsoas

Long adductor muscle

b

Levator muscle of scapula

Erector muscle of spine

Piriform muscle

Great adductor muscle

Semimembranous muscle

Soleus muscle

Trapezius, descending part

Latissimus dorsi

Quadratus lumborum

Biceps muscle of thigh

Semitendinous muscle

Gastrocnemius

Posterior tibial muscle

▶ **Fig. 6.1 (a, b)**   Postural and phasic muscles (as per Janda).

6.6 Muscles that Tend toward Weakening

- Deltoid.
- Lower part of trapezius.
- Anterior serratus.
- Gluteal muscles.
- Rectus abdominis.
- Deep neck flexors.
- Suprahyoid muscles.
- Vastus muscles.
- Anterior tibial muscle.
- Toe extensors.
- Peroneal muscles.
- Extensors of the upper extremities.

It appears that muscle fiber function is not genetically determined, but is governed by the activity the muscle must perform. This applies to both postural and phasic muscles. The English physical therapist Chris Norris [in[41]] writes that the number of postural or phasic muscle fibers is determined by the level of muscle training.

Lin et al [in[41]] demonstrated that postural and phasic muscle characteristics depend on the innervation of the muscle (or on the impulses the muscle receives). This was demonstrated by transplanting a phasic muscle nerve into to a postural muscle.

This likely also explains why different muscle properties are found in malpositions (e.g., due to differences in leg length) or excessive strain on certain muscle groups (e.g., due to monotonous motion patterns while working).

For some muscles, classification into postural or phasic is questionable. This applies to scalene, oblique abdominal, gluteal, deep neck, and peroneal muscles.

Another remarkable fact is that the postural muscles are found in the concavities of the spine and of the extremities.

From cranial to inferior:

- Neck extensors.
- Smaller and greater pectoral muscle.
- Lumbar section of erector muscle of spine.
- Iliopsoas for the hip.
- Hamstrings (ischiocrural muscles) for the knee.
- Peroneal muscles for the foot.
- Flexors of the upper extremities.

Janda's explanation for the development of these motion patterns is based on evolution. These are mostly muscles that support gait.

According to Waddell [in[41]], postural muscles are muscles that have a support function. Their ability to maintain continuous tension supports posture. Phasic muscles are more dynamic and responsible for movement. Waddell considers postural and phasic muscles antagonists.

This leads to another observation by Janda, the crossed syndrome.

6.7 Crossed Syndrome

The shoulder girdle and the pelvic girdle often exhibit a very special posture pattern.[40, 41, 107]

Upper Crossed Syndrome (▸Fig. 6.2a)

- Occiput and C1–C2 in hyperextension.
- Protracted chin.
- Tension on lower cervical spinal column (CSC) and upper thoracic spinal column (TSC).
- Rotation and abduction of shoulder blades.
- Forward orientation of glenoid cavity of scapula.
- Levator muscle of scapula and descending part of trapezius pull shoulders up.

The following muscles are involved:

Hypertonic Muscles
- Smaller and greater pectoral muscles.
- Descending part of trapezius.
- Levator scapulae.
- SCM.

Hypotonic Muscles
- Ascending part of trapezius.
- Anterior serratus.
- Rhomboid muscles.

This results in tensions in the cervical spine as well as pain in the shoulders and arms.

Lower Crossed Syndrome (▸Fig. 6.2b)

- Anteversion of the pelvis.
- Hip flexion.
- Lumbar spinal column (LSC) lordosis.
- L5–S1 stress.

The following muscles are involved:

Hypertonic Muscles
- Iliopsoas.
- Rectus femoris.
- TFL.
- Adductors.
- Erector muscle (erector spinae) of lumbar spine (LSC).

Hypotonic Muscles
- Abdominal muscles.
- Gluteal muscles.

The two syndromes together result in kypholordosis of the spine.

Note: This crossed syndrome can be applied to all other planes.

Example: Hypertonic hamstrings and foot flexors with hypotonic quadriceps and triceps muscles of calf lead to a flexed knee position. Hypertonic short adductors and quadratus lumborum muscles with hypotonic abductors and biceps muscle of thigh lead to pelvis translation.

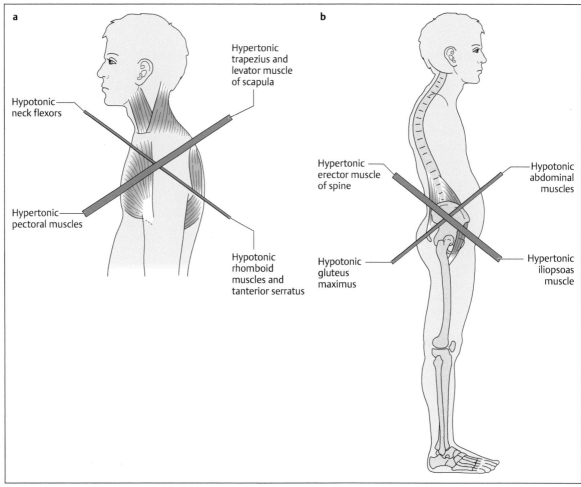

▶ **Fig. 6.2 (a, b)**   Upper and lower crossed syndromes (as per Janda).

6.8   Practical Implications

Some muscles tend toward hypertonicity and contraction; their functional antagonists tend toward hypotonicity and weakening. This leads to malposture. Posture analysis provides indications of hypertonic and hypotonic muscles.

Before a hypotonic muscle can be strengthened, hypertonic muscles must be adequately detonified and stretched. The focus should be on muscle groups and motion patterns rather than on isolated muscles and motions. Agonists and antagonists depend on motion patterns.

Muscle characteristics (postural or phasic) can be influenced through adequate training. The number of red or white muscle fibers is determined by function.

Stereotypes and motion patterns develop during childhood. Trauma, psychological stress, and lifestyle habits contribute to their development. Prolonged inactivity transforms phasic muscles into postural muscles.

7 Zink Patterns

The American osteopath J. Gordon Zink, who taught for many years at the College of Osteopathic Medicine at Des Moines University in Iowa, spent a major part of his life studying fasciae and the impact of fascial imbalance on posture and circulation.

Michael Kuchera, who had the pleasure of working with Zink, reports (during a seminar in May 2004 in Berlin) that at the end of his career, Zink was an osteopath known for his brief treatments and quick results.

He developed a diagnostics procedure that enabled him diagnose and verify treatment success for a dysfunctional region very quickly and with very little manipulation.

Zink's research emphasis was on posture, fascial tensions, and, above all, their impact on lymph circulation. He discovered that certain posture patterns exhibited special fascial tension patterns. He employed this discovery in his diagnosis and treatment.

During his research, he examined **nonsymptomatic** as well as **symptomatic people** and made some interesting discoveries. Zink found fascial torsion patterns even in people who viewed themselves as perfectly healthy and who did not indicate any symptoms. People without fascial torsion patterns are extremely rare.

In all other **asymmetric** people, Zink found special torsion patterns. He noticed that the fascial pattern reversed at the functional junctions of the spine—occipitoatlantoaxial (OAA), cervicothoracic, thoracolumbar, and lumbosacral.

Fascial pattern refers to a region's ease of rotation (ease-bind). This is also an indicator for fascial bias in the direction of unrestricted movement.[40,41,81,82]

Zink found the following pattern (▶ **Fig. 7.1a**) in 80% of **nonsymptomatic** people:
- OAA: left torsion.
- Superior thorax aperture: right torsion.
- Inferior thorax aperture: left torsion.
- Pelvis: right torsion.

Since this fascial pattern was the one most frequently found in healthy people, Zink called it "common compensatory pattern" (CCP).

In the remaining 20% of **asymptomatic people**, Zink found the opposite pattern (▶ **Fig. 7.1b**):
- OAA: right torsion.
- Superior thorax aperture (inlet): left torsion.
- Inferior thorax aperture (outlet): right torsion.
- Pelvis: left torsion.

This pattern is called "uncommon compensatory pattern" (UCCP). When fascial bias reverses at the respective anatomical junctions, the person has achieved homeostatic postural adaption. The organism successfully compensated even if it was not able to achieve the "ideal" adaption pattern without torsions.

None of these three patterns present in patients, that is, people who indicate symptoms. People who exhibit

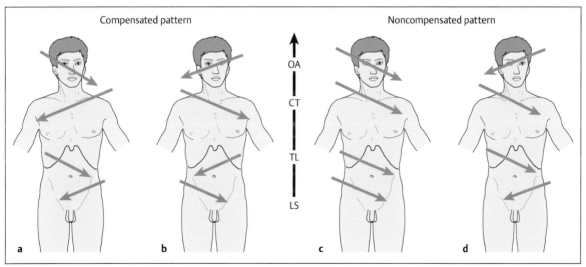

▶ **Fig. 7.1 (a–d)** Zink patterns.

neither the ideal fascial pattern nor one of the two compensatory torsion patterns (CCP or UCCP) frequently present with fascial bias in the same direction at two or even more junctions. These patterns are called "non-compensated facial patterns" (NCP; ▶ **Fig. 7.1c, d**).

Zink viewed microtraumas and macrotraumas as the reason for the body's inability to adapt to the laws of gravity.

Two facts are noteworthy about this model:

* Reversal of fascial bias takes place in areas where anatomical or functional diaphragms are found. We know these diaphragms play a key role in endolymphatic circulation as an active pump.
* These reversal areas are also the regions where lordosis transforms into kyphosis or vice versa. These regions are also reversal areas for scoliotic curvatures.

Note: If we continue to explore the concept of diaphragms and junctions, we inevitably arrive at a discussion of the sphenobasilar synchondrosis (SBS) and the cerebellar tentorium. We all know about the significance of the tentorium for cranial circulation. Cranial osteopathy also teaches us the importance of the SBS for postural adaption. If the information presented so far in this book has not illustrated this concept, we hope to do so in the chapters that follow.

The superior thoracic aperture and the cervicothoracic diaphragm are functional diaphragms. The anatomical thoracic inlet consists of the superior end of the manubrium of sternum, the first two ribs, and vertebra T1. The functional thoracic inlet is also the clinical thoracic inlet. It consists of the manubrium of sternum, the sternal angle (Louis' or Ludwig's angle), the first two ribs on both sides, and the first four thoracic vertebrae. This thoracic aperture contains both apexes of the lung as well as vessels, nerves, trachea, and esophagus. These constitute the superior mediastinum. These structures are enveloped by the suprapleural membrane (Sibson's fascia). The Sibson fascia derives from the fasciae of the two long muscles of neck (longus colli) (which reach down to T4–T5) and the fascia covering the scalene muscles. It covers the apexes of the lung, is attached to the vessel trunks of the thoracic inlet, and merges with the cupula of pleura. The Sibson fascia constitutes the actual cervicothoracic diaphragm.

7.1 The Composition of Zink Patterns

The next step in our endeavor to compare the different concepts and identify analogies is to describe the muscle groups responsible for torsion patterns and the segments involved in this process (▶ **Fig. 7.2**).

Occipitoatlantoaxial Complex

■ Vertebrae

* Occiput.
* Atlas.
* Axis.

■ Responsible Muscles

* Rectus capitis (posterior major and minor, lateral, anterior).
* Superior and inferior oblique muscle of head.
* Sternocleidomastoid (SCM) and superior part of trapezius.

We consider the SCM to be one of the muscles that play a role with the OAA joints, because its main function relates to the head.

The trapezius is involved in both the OAA and the superior thoracic aperture.

■ Segments

Cervical plexus.

■ Special Osteopathic Considerations

* The atlas is the base of the head. All cranial problems impact the OAA complex and vice versa.
* The OAA is an important area for the cranial part of the parasympathetic nervous system.
* The suboccipital muscles in general and the SCM (because of its attachment to the suture) can irritate the occipitomastoid (OM) suture.
* Hypertonicity can impact the jugular foramen. In addition, the nodose ganglion (inferior ganglion of vagus nerve) is wrapped in fascia between the lateral mass of atlas and the jugular foramen.
* The OAA, in addition to the lumbosacral junction and the lower ankle joint, is the most important adaption zone for posture.
* The suboccipital muscles contain a high number of muscle spindles and are therefore extremely important for posture.

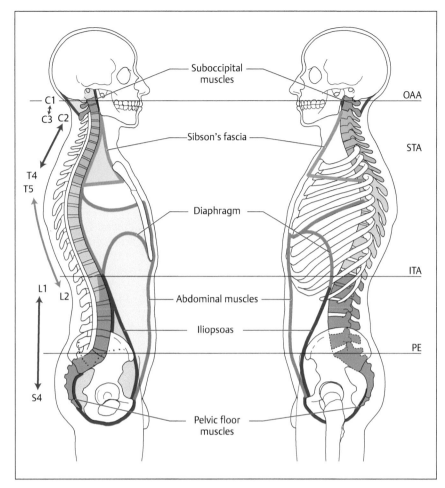

▶ **Fig. 7.2** Myofascial components and spinal segments of Zink patterns.
OAA, occipitoatlantoaxial complex;
STA, superior thorax aperture;
ITA, inferior thorax aperture;
PE, pelvis.

Superior Thorax Aperture

■ Vertebrae

- C3–T4 (T5).

■ Muscles

- Long neck muscles.
- Upper three to four intercostal muscles.
- Scalene muscles.
- Long muscle of neck (longus colli).
- Scapular muscles.

■ Segments

- Brachial plexus.
- Thoracic segments of T1–T5.

■ Special Osteopathic Considerations

- The superior thorax aperture is the gateway for venolymphatic circulation. The fasciae of the neck wrap all vessels in the superior thorax aperture.
- The stellate (cervicothoracic) ganglion lies in front of the head of the first rib.
- The sympathetic nerves supplying all head and thorax organs come from segments T1–T5.
- There is a functional connection between the upper thoracic spine (thoracic spinal column [TSC]) and the cervical spine (cervical spinal column [CSC]).
- The cervicothoracic junction represents a transition from a less mobile to a more mobile zone.
- Interrelationship between the upper extremities and the cervicothoracic junction.

Inferior Thoracic Aperture

■ Vertebrae

- T6–L3.

■ Muscles

- Diaphragmatic muscle.
- Abdominal muscles.
- Last seven intercostal muscles.

■ Segments

- T6–T9: greater splanchnic nerve.
- T9–T12: lesser splanchnic nerve.
- Pelvic splanchnic nerves.

■ Some Osteopathic Considerations for this Region

- Significance of diaphragm for thoracic respiration, circulation, organ function, and posture.
- Functional unity between diaphragm, quadratus lumborum muscles, and iliopsoas.
- Sympathetic nerve supply for all abdominal organs.
- Connection to the CSC via the phrenic nerve, which originates in segments C3, C4, and C5.
- Diaphragm plays a key role for abdominal and thoracic pressure ratios and therefore for all bodily functions.

Example: Increased abdominal pressure pushes the diaphragm upward to maintain constant pressure gradients between thoracic and abdominal cavities. This increases pressure in the thorax, which eventually impacts respiration and circulation. Increased physical activity requires increased activation of the accessory muscles of respiration. Both the changed pressure ratios and the strain on the accessory muscles of respiration change spine posture. When the diaphragm functions in this raised position for a longer period, this not only changes the motion axis of the organs, but also the orientation of the respiratory motion in the diaphragm. This in turn affects the entire respiratory-dependent mobilization of the organs.

- The iliopsoas and the quadratus lumborum are important muscles for pelvic and lumbar spine (lumbar spinal column [LSC]) posture. Their nerve supply originates in the upper lumbar spine.

- The thoracolumbar junction is a key region for spine torsions.

Pelvis

■ Vertebrae

- L4, L5.
- Sacroiliac joints.

■ Muscles

- Iliopsoas muscle.
- Gluteal muscles.
- Pelvic floor muscles.

■ Segments

- L4–S4.
- Lumbosacral plexus.
- Sacral parasympathetic nerves.

■ Some Osteopathic Considerations

- The lumbosacral junction is a hinge zone for posture, just like the OAA and the ankle joints.
- Functionally, L4 and L5 belong to the pelvis. Their action is connected to the ilium and the sacrum by the iliolumbar ligaments.
- Lumbosacral junction stability depends on the integrity of all pelvic joints.
- The sacroiliac joints are very susceptible to traumatic dysfunction. Frequently, creeping dysfunctions can develop after landing on one or both legs without sufficient suspension or a fall on the back or the buttocks (toddlers).
- Differences in leg length will sooner or later lead to pelvic torsion (±70% of the population have legs of different lengths!).
- The craniosacral connection was discussed in an earlier section. In this context, we would like to mention that Chapman (Chapman's reflex) views the pelvis as a key region for endocrine imbalances.
- Connections to the organs are provided by fascial attachments and by nerve connections via the sacral parasympathetic nerve.

7.2 Practical Applications of the Zink Pattern

The Zink pattern can be employed diagnostically and therapeutically. More information about this can be found in the practical part of this book (see Chapter 10 e.g.).

Each junction (OAA, cervicothoracic junction [CTJ], diaphragm, and pelvis) is of special significance for a specific area.

Occipitoatlantal Axis

- Head:
  Dominant cranial problems lead to suboccipital tensions and dysfunction. (*Example:* problems with temporomandibular joint [TMJ], sinuses, eyes, etc.) *Note:* We intentionally do not use the terms "primary lesions" or "primary dysfunction" because we believe that each person acquires certain patterns during childhood or earlier that increase susceptibility for certain dysfunctions. This concept can also be found in typology (Vannier) and in homeopathy.

Superior Thorax Aperture

- Lower cervical spine (CSC).
- Upper extremities.
- Upper thoracic spine (TSC) and ribs.
- Thoracic and cervical organs.

Note: It goes without saying that a dominant thoracic organ problem also involves irritation of the diaphragm with its associated segments.

With few exceptions, however, test results for the superior thorax aperture will be more pronounced.

Inferior Thorax Aperture

- Vertebral segments T6–L3.
- Last six ribs.
- Upper abdominal organs.
- Cervical spine (CSC) segments C3–C5 (phrenic nerve).

Note: The same applies here as for the superior thorax aperture. Because of its importance for the entire organism, the diaphragm is often involved. Rotation tests enable comparisons of the torsion patterns at the different junctions.

- A dominant test result for the inferior thorax aperture implies that structures listed above play a main role in this pathological process.

Pelvis

- Vertebrae T12–L5.
- Sacroiliac joint, symphysis.
- Lower extremities.
- Lower abdominal organs.

Note: The quadratus lumborum and the iliopsoas connect the thoracolumbar junction and the pelvis. These two regions impact each other in the same way as the upper thoracic spine (TSC) and the OAA region.

Since we understand the importance of diaphragms for circulation, it is worthwhile to include them in treatment of tensions to influence the pressure ratios in the cavities and to improve venolymphatic circulation.

Achieving longer-lasting improvements requires treating the structure(s) in the associated segment that prevent(s) optimal diaphragm function. Frequently, manipulating one vertebra or treating one organ complex suffices.

In addition to researching torsion patterns, Zink also developed his own method for testing the effectiveness of his treatment. After treating the body region that required therapy, he placed one hand on the abdomen of his standing patients and exerted slight pressure. He then invited his patients to spontaneously report any heat sensation spreading from the cervical area down along the spine and where this heat sensation stopped. The area where the heat sensation stopped required more treatment.

This test is based on the fact that increased intra-abdominal pressure backs up venous blood toward the azygos system and the venous plexus of the spine. This causes a slight hot flash in the areas of increased circulation. Increased muscle tonicity and blockage in the spine slow down circulation and increases in tissue temperature.

We find the Zink patterns to be an interesting diagnostic tool. They enable us to locate the impacted spine segment and provide additional information about the dominant muscle chain.

Example: Right torsion of the thorax aperture (▶**Fig. 7.3**) positions the left shoulder anteriorly and the right shoulder posteriorly. If the left shoulder offers more resistance to being pushed backward than the left shoulder does to being pushed forward, then the left anterior chain is dominant.

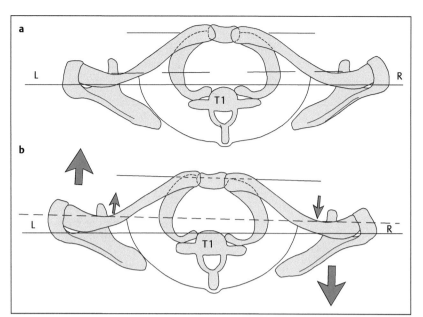

▶ **Fig. 7.3 (a, b)** Superior thorax aperture torsion.

8 Myofascial Chains: A Model

As noted in the introduction, we believe that muscles—as the organ of myofascial chains—play an important role in all bodily functions. Their main tasks may be locomotion and maintaining balance, but we should also consider their contributions to other vital functions. They are important for respiration, digestion, and circulation. Their significance becomes obvious in the case of dysfunctions. Still's assertion that fasciae are where one should look for the origins of disorders and to begin treatment only underscores the importance of fasciae.[140]

Myofascial tissue is part of the connective tissue. It contains subcutaneous and deep fasciae, skin, muscles, tendons, and ligaments. R. Louis Schultz and Rosemary Feitis refer to the fascial system as an endless web that connects everything to everything[132]

Fascial connections are not random or anarchic, but are arranged by function. The spine plays a special role. It serves as an anchor for all fascial connections, comparable to the mast of a ship to which ropes are tied. The ropes stabilize the mast, but the mast holds the sails. As long as the ropes are taut and the mast is securely anchored, the sails can function. Our trunk consists of several fascial layers that are connected to the spine and that balance each other.

Three anterior and three posterior (muscle) fascia layers could be differentiated for the trunk:
- An outer layer consisting of:
  - Posterior: latissimus dorsi and trapezius.
  - Anterior: pectoral muscles and anterior serratus.

The main task of these muscles is to mobilize the arms.
- A middle layer consisting of:
  - Posterior: paravertebral muscles and the two posterior serratus muscles.
  - Anterior: long muscle of neck (longus colli), intercostal and abdominal muscles, psoas.

These muscles directly influence the spine (even if the intercostal and abdominal muscles use the ribs as a lever).
- A deep layer consisting of fascial structures:
  - Posterior: nuchal ligament and ligamentous apparatus of the vertebral arches.
  - Anterior: central tendon of diaphragm with serosa of the organs.

These three anterior and three posterior myofascial layers can balance the spine (the mast). If one side is hypertonic, the other side yields a little. This causes the mast to lean a little, but it is still stable. This is another example of the interplay between agonists and antagonists. We can apply the same model in the frontal plane. Myofascial structures on one side must adapt to tensions on the other side to stabilize the spine.

We are convinced that when it comes to maintaining balance, and especially when a position needs to be held over a longer period, the organism will employ all available means while minimizing the impact on other bodily functions. Thoracic respiration as well as cell respiration and venolymphatic circulation must continue to function.

The curvatures of the spine contribute to its stability. It can be assumed that vertebrae, when under strain, position the spine in a way that allows its physiologic curvatures to counteract the strain. Asymmetric strain (e.g., when carrying weight in one hand) leads to scoliotic posture.

The individual spine segments rotate around Littlejohn's vertebral pivots (see Chapter 5. These vertebral pivots can sometimes be located one segment higher or lower. As a rule, however, they are C2, C5, T4, T9, L3, and L5/S1.

Muscles need stable support to perform their work. This support is provided by other muscles, which leads to the formation of muscle chains.

In upright posture, the feet are the fixed points for muscle chains. Therefore, the feet are very important for posture.

Another factor that contributes to stability as well as enables harmonious motions in all planes is the arrangement of muscles into lemniscate shapes. A lemniscate, as per Wahrig,[165] is "an arrangement in the shape of a figure eight on its side."

In fact, except for the rectus abdominis, all muscles run along a more or less diagonal or curved course. Muscles follow each other in chains in a manner that creates loops. These loops transition harmoniously from one plane to the next.

Littlejohn's pivots and the joints of the extremities are located more or less at the crossing points of lemniscates or in the center of a loop. This illustrates that Littlejohn's model is not only structural, but also very functional.

The arrangement of muscles into lemniscates enables energy-efficient fluid motions in all planes. It allows for the transformation of potential energy into kinetic energy and makes use of the locomotor system's elasticity. This creates a spiral or coiled spring effect (see Gait Analysis).

It also provides the additional benefit of decreasing pressure on the vessels, thorax, and abdomen.

Note: The greater the load we must transport, the greater the effort required of our muscles, because we can no longer take advantage of the momentum of the motion. At the same time, strain on joints, respiration, and circulation increases. Muscle contractions and joint blockages have the same effect.

8.1 Muscle Chains

In the previous chapters, we introduced several muscle chain models. Some of these display certain similarities, for example, Busquet and Chauffour, who both come from the "French school." Others are very distinct, for example, Myers and Denis-Struyf. Each of these authors described their model from a certain perspective.

Rolfing practitioners emphasize different aspects than osteopaths or physical therapists. We also described the mechanical aspects of cranial osteopathy, Zink patterns, and Littlejohn's model of the spine.

We also showed how one of the main functions of the locomotor system, walking, reproduces the behavior of the spine and the pelvis. Sutherland, Zink, and Littlejohn described this in their models.

We take it as a given that these patterns are created by muscles. This in no way contradicts Sutherland's cranial theory. Regardless of whether a pattern is triggered by the head, trunk, or extremities, the rest of the body will adapt to the same pattern (for economic reasons and to avoid taxing the brain). From a cranial perspective, this is very important for the primary respiratory mechanism (PRM) to develop without tension as much as possible. This explains why the Sutherland technique includes the segment or the cranium into the treatment of a lesion pattern: it enables unrestricted flexion and extension of the PRM.

The muscle chain model we propose differs from other models in two important aspects:

- We are convinced that flexion and extension alternate in the spine and the upper and lower extremities (▶**Fig. 8.1**). Flexion is defined as moving the two ends of a curve toward each other. Extension is defined as moving the two ends of a curve further apart.

The spine consists of three curvatures: two are concave posteriorly and one is concave anteriorly. Therefore, cervical spine (cervical spinal column [CSC]) flexion is a posterior flexion, thoracic spine (thoracic spinal column [TSC]) flexion is an anteflexion (anterior flexion), and lumbar spine (lumbar spinal column [LSC]) flexion is a posterior flexion again. This perspective of flexion and extension of the spine is interesting because it concurs with Sutherland's model. Cranial flexion corresponds to

extension of the spine, which represents extension of the three curves. Cranial extension is the opposite.

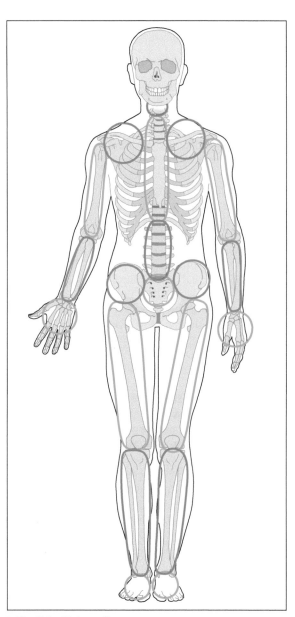

▶ **Fig. 8.1** Motor units.

The upper extremities also present consistent reversal of flexion and extension (upper arm extended, elbow flexed, fist extended and fingers flexed; e.g., arm position when writing).

In our view, the neutral lower arm position is halfway between pronation and supination, with a slight flexion of the elbow.

- We think that there are only two muscle chains in each half of the body:
  - One flexion chain.
  - One extension chain.

As described by Sutherland, external rotation and abduction are associated with flexion, and internal rotation and adduction are associated with extension.

This creates the following combinations:

- Flexion + abduction + external rotation.
- Extension + adduction + internal rotation.

> *Please note:* We would like to emphasize again that cranial flexion corresponds to extension in the parietal plane.
> The arrangement of muscles into lemniscates provides for continuity of myofascial chains between the individual spine segments. This creates connections between left and right. The same applies for the extremities.

Inhibition of antagonists and the crossed stretch reflex constitute the neurophysiological basis for the development of torsion patterns.

Before describing muscle chains, we would like to illustrate the functional motor units of the skeleton.

■ Cranium

- Sphenoid with facial and frontal bones.
- Occiput with temporal bones, parietal bones, and mandible.

■ Spine

- Atlas and axis.
- C3–T4.
- T4–T12.
- T12–L5.
- Sacrum.

■ Lower Extremity

- Ilium.
- Thigh.
- Lower leg.
- Upper ankle joint.
- Lower ankle joint and foot.

■ Upper Extremity

- Shoulder blade.
- Upper arm.
- Lower arm.
- Wrist.
- Fingers.

These individual units work together like a cogwheel.

Before we assign muscles to muscle chains, we would like to point out again that the brain does not know individual muscles, only functions. Motions are performed by muscle groups (agonists and synergists).

For motions that do not take place in one consistent plane, the participating muscles can change. Polysegmental muscle innervation also makes it possible for only part of a muscle to participate in the motion. It can be difficult to assign individual muscles to a motion, especially in the extremities and in the distal areas of the arms and legs. If a clear diagnosis cannot be obtained through visual examination, therapists sometimes need to palpate and compare the individual compartments.

The practical part of this book illustrates some simple tests to identify the dominant muscle chain.

Flexion Chain

Dominant flexion chains (▶ **Figs. 8.2, 8.3, 8.4, 8.5**) are found together with a cranial mechanism in extension (internal rotation).

■ Cranium

- Occipital bone posterior.
- Sphenobasilar synchondrosis (SBS) low.
- Sphenoid: body low.
- Greater wing of sphenoid bone posterior and medial.
- Peripheral cranium bones in internal rotation.

■ Spine

- **Occipitoatlantoaxial (OAA):** Occiput is in flexion; atlas is relatively anterior.
  Responsible muscles: rectus capitis posterior and long muscle of head (longus capitis).

Note: The central tendon can also pull the SBS into extension. It is not a muscle, but the weight of the organs can create traction toward inferior. This is the case with this pattern because the thorax is in expiration position and cannot assist in lifting the organs.

- **C3–T4:** In extension, lordosis is increased globally.
  Responsible muscles: deep paravertebral muscles between C3 and T4, semispinal muscle of head, longissimus muscle of head, splenius muscle of head (splenius capitis), and splenius muscle of neck (splenius cervicis).

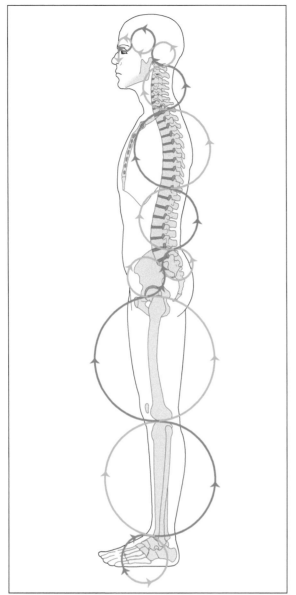

▶ **Fig. 8.2** Behavior of individual motor units with dominance of flexion pattern (*light red*) and extension pattern (*dark red*).

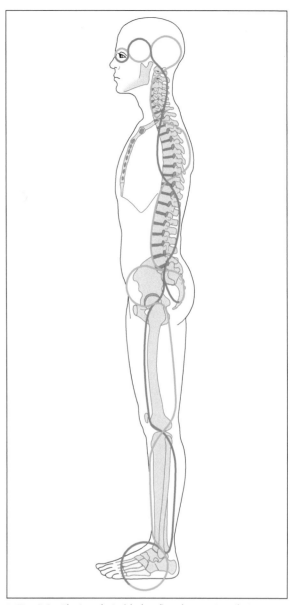

▶ **Fig. 8.3** Flexion chain (*dark red*) and extension chain (*light red*).

- **T4–T12:** Thoracic vertebrae are in flexion and ribs are in the expiration position.
  Responsible muscles: intercostal and abdominal muscles.

  Note: It may surprise some readers that we view abdominal muscles as thoracic muscles. Embryologically, they belong to the thoracic segments from which they are innervated (T5–L1). They pull the thorax into flexion via their connection with the last seven ribs.
- **T12–L5:** The lumbar spine is extended.
  Responsible muscles: lumbar paravertebral muscles and quadratus lumborum.

Note: The quadratus lumborum maintains continuity for this chain through its connection with the 12th rib and the abdominal fascia.
- **Sacrum:** The sacrum performs a nutation. Its base moves forward and downward and the coccyx moves backward and downward.
  Responsible muscles: multifidus muscles in the lumbosacral area.

Note: The thoracolumbar fascia also participates in this mechanism. Its deep layer provides attachment for the multifidus muscles and the quadratus lumborum.

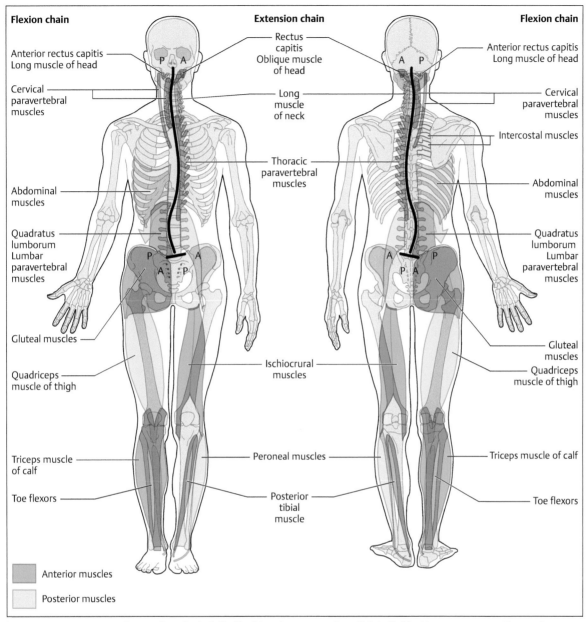

Fig. 8.4 Anterior view: flexion chain (*right half of body*) and extension chain (*left half of body*). Posterior view: flexion chain (*right half of body*) and extension chain (*left half of body*).

■ Lower Extremity

- **Ilium:** The ilium rotates posteriorly while being simultaneously pulled by the abdominal and gluteal muscles.
  Responsible muscles: abdominal muscles, gluteal muscles, and tensor fasciae latae.
- **Hip:** The hip is extended.
  - Responsible muscles: gluteal muscles.
    Note: There is a continuous chain between the abdominal and gluteal muscles via the iliac crest on one side and the thoracolumbar fascia with the quadratus lumborum and the gluteal muscles on

the other side. For the gluteal muscles to rotate the iliac posteriorly, they need secure support from the femur. This is provided by two mechanisms:

- The gluteus maximus connects with the tensor fasciae latae via the iliotibial tract. The tensor fasciae latae prevents external rotation of the hip. This allows the gluteus maximus to apply traction to the ilium.

The deep layer of the gluteus maximus connects with the vastus lateralis, which is activated by the same motion pattern. Traction from the vastus lateralis provides additional stabilization to the gluteus maximus.

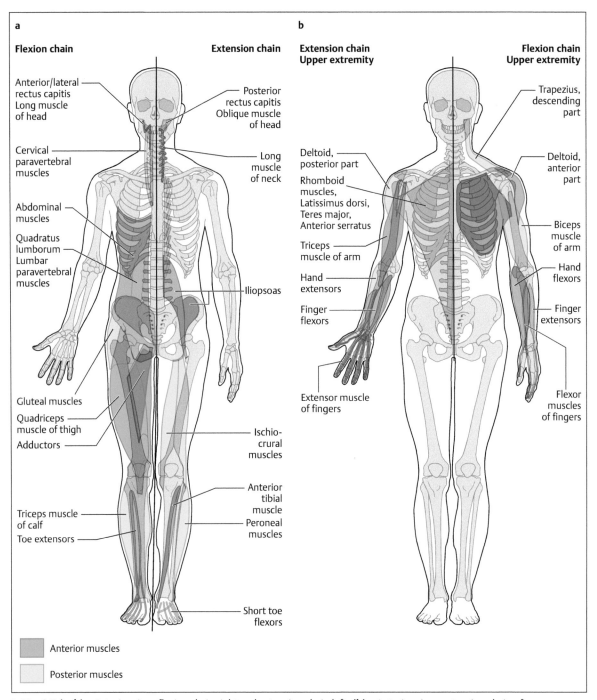

a

Flexion chain   **Extension chain**

Anterior/lateral rectus capitis Long muscle of head

Posterior rectus capitis Oblique muscle of head

Cervical paravertebral muscles

Long muscle of neck

Abdominal muscles

Quadratus lumborum Lumbar paravertebral muscles

Iliopsoas

Gluteal muscles
Quadriceps muscle of thigh
Adductors

Ischio-crural muscles

Anterior tibial muscle

Triceps muscle of calf
Toe extensors

Peroneal muscles

Short toe flexors

Anterior muscles

Posterior muscles

b

Extension chain Upper extremity   **Flexion chain Upper extremity**

Trapezius, descending part

Deltoid, posterior part
Rhomboid muscles, Latissimus dorsi, Teres major, Anterior serratus

Deltoid, anterior part

Triceps muscle of arm

Biceps muscle of arm

Hand extensors

Hand flexors

Finger flexors

Finger extensors

Extensor muscle of fingers

Flexor muscles of fingers

▶ **Fig. 8.5 (a, b)** Anterior view: flexion chain right and extension chain left. **(b)** Anterior view: extension chain of upper extremity right and flexion chain of upper extremity left.

– The posterior rotation of the ilium raises the ramus of pubis and stretches the adductors. The adductors will reclaim their lost length at the other end, at the femur. Posterior rotation of the ilium pulls the leg adductors into adduction and internal rotation. This creates the following

position for the lower extremities: **extension + adduction + internal rotation**.
• **Knee:** The knee is extended.
  Responsible muscles: quadriceps muscle of thigh.
• **Upper ankle joint:** The upper ankle joint is in plantar flexion. The talus is pushed forward between

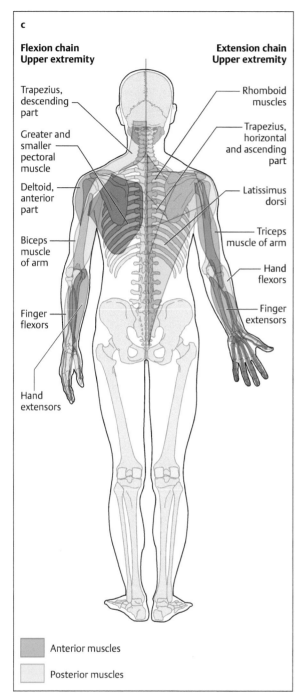

c

Flexion chain Upper extremity

Extension chain Upper extremity

Trapezius, descending part

Greater and smaller pectoral muscle

Deltoid, anterior part

Biceps muscle of arm

Finger flexors

Hand extensors

Rhomboid muscles

Trapezius, horizontal and ascending part

Latissimus dorsi

Triceps muscle of arm

Hand flexors

Finger extensors

Anterior muscles

Posterior muscles

▶ **Fig. 8.5 (c)** Posterior view: extension chain of upper extremity right and flexion chain of upper extremity left.

the ankle fork (mortise formed by the lateral and medial malleolus) and the calcaneus.
Responsible muscles: triceps muscle of calf and flexors.
- **Lower ankle joint and foot:** Dominance of the flexion chain results in eversion of the foot and lowering of the foot arches. The talus plays the main role in this process. Since it does not have muscle insertions, pressure coming from the ankle fork

pushes it medially forward. This shifts the weight to the inner edge of the foot. The cuboid bone rotates externally and the navicular bone rotates internally. Responsible muscles: long flexor muscle of toes, anterior tibial muscle, long extensor muscle of great toe, and long extensor muscle of toes.

■ Upper Extremity

- **Shoulder blade:** The shoulder blade is in abduction; the glenoid cavity of scapula is oriented forward and outward. This presents as rolled in (hunched) shoulders (Janda's upper crossed syndrome). Responsible muscles: descending part of trapezius and smaller pectoral muscle.
Depending on which muscle traction dominates, the shoulder is either depressed or raised.
- **Upper arm:** The arm is in adduction–internal rotation and extension. The greater pectoral muscle is placed in traction because the thorax is in the expiration position. The muscle reclaims its lost length by moving the arm into adduction–internal rotation. The anterior shoulder tenses the latissimus dorsi. The latissimus dorsi attempts to regain its normal length by extending the shoulder.
Responsible muscles: greater pectoral muscle, latissimus dorsi, teres major, and subscapular muscle.
- **Lower arm:** The elbow is flexed and the lower arm is pronated.
Responsible muscles: biceps muscle of arm, brachial muscle, pronator muscles.
- **Hand:** The wrist is in extension.
Responsible muscles: hand extensors.
- **Fingers:** The fingers are flexed.
Responsible muscles: finger flexors.
In this case, we find a reversal of flexion and extension as well as a predominance of the extension-adduction–internal rotation component. However, unlike the lower extremities, which exhibit global extension, this area exhibits flexion behavior. We think this is a vestige of archaic reflexes, such as can be found in spastic hemiplegia.

Extension Chain

Extension chains (▶**Figs. 8.2, 8.3, 8.4, 8.5**) are found together with a cranial flexion pattern.

■ Cranium

- Occipital bone anterior.
- SBS high.
- Sphenoid: body high.
- Greater wing of sphenoid bone anterior and lateral.
- Peripheral cranium bones in external rotation.

■ Spine

- **OAA:** Occiput is in extension.
  Atlas is relatively posterior.
  Responsible muscles: major and minor rectus capitis posterior, inferior and superior oblique muscle of head, and sternocleidomastoid (SCM).
  Note: The descending part of the trapezius can move the occiput into extension. Its main function, however, is focused on the shoulder.
- **C3–T4:** Cervical spine is in extension.
  Responsible muscles: long muscle of neck (longus colli).
- **T4–T12:** Thoracic spine is extended.
  Responsible muscles: thoracic paravertebral muscles, superior and inferior posterior serratus muscles, and thoracic fascia.
  Note: Extending the thoracic spine places the thorax into the inspiration position. This is made possible by reciprocal inhibition of the abdominal muscles. It places the diaphragm in its uppermost position, where it can function optimally.
- **T12–L5:** Lumbar spine lordosis is decreased.
  Responsible muscles: iliopsoas.
- **Sacrum:** The sacrum performs a counternutation. Its base moves backward and the coccyx moves forward.
  Responsible muscles: pelvic floor muscles.
  Note: This raises the pelvic floor and improves its function.

■ Lower Extremity

- **Ilium:** In the sacroiliac joint (SIJ), the ilium rotates anteriorly.
  Responsible muscles: iliopsoas, sartorius, rectus femoris, and adductors.
- **Hip:** The hip is flexed.
  Responsible muscles: rectus femoris, sartorius, adductors (except great adductor), and iliopsoas.
  Note: Anterior ilium rotation and hip flexion stretch the gluteus maximus. This muscle compensates by increasing abduction and external rotation.
  The piriform muscle helps rotate the sacrum toward posterior and at the same time rotates the thigh externally. This results in flexion, external rotation, and abduction of the leg. This fits with the cranial flexion model described by Sutherland.
- **Knee:** The knee is flexed.
  Responsible muscles: ischiocrural muscles (hamstrings).
  The anterior rotation of the coccyx shifts the ischial tuberosity toward posterior. This places tension on the ischiocrural muscles, which can be reduced by knee flexion.
  Note: In the standing position, knee flexion is often inconspicuous. The knee is frequently in recurvation. This is due to the relative relaxation of the

sacrotuberal ligaments created by counter-rotation of the ilium and sacrum. This causes the entire pelvis to acquire a tendency toward anteversion. The body balances itself by shifting the buttocks backward. Such patients present with "false hyperlordosis." The lower lumbar spine is in flexion and the lower thoracic spine compensates by going into lordosis. Typical examples are pregnant women and potbellied men.

- **Upper ankle joint:** The foot is in posterior extension. The talus is pushed backward between the ankle fork and the calcaneus.
  Responsible muscles: anterior tibial muscle, posterior extensor muscles of the toes.
- **Lower ankle joint:** The foot goes into inversion. The plantar muscles of the foot increase the arches of foot. Toes are flexed. Depending on which flexors dominate, this can result in hammer or claw toes.
  Responsible muscles: flexors, peroneal muscles, and posterior tibial muscle.

■ Upper Extremity

- **Shoulder blade:** The shoulder blade is in adduction and rests on top of the ribs. The shoulder is pulled back and the glenoid cavity of the scapula is oriented toward lateral.
  Responsible muscles: trapezius, rhomboid muscles, and anterior serratus.
  Note: The thorax is in inspiration position and the thoracic spine is in extension. Both contribute to this presentation.
- **Upper arm:** The arm is flexed or less extended than in the flexion pattern.
  Responsible muscles: clavicular part of the greater pectoral muscle, deltoid, and coracobrachial muscle.
  Note: If the shoulder is stabilized toward posterior by the shoulder blade fixators, the smaller and greater pectoral muscles help pull up the ribs. The latissimus dorsi is relatively relaxed due to the posterior positioning of the shoulder. This allows the greater pectoral muscle together with the anterior part of the deltoid and coracobrachial muscle to pull the arm forward. The orientation of the glenoid cavity toward lateral places the arm into external rotation. If the deltoid adds some abduction, it results in the following position: flexion–abduction–external rotation.
- **Lower arm:** The elbow is extended and the lower arm is supinated.
  Responsible muscles: triceps muscle of arm, supinator, and brachioradial muscle.
- **Hand:** The wrist is flexed (or less extended).
  Responsible muscles: hand and finger flexors.
- **Fingers:** The fingers are extended.
  Responsible muscles: finger extensors.

8.2 Summary and Conclusion about Flexion and Extension Chains

Flexion Chain

This pattern can dominate bilaterally or unilaterally. Bilateral patterns present as the kypholordotic posture with extended legs and a tendency toward fallen arches. The shoulders are pulled forward and the arms are flexed and in internal rotation. The thorax is sunken and the abdomen more or less protrudes despite a taut abdominal wall.

On the cranial level, this pattern fits the extension pattern described by Sutherland with the SBS in extension and the peripheral bones in internal rotation. The sinuses are narrower and the cerebellar tentorium is more oblique. The head is narrower and the face is more elongated.

The diaphragm is lowered because of the low thorax position. This creates traction on the central tendon, which accentuates the cranial extension position.

The low position of the diaphragm provides less support to the abdominal organs, which favors prolapses.

Notably, this position matches the asthenic, passive type. Some authors describe the extension phase of the craniosacral mechanism as a passive phase. It represents the return from the active flexion phase. The flexion posture corresponds to the "relaxation posture." This posture is forced on the organism by gravity.

Spinal curvatures are increased, which leads to ligament tension. Nutation of the sacrum and posterior rotation of the ilia tighten the lumbosacral junction ligaments. Rotation of the pelvis toward posterior and extension of the hip tighten the anterior ligamentous apparatus of the hip joint.

Extension of the knee locks the knee via the cruciate ligaments. Only the foot is "unlocked" and becomes a weak point, along with the diaphragms. This physiologic self-locking of the spine and the lower extremities requires less muscle activity for stabilization. This may explain the flaccid muscle tone and the asthenic type.

Extension Chain

This pattern can present bilaterally or unilaterally. The extension pattern (cranial flexion) involves an extended spine and flexed extremities. The organism is ready for action or is active. Cranial flexion is the active phase of the craniosacral rhythm PRM.

The SBS is in flexion (high) and the peripheral cranial bones are in external rotation. The cranial foramina are open and the cranial (dural) venous sinuses are wide. Everything is prepared for good circulation.

The cerebellar tentorium is positioned high, similar to the thoracic and pelvic diaphragms. Even the plantar aponeurosis is arched and ready for the propulsion phase of walking.

The inspiration position of the thorax and the high position of the thoracic diaphragm support the abdominal organs and prevent excessive pressure on the lower abdomen. The high position of the thoracic diaphragm reduces traction on the central tendon. This allows the SBS to move into flexion.

8.3 Torsion

Torsion patterns occur when a dominant chain develops on one side of the body, resulting in a "crossed extension reflex." This creates a torsion pattern and scoliotic posture.

If this pattern develops during early childhood, it creates a large, C-shaped curve, because the lordoses are not yet fully developed. The diagonal arrangement of muscle fibers and the continuity of fascial layers between the two halves of the body facilitate torsions. This is especially evident on the trunk. For example, the fibers of the following muscles all run in the same direction: latissimus dorsi and gluteus maximus posteriorly; greater pectoral muscle and external oblique muscles of abdomen anteriorly.

This arrangement of muscle fibers developed to meet a functional need. As discussed earlier, while walking, the pelvic and shoulder girdles move in opposite directions. This creates trunk torsion. Structure has adapted to function. These diagonal chains can be traced into all the extremities.

For example, the posterior chain can be traced via the latissimus dorsi and gluteus maximus toward inferior via the vastus lateralis, which extends from the vastus lateralis to the medial side of the knee through the medial patellar retinaculum. This is a posterior chain that transitions to an anterior chain.

Another similar anterior chain can be described as follows: Starting, for example, at the left greater pectoral muscle, we reach the right ilium via the right external oblique muscle.

The right adductors provide continuity to the right leg. The short head of the biceps muscle of thigh continues to the middle part of the great adductor to the head of fibula.

The anterior continuation of the great adductor is the vastus medialis, which connects to the other side of the leg, similar to the vastus lateralis. From here, the chain can be continued via the anterior tibial muscle or the peroneal muscles.

The connections between individual muscles and the continuous transition from one side to the other and from posterior to anterior create a loop-shaped network comparable to lemniscates.

Scoliosis and scoliotic posture represents a holistic process that takes place in three body planes.

The anteroposterior curvatures of the skeleton are respected. It is as if the entire trunk rotated around a vertical axis, while the feet stayed in place. We think it very likely that spine mechanics and muscle sensibility play an important role in the genesis of scoliosis and other contortions of the spine. These problems are holistic in nature, with the nervous system and the organ systems playing a part and maybe even being the cause.

Sutherland provides a craniosacral explanation for the development of spine contortions. Busquet and others add a visceral theory. Posturologists view the locomotor system and especially the feet as having a key role. Most likely, all of them are correct.

Therapists should consider all three views and incorporate them into their treatment plans. It is essential to remember that muscles always play an active role. **In keeping with the law of function and structure, muscles adapt to their circumstances.**

Louisa Burns[163] and other researchers showed that this process starts very early. For this reason, although looking for the cause of scoliosis makes sense, treatment of myofascial chains should not be ignored.

The same applies to all malpositions, whether they result from trauma or from excessive or imbalanced strains in daily life.

8.4 Special Characteristics of Some Muscles and Muscle Chains

The following is not a detailed anatomy presentation, but rather a brief description of the essential and any special characteristics of the following muscles and muscle chains:

- SCM.
- Scalene muscles.
- Thoracic diaphragm.
- Iliopsoas.
- Hip rotators.

Sternocleidomastoid

The SCM (▶ **Fig. 8.6**) has two muscle components that insert at the manubrium of sternum and the clavicle inferiorly and at the superior nuchal line cranially. The SCM's cranial insertion is located on the occipitomastoid (OM) suture, which Sutherland viewed as especially important for cranial mobility. Restrictions in the OM suture limit the movement of the PRM. For these reasons, the SCM has a special role.

▪ Functions

Bilateral
- Both SCMs together flex the CSC to pull the chin toward the chest.
- If the head is hyperextended, the SCMs pull the chin forward or assist in extension of the neck muscles.

- SCMs prevent hyperextension of the cervical spine in the event of a sudden thrust from behind, for example, whiplash.
- SCMs are inspiration muscles.
- SCMs are important for spatial orientation.

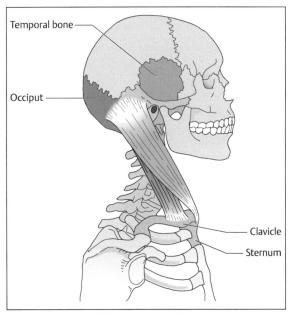

▶ **Fig. 8.6** Sternocleidomastoid (SCM).

Unilateral
- In unilateral tension, the SCMs tilt the head and rotate it to the other side while raising the chin.
- Together with the trapezius, the SCM performs a perfect sidebend.
- In scoliosis, the SCM, together with the trapezius, raises the head.

Innervation
- Accessory nerve.
- CSC segments C1–C3.

The SCM tends toward contraction (postural muscle). Its course and the many adaptation possibilities make it impossible to compare the length of the SCM. It is examined by palpating the muscle for trigger points or indurations.

Scalene Muscles

The scalene muscles (▶**Fig. 8.7**) normally consist of three muscles: anterior, middle, and posterior. Sometimes, there is a fourth, called the smallest (minimus) scalene muscle. In most cases, this fourth muscle is missing and is replaced by vertebropleural ligaments.

The anterior scalene muscle originates in the transverse processes of cervical vertebrae C3–C6 and inserts at the first rib, at the scalene tubercle.

The middle scalene muscle originates at the transverse processes of cervical vertebrae C2–C7 and then also inserts inferiorly at the first rib.

The scalene hiatus or thoracic inlet is located between the anterior and middle scalene muscles. The subclavian artery and the brachial plexus pass through this gap. Spasms of the scalene muscles can irritate these structures.

The posterior scalene muscle inserts at the posterior tubercle of cervical vertebrae C4–C6 and then continues to the second rib.

The smallest scalene muscle inserts cranially at the anterior tubercle of the last two cervical vertebrae and then continues to the cupula of pleura. The scalene muscles are susceptible to spasms, but can also contract and fibrose, depending on their function. Trigger points can imitate the symptoms of neuralgia of the median nerve. Scalene muscles are to the cervical spine what the iliopsoas is to the lumbar spine. They are primarily flexors of the cervical spine, but can also help create lordosis in the cervical spine when necessary. This functional ambivalence possibly explains their susceptibility to spasms.

The scalene muscles are part of the prevertebral muscles, together with the long muscles of head (longus capitis) and neck (longus colli). They are wrapped by

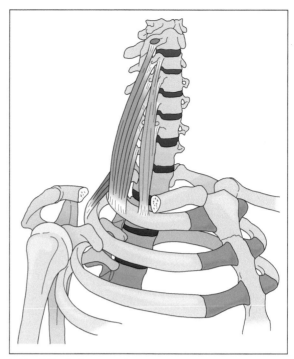

▶ **Fig. 8.7** Scalene muscles.

the deep neck fascia and are part of the Sibson fascia, which forms the upper thoracic diaphragm. This provides them with a connection to the central tendon and the visceral compartment.

■ Functions

Bilateral
- The anterior scalene muscles can flex the cervical spine.
- Together, the scalene muscles stabilize the cervical spine in the frontal plane.
- The scalene muscles are important muscles of inspiration. Electromyography studies have shown that they become active at the same time as the diaphragm. By pulling the superior thorax aperture and with it the cupula of pleura upward, the scalene muscles prevent the diaphragm from pulling the lungs toward inferior during inspiration.

The scalene muscles are responsible for thoracic high (clavicular) breathing.

Unilateral
- Unilaterally, the scalene muscles are sidebenders for the cervical spine.

Innervation
- C3–C8.

Diaphragm

Dr. Still said something like this about the diaphragm (▶ **Fig. 8.8**): "Through you we live and through you we die".[140] This is all the more applicable since the diaphragm does indeed impact all vital functions.

- Pressure changes during inspiration and expiration regulate the exchange of gases in the lungs.
- Breath-induced pressure changes also activate cell metabolism. Inspiration creates centrifugal pressure that is countered by peripheral muscles. This produces rhythmic pressure changes that influence diffusion and osmosis. Inspiration draws the blood toward the thorax, compresses the abdominal organs, and widens the venous sinus of the cranium and the veins in the neck.
- The upward and downward motion of the diaphragm mobilizes all organs in a rhythmic fashion around the physiologic motion axis of the organs.
- If necessary, the diaphragm helps with posture. Changes in the abdominal and thoracic pressure ratios can modulate spine posture. This allows the diaphragm to maintain trunk stability and, at the same time, simplify the motion of the extremities.
- Let us not forget all the vascular and nerve structures that pass through the diaphragm.

Because of its multitude of functions, the diaphragm displays some level of dysfunction in all patients. The diaphragm separates the thoracic from the abdominal cavity and consists of two parts:

- A fibrous part, the central tendon of diaphragm, to which the organs attach.
- A peripheral muscular part that is responsible for motion. This part inserts at the last five ribs and the first three lumbar vertebrae. Nerves, vessels, and organs pass through openings in the diaphragm. The muscle fibers run approximately from cranial medial to inferior lateral, from the central tendon of the diaphragm to the periphery.

Innervation
- Motoricity: Both phrenic nerves (C3–C4–[C5]).
- Sensibility: The central tendon of diaphragm and the posterior part of the muscular part are supplied by the two phrenic nerves on both sides.
- The lateral muscular part is sensibly supplied by segments T7–T10.

■ Respiratory Motion and Its Influence on the Locomotor System

The following muscles participate in respiration.

Inspiration

- Primary inspiratory muscles:
  - Diaphragm.
  - Scalene muscles.

In basal respiration, only these two muscles are usually active.
- Accessory muscles of respiration:
  - SCM.
  - Trapezius.
  - Greater pectoral muscle.
  - Smaller pectoral muscle.
  - Quadratus lumborum.
  - Iliopsoas.
  - Anterior serratus.

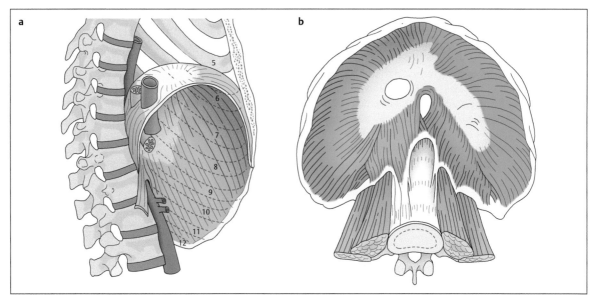

▶ **Fig. 8.8 (a, b)** Diaphragm.

– Rhomboid muscles.
– Longissimus muscle (of erector muscle of spine).
– Intercostal muscles.

Recruitment of these muscles depends on the depth of inspiration. The intercostal muscles are recruited first, from cranial to inferior.

During inspiration (▶**Fig. 8.9**), the crura of diaphragm pull the central tendon of diaphragm downward. This lowers pressure in the chest and causes air to be inspired. At the same time, pressure in the abdomen and on the abdominal wall increases. These changes are proportional to the depth of inspiration.

The central tendon of diaphragm is moved downward until it is slowed by abdominal pressure. At this point, the costal fibers of the diaphragm pull up the ribs, causing the thorax and sternum to rise. The scalene muscles support the diaphragm in this motion. The intercostal muscles stabilize the ribs against each other. Deep inspiration recruits the other muscles of inspiration.

Raising the chest and widening the ribs requires the spine to be stabilized. This task falls to the iliopsoas and the quadratus lumborum in the lumbar spine and the longissimus muscle (of erector muscle of spine) in the thorax region.

The quadratus lumborum and the iliopsoas also stabilize the last two ribs and the upper lumbar spine. This provides staple support to the crura of diaphragm.

The shoulder blade fixators stabilize the scapula and enable the anterior serratus and the pectoral muscles to raise the ribs.

The scalene muscles extend the cervical spine. At the end of a deep inspiration, the SCM is activated. It pulls up the sternal (clavicular) notch and prevents flexion of the occiput to keep the gaze directed forward.

The abdominal muscles work eccentrically. They control the descent of the abdominal organs.

What happens in the pelvis, cranium, and extremities during inspiration? The downward motion of the central tendon of diaphragm pushes the abdominal organs down and forward.

This exerts pressure on the pelvic floor and the abdominal muscles. The pressure on the pelvic floor pulls the pubic bones backward, the apex of the sacrum and the coccyx forward, and the ischial tuberosity toward medial. This pulls the wings of ilium toward anterior and outward. The traction applied to the sacrum by the pelvic floor mobilizes the base of the sacrum toward posterior and into counternutation. These motions are supported by the iliopsoas, which

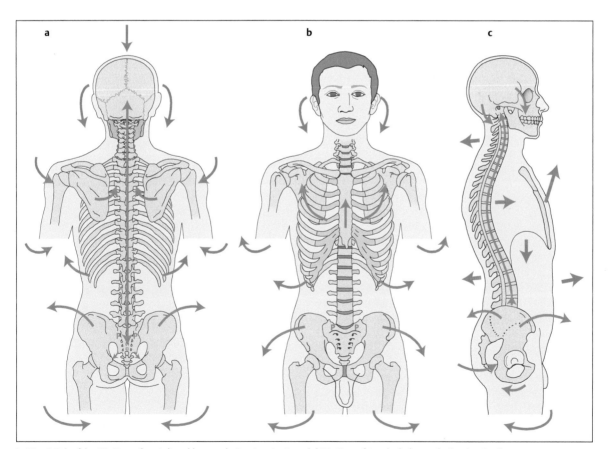

▶ **Fig. 8.9 (a, b)** Motion of peripheral bones during inspiration. **(c)** Motion of trunk skeleton during inspiration.

pulls the lumbar spine into flexion and pushes the pubic bones backward.

This means the pelvis performs a motion described earlier as the extension pattern. It conforms to the flexion motion of the craniosacral rhythm.

The lower extremities perform a flexion–external rotation–abduction motion. The extension of the thoracic spine and adduction of the shoulder blades rotate the shoulder joint outward. This facilitates the flexion–abduction–external rotation of the shoulders.

Inspiration raises the superior thorax aperture and tightens the fasciae of the neck like a tent roof. This pulls the temporal bones into external rotation. The SCM muscles and the trapezius muscles pull the occiput into extension, which corresponds to craniosacral flexion.

The nuchal ligament passively supports this effect. The extension of the cervical spine places it in tension. One way to avoid this tension is to move the occiput down and forward, that is, into cranial flexion.

The downward motion of the diaphragm and the tension it creates on the central tendon is neutralized by raising the chest. This enables the SBS to move toward cranial.

Inspiration therefore completely matches the flexion pattern of the PRM described by Sutherland. The flexion phase, like inspiration, is an active phase. Expiration is the opposite phase.

Expiration

- At rest, the expiration phase is normally a passive process. Tissue elasticity returns the structures to their original position.
- During deep respiration, the abdominal muscles are the primarily active muscles. Some authors also consider the internal intercostal muscles and the transverse muscle of thorax to be expiration muscles (Mac Conail, Basmajian[164]).

The diaphragm and the scalene muscles, as well as the accessory muscles of respiration, relax if they were activated by deep inspiration. Deep expiration activates the abdominal muscles. This compresses the contents of the abdomen and pushes it upward. At the same time, the chest is pulled toward inferior.

In the SIJ, the ilium performs a posterior rotation and inflare. The extremities rotate internally. The expiration position of the chest causes the ribs to pull the upper thoracic spine into flexion and the cervical spine into lordosis. The cranial bones return to their original position.

Compared to the inspiration position, expiration represents extension–internal rotation. The position of the occiput corresponds to the position of the sacrum.

Note: It should be noted that the head remains horizontal during both inspiration and expiration. We believe that this represents a conjugated action of the SCM muscles, trapezius muscles, and suboccipital muscles.

Iliopsoas Muscle

The iliopsoas muscle (▶**Fig. 8.10**) is perhaps the most interesting muscle of the entire myofascial apparatus. It is certainly the muscle whose function gives rise to the most controversial discussions. Based on its insertion and especially its course, it can coordinate the positions of the hip, pelvis, and lumbar spine with each other.

Basmajian[164] views the iliopsoas as the most important muscle in the body for posture. It can adjust the spine and the pelvis in the frontal as well as in the sagittal plane.

Lewit[86] writes that the psoas often causes abdominal pain in the iliac fossa or imitates gall bladder or kidney colic. Because of its insertion at T12 and at the psoas arcade of the diaphragm, the psoas is directly involved in respiration.

Bogduk[14] says that psoas spasms put great strain on the lumbar vertebral disks. Fryette,[56] Kuchera,[82]

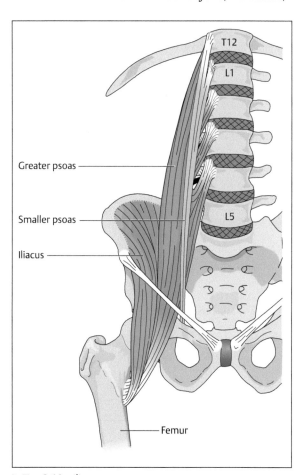

▶ **Fig. 8.10** Iliopsoas.

DiGiovanni and Schiowitz,[49] and others describe the psoas syndrome as the main reason for acute lumbago.

The psoas is classified as a postural muscle, meaning it contains primarily type I fibers. Contracted or spastic iliopsoas are indeed both found with similar frequency. Lewit[86] states that contraction of the psoas causes pain at the thoracolumbar junction and contraction of the iliacus muscle causes pain in the SIJ.

Psoas hypertonicity can cause nerve irritations of the lumbar plexus. The psoas inserts at the vertebral bodies of T12–L4 (L5) and the vertebral disks between those vertebrae as well as at the transverse processes of L1–L4. The lumbar plexus passes between the two muscle bellies. The iliacus muscle has its origin in the iliac fossa.

Both muscles unite and extend below the inguinal ligament to the lesser trochanter of the femur. The smaller psoas muscle originates at the muscle belly of the greater psoas muscle and its inferior insertion is at the linea pectinea and at the inguinal ligament.

The iliopsoas is wrapped by a tight fascia, the iliac fascia. It represents the inferior extension of the diaphragm fascia. The iliac fascia is connected to the inguinal ligament at the pelvis.

The iliopsoas is the slide rail for the kidney and is also in contact with other organs. It runs from posterior–medial–cranial to inferior–anterior–lateral. At the level of the linea pectinea, its fibers change course and run posterior–lateral.

The iliopsoas runs in front of the hip joint and is separated from that joint by a bursa. The reversal of fiber direction at the pubic bone causes the muscle to rotate the ilium anteriorly when stressed. This means the psoas supports the traction of the iliacus muscle.

■ Functions

Bilateral
- Both iliopsoas muscles are the strongest hip flexors in the body. When the legs are fixed, they rotate the wings of ilium forward and create pelvic anteversion.
- They are lumbar vertebrae flexors when the pelvis is prevented from tilting forward.

Unilateral
- The iliopsoas muscles sidebend the lumbar spine ipsilaterally. If the spine can go into lordosis while this happens (in easy flexion as per Fryette), the vertebrae rotate into the convexity. If the pelvis is not able to tilt forward (because of tension in the abdominal muscle or the pelvic floor), the psoas causes the lumbar spine to flex, sidebend, and rotate ipsilaterally.

Innervation
- Lumbar segments L1, L2 (L3).

Hip Rotators

The hip rotator muscle group (▶**Fig. 8.11**) consists of the following muscles:
- Piriformis.
- Gemellus muscles.
- Internal obturator.
- External obturator.

These muscles are all close to a joint. Their lever is too short for powerful motion. They serve more of a proprioceptive function for the hip joint. They adapt the rotation of the femur to the rotation of the ilium with the goal of optimally centering the head of femur into the acetabulum. Together with the pelvic floor muscles, they provide a kind of hammock for the pelvis.

During the stance phase of gait and in one-legged stance, the piriformis and the gluteus maximus stabilize the diagonal axis of the sacrum. The piriformis is a postural muscle with a tendency toward contraction. It exits the pelvis through the greater sciatic notch. In this area, the piriformis is in close vicinity of the gluteal nerves, the pudendal nerve, the sciatic nerve, and the vessels that supply the pelvic floor. Piriformis contraction can irritate those structures and cause pseudoneuralgias and functional problems of the perineum. The leg is then rotated outward and shortened. Pain radiates to the SIJ, the buttocks, and the back of the thigh. In rare cases, pain can radiate to below the popliteal cavity. Prolonged sitting or crouching with knees pressed together causes pain because it stretches the piriformis (in the presence of piriformis lesions).

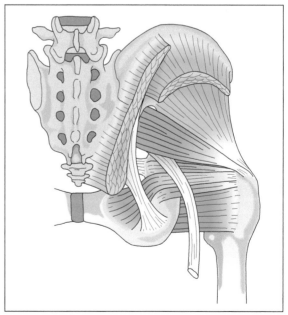

▶ **Fig. 8.11** Hip rotators.

■ Functions

As mentioned earlier, the hip rotators serve a proprioceptive function for the hip joint. They rotate the hip externally and are abductors and mild extensors. When the hip is flexed more than 60°, the piriformis becomes an internal rotator for the hip.

Summary

We could continue this list of interesting muscles and muscle groups, but we feel this overview suffices.

Before concluding this chapter, we would like to briefly mention the anterior muscles:

- Hyoid muscles play a very minor role as mobilizer of the cervical spine. They are primarily active during motions of the lower jaw (mouth opener), where the lower hyoid muscles stabilize the hyoid bone. They play a role in swallowing, yawning, talking, and breathing. Their main function likely is to prevent the trachea and the esophagus from collapsing during head and neck motions.
- For these muscles to be able to flex the neck, the muscles of mastication must close the mouth. The main flexors for the cervical spine are the prevertebral muscles and the SCM (when the head is flexed).
- The intercostal muscles stabilize the trunk and contribute to trunk rotations. For this function, they are synergists to the oblique abdominal muscles.

Their main function is to assist the respiratory muscles. This characteristic dominates even while these muscles perform support functions.

The abdominal muscles, and especially the rectus abdominis, are antagonists to the longissimus muscle of thorax, which underscores their affiliation with the thoracic muscles.

They are active in almost all motions of the trunk and the lower extremities. These muscles act as less of a mobilizer and more of a stabilizer of the trunk. They compress the abdominal organs and the thorax and this provides support to the spine.

While walking, the abdominal muscles and the multifidus muscles are active in advance of the muscles in the lower extremities (the transverse abdominal muscle acts first).

Except for the hip rotators, all other muscles described in this section (SCM, scalene, diaphragm, and iliopsoas) can support other muscles during flexion as well as during extension of the spine.

- The SCM extends the upper cervical spine and flexes it if the lower cervical spine is in flexion.
- The scalene muscles are flexors for the cervical spine.

If the paravertebral muscles of the neck place the cervical spine into lordosis, the scalene muscles change their function and support the paravertebral muscles.

- The diaphragm can flex or extend the thoracolumbar junction, as needed.
- The iliopsoas can place the lumbar spine into lordosis or help extend it.

If the abdominal muscles and the pelvic floor place the pelvis in retroversion, the psoas places the lumbar spine into kyphosis.

The importance of the hip rotator muscles is often underestimated. During gait, weight is shifted from the sagittal plane to the frontal plane. From flexion–extension of the spine, the motion transforms into abduction–adduction in the pelvis to maintain balance. The hip rotators help stabilize the pelvis and assure good congruency of the head of femur in the joint socket. For this reason, these muscles are often strained in all types of pelvic dysfunctions.

9 Posture

This chapter focuses on the impact of posture on the organism. Posture problems are often overlooked as potential causes of locomotor dysfunctions, especially of the spine. Manual therapists are very familiar with the importance of the musculoskeletal system for the entire organism. Korr[10] talked about the "primary machinery of life" when describing the locomotor system. Kuchera[12] views myofascial tissue as having vital functions:

- Protection from thermal, mechanical, and chemical stimuli.
- Support and posture.
- Connecting link between the individual systems.
- Pathway for vessels and nerves.
- Respiration for cell respiration and gas exchange in the lungs.
- Mobilization.

Still[26] was convinced that dysfunctions of the locomotor system, and especially of the spine, are the cause of all physical ailments and that treatment can only be successful if normal spine function can be achieved. This makes sense considering that the sensibility of the entire body reaches the spine segments.[8,9,24,25] This also certainly explains why so many people have back pain.

In the medical world, there is no question that mental or emotional problems can manifest as physical ailments. Studies seem to confirm that about one-third of chronic back problems have mental or emotional causes. A significant number of organic disorders are caused or at least influenced by emotional stress (e.g., stress ulcers). Upledger's theory of emotional cysts is an interesting model to explain how emotions can cause physical dysfunctions that manifest as palpable tissue changes ("emotional cysts"). Even if this theory has not been proven scientifically, treatment successes seems to prove him right. The mechanisms by which emotions trigger physical ailments are not yet understood. Several explanation models are possible:

- Neuronal connections could explain functional disorders of the spine (which are always present).
- Neuroendocrine feedback loops could explain hormonal imbalances like the kind found in fibromyalgia patients.
- Biomechanical and electromagnetic phenomena caused by changes in the areas of tension in myofascial tissue.[22]

In this context, it is interesting to note that piezoelectric phenomena and electromagnetic fields have been measured in myofascial tissue.[22] Newer studies showed that contractile cells occur in fasciae. This supports the conclusion that fasciae react independently. These phenomena add a new dimension to Buckminster Fuller's tensegrity model. There are now medical devices that produce an electromagnetic field to treat poorly healing bone fractures. The frequency used by these devices can demonstrably stimulate the healing process. Interestingly, this frequency is precisely the same as the electromagnetic field produced by a human hand.[22]

If one considers the interrelationships between the areas of the body that are explained by neurologic reflex arcs (viscerosomatic, somatovisceral, viscerovisceral, and somato-somatic),[10,12] then one can understand why Still viewed fasciae as the hunting grounds where the osteopath needs to search for the cause of ailments and should start treatment.[26] Therefore, it is important for manual therapists who work holistically to find the cause of the patient's complaints. These could be located in visceral as well as in cranial or parietal areas.

9.1 Factors Impacting Posture

Posture results from the musculoskeletal effort needed to counter the force of gravity. Any deviation from ideal posture results in increased stress for the entire organism.

Kappler (1982) defines perfect posture as a condition in which body mass is distributed in a way that enables muscles to retain their normal tonicity and ligament tensions to neutralize the impact of gravity.

When a person is standing upright, posture primarily depends on three factors:

- How levelled is the ground on which the person is standing?

- What is the condition of their feet as the contact point with the ground?
- The base of the sacrum as the foundation of the spine, since the spine keeps the organs of equilibrium in balance.

Note: This is true if one considers that malpositions of the occipitoatlantoaxial (OAA) complex cause the sacrum to adapt. If the base of the sacrum is horizontal, then the OAA complex also has to be balanced. However, since cranial dysfunctions can also be primary, we tend to add the OAA complex as a fourth factor that impacts posture.

The three arches of the foot must be optimally balanced on both sides. Ideally, the tibia should be positioned vertically above the foot (in the frontal plane) for the weight of the body to be distributed harmoniously among all three arches. This assures optimal power transmission toward the pelvis. These descriptions are beginning to illustrate the potential impact of myofascial traction on posture.

The iliolumbosacral junction consists of the lumbosacral junction and the two sacroiliac joints. Stability is provided by the configuration of joints, ligaments, and muscles. Optimally directed forces provide sufficient compression to the joints to not require muscle power to stabilize the pelvis.

Basic muscle tonicity and ligaments assure joint surface congruency. The three forces that meet in the lumbosacral junction neutralize each other. The force of gravity impacting the base of the sacrum is neutralized by the two forces ascending from the legs. This mechanism only functions if the base of the sacrum is horizontal. Even a minimal tilt of the promontory of sacrum changes the force lines and leads to instability. If this happens, muscles are recruited to reestablish stability. This automatically impacts the entire locomotor system. It changes the position of the pelvis, which in turn changes the position of the spine and the lower extremities.

Robert Irvin conducted a study [in[155]] that found that persons with chronic back pain who had been treated by classical osteopathy without durable success experienced a 70% improvement of general symptoms if, in addition to this treatment, the base of their sacrum was leveled with orthotics.

The most frequent malpositions are:
- Fallen arches (pes planus).
- Valgus of the hindfoot (flatfoot, pes valgus), talipes valgus.
- Lateral tilt of base of sacrum.

All three deformities can be corrected by orthotics. In a radiology study [in[155]] conducted by Irvin, he discovered that 98% of all X-rayed people presented with a tilt of the base of sacrum of 1.2 mm on average in the frontal plane.

A tilt of the base of the sacrum (in the frontal plane) can have many causes:
- Sacrum dysfunction: one anterior base of the sacrum is also lower.
- Ilium dysfunction: rotation of the ilium toward anterior also raises the base of the sacrum on the same side; rotation toward posterior also lowers the base of sacrum on the same side.
- Leg length differences: anatomical or acquired because of trauma, surgeries, and foot malpositions.

Adaptations of the spine to a tilted base of the sacrum are always three-dimensional and can result in either a C-shaped (rarely) or S-shaped scoliosis. Adaption in the shape of an S-shaped curve is the most economical and is also the simplest way to maintain balance. In newborns and small children, however, we only find C-shaped scoliosis.

Rotation and sidebending in scoliosis and scoliotic posture are always opposing (neutral position-sidebending-rotation, [NSR] according to Fryette—see Chapter 3). Functional scoliosis (scoliotic posture) can progress to structural scoliosis (structure adapts to function).

The organism attempts to compensate posture imbalances by adapting the body segments above and below the interference field in opposite directions. This results in alternating rotation sidebending. These changes are created in the junction zones.[12]

Zink patterns are one example: Littlejohn's model of biomechanics of the spine provides a mechanical explanation.

Treatment of scoliosis and kypholordosis depends on whether the curvatures are functional or structural. For functional, nonfixed curvatures, the goal is improved posture. For structural imbalances, the primary goal is to alleviate pain and enable optimal functioning of all structures and systems. In every case, all causes of the structural imbalance should be considered:
- Eyes.
- Vestibular organs.
- Cranium and OAA complex.
- Temporomandibular joint.
- Organs.
- Spine–pelvis.
- Feet.

Fibrosis, retractions, and adhesions must be specifically treated over a longer period. Dynamic orthotics are often very effective because they can stimulate specific hypoactive muscle chains. They are also able to imitate weight shift that influences the equilibrium via the vestibulospinal tracts.

Frequently, structural changes of the feet must be stabilized by static orthotics to prevent nociceptive reflexes from muscles that are under excessive strain. Leg length differences that are greater than 3 mm should be equalized[11] regardless of whether they are anatomical or acquired.

9.2 Impact of Gravity on the Locomotor System

Gravity continuously influences the locomotor system as soon as a human becomes upright. According to Fryette, "Gravity kills the men."[9] However, gravity helps stabilize the locomotor system if it is in balance, for example, by locking the sacroiliac joints via the nutation component. This process is induced by gravity if the gravitational line runs between the sacroiliac joint and the acetabulum through the shaft of femur.[15,16,20] However, posture imbalances caused by trauma or myofascial tension disrupt the normal course of the gravitational line.[23]

This requires the organism to adapt. These adaptations are carried out by contractile elements (at least during the initial phase). Posture changes occur to prevent gravity from having any or little negative impact. However, this condition limits the opportunities for further adaptations by the organism and, in the worst-case scenario, can be the reason for pain in any area of the spine or the extremities. The reason for that can be found in the extreme sensibility of muscle spindles and the way muscles function as chains.

For example, intense or repeated supination trauma (supination outward rotation injury or ankle sprain) can lead to valgus position of the calcaneus if not treated properly. It results in the weight of the body being shifted to the medial longitudinal arch of the foot. This can lead to internal rotation of the ankle fork and could cause internal rotation of the leg and anteversion of the pelvis on that side. The pelvic torque causes the spine to adapt all the way up to the occipitoatlantoaxial (OAA) joints.[15,20] If this posture disorder is accompanied by disorders of the organs, for example, gastritis, it can cause blockages in the medial thoracic spine (T5–T9) or motion limitation in the OAA joints. These dysfunctions can cause pain in the thoracic spine, neck, and head, as well as tinnitus, vertigo, etc. If this condition persists for longer periods, it results in sensitization at the level of the spinal cord (chronic lowering of stimuli threshold). This allows even extremely mild stimuli (cold, stress, physical exertion) to trigger a recurrence of the stomach problem, headaches, etc. Treatment of the patient encompasses elimination of all stimuli, including posture imbalance. If any source of stimulation remains, then any negative stimulus can trigger the entire clinical presentation again at any time, because the sensitized segment was not normalized.

In addition to the musculature as an implementing organ, posture receptors are extremely important for maintaining upright posture.[2,3] The sensitivity of muscle spindles enables extremely quick and precise adaptions to sudden shifts in the body's center of gravity.

These mechanisms occur subconsciously and possibly according to certain patterns. This process is very significant because it is ongoing and places very little demand on the body (law of economics and freedom from pain).

It is not yet fully understood exactly which muscles participate and to what extent in the posture process. They must be the type of muscles that can respond quickly to changes to reestablish posture equilibrium. Phasic muscles are suited to this task because they contain plentiful receptors. However, posture imbalances that persist for a longer term recruit muscles that can maintain tension for longer periods. These are muscles that contain a predominance of tonic muscle fibers. This is a very simplified illustration. The actual process is likely to be much more complex.

The central nervous system adapts posture entirely to momentary needs. However, the following should be noted:

- Normally, the factors that counteract gravity are passive. The skeleton with its bones, joints, and ligaments is designed to automatically "lock" in upright posture and requires only minor adjustments to maintain balance.[5,6]
- The spinal curvatures are increased, which causes tightening of the ligaments.
- The sacrum is rotated toward anterior and the hip bone is rotated toward posterior, which leads to tightening of the posterior iliosacral, sacrotuberal, and sacrospinal ligaments. This stabilizes and compresses the sacroiliac joints.
- The pelvis is tilted toward posterior, which tightens the coxofemoral ligaments.
- The feet develop a tendency toward fallen arches (flatfoot or pes planus), which tightens the plantar aponeurosis and all ligaments.[15]

Overall, this corresponds to the expiration or flexion pattern. In this ideal case, the central line of gravity runs in the frontal plane from the anterior edge of the foramen magnum through the entire spine to exactly between both feet. In the sagittal plane, the line runs through the outer ear canal through the center of the humeral head, through the greater trochanter, in front of the head of fibula and in front of the lateral malleolus.

Gravity pushes the thorax along with the diaphragm and its attached organs downward. This effect is neutralized by the fact that the lungs always retain a certain amount of air (residual volume) and that the colon inflates. Together, these provide a kind of air cushion for the thorax and prevent ptosis.

9.3 Hinge Zones

Osteopaths, chiropractors, and posturologists are equally conscious of the importance of posture for the health of the organism. Each of these three professions has different explanations for the causes of imbalance and utilizes different treatment approaches. They are aware of the importance of the spine, but locate the main causes of imbalance in different regions of the body. Their treatment success confirms their methods.

We posed the following question to ourselves: why are the pelvis and the OAA complex so important for the osteopath, the atlas so important for the chiropractor, and the feet so important for the posturologist? What do these three regions have in common that so profoundly influences posture? Not entirely to our surprise, we found one possible interesting answer in the anatomy and biomechanics of each of those regions of the body.

The OAA complex, the iliolumbosacral junction, and the hindfoot feature two important commonalities:

- Each of these three areas contains a bone whose motion depends on the amount of pressure exerted on it. Direct mobilization of this bone by muscles is secondary.
  - The atlas acts like a meniscus between the occiput and the axis.
  - Globally, it acts opposite to the occiput and C2.
  - The sacrum performs motions that are relatively opposite to those of the spine and the ilia. This action is forced upon the sacrum by pressure coming from the spine.
  - The talus has no muscle insertions. Its behavior depends entirely on pressure. Its direction of motion is forced upon it by the orientation of the ankle fork and the position of the calcaneus.
  - The behavior of these three bones can be compared to a ball in a ball joint.
  - The ball enables harmonious motions and makes it possible to shift pressure in a different direction.

- In all three regions, pressure ratios are redistributed.
  - The weight of the head is distributed via the atlas to the vertebral bodies and the zygapophyseal (facet) joints of C2 (Mitchell: cervical spine facets have a weight-bearing function; ▶ **Fig. 9.1**).
  - At the lumbosacral junction, gravity is shifted to a different plane.
  - Weight is transferred from the promontory of the sacrum in the direction of the two hip joints (▶ **Fig. 9.2**).
  - The talus shifts the weight of the body while standing and walking onto the tuberosities of the heel bone (calcaneus) and toward the cuboid bone

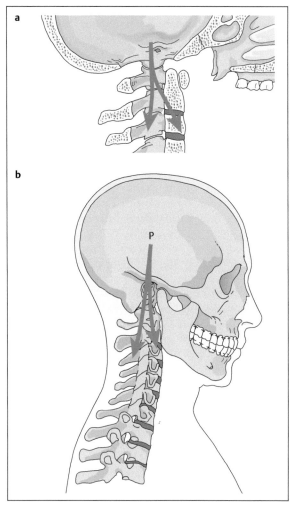

▶ **Fig. 9.1 (a, b)** Weight shift from head to vertebral body and zygapophyseal (facet) joints of the axis (in the sagittal plane).

and navicular bone of foot, that is, to the outer or inner edge of the foot (▶ **Fig. 9.3**).

Notes: Weight is shifted in different planes in these three regions:

- OAA: in the sagittal plane—facets and vertebral bodies of C2.
- Lumbosacral junction: in the frontal plan—toward both hip joints.
- Foot: in the horizontal plane—from talus to calcaneus and to cuboid and navicular.

This once again illustrates how structure adapts to function. While walking, weight shifts:

- Posteroanteriorly in the spine.

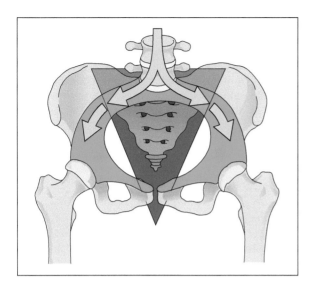

▶ **Fig. 9.2** Weight shift in the frontal plane from the spine to both hip joints.

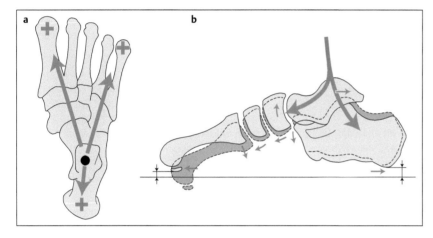

▶ **Fig. 9.3 (a, b)** Weight shift in the horizontal plane in the upper ankle joint.

- From left to right and vice versa in the pelvis.
- From the calcaneus to the first and fifth metatarsal heads in the foot.

Dysfunctions or structural changes in those areas cause power transmissions to be misdirected, which results in changes in muscle strain. This leads to the development of changes in muscle tracks, which causes the entire locomotor system to adapt and creates a different posture pattern.

9.4 Maintaining Equilibrium

Roughly speaking, the equilibrium system of the body can be categorized as follows:
- Afferent pathway: receptors and sensible pathways.
- Control center: cortex, cerebellum, reticular formation, and subcortical nuclei (basal nuclei, basal ganglia).
- Efferent pathways: pyramidal tract and parapyramidal tract.[24,25,28]

The afferent pathway consists of the anterior funiculi of spinal cord (anterior and lateral spinothalamic tracts) and the posterior funiculi of spinal cord (fasciculus gracilis medullae spinalis or Goll column and cuneate fasciculus of spinal cord or Burdach column). The anterior funiculi of spinal cord primarily conduct sensations of pressure, touch, temperature, and pain via the thalamus to the cortex. These tracts also contain fibers to subcortical centers such as the reticular formation, the olive, and the tectal plate. These are afferents for the pyramidal tract. The posterior funiculi of spinal cord are responsible for transmitting proprioception and epicritic surface sensibility. They also exhibit connections to cortical and subcortical motoricity centers.

While the pyramidal tract of the efferent pathway is responsible for target motoricity, the parapyramidal tract has the main role in automatisms. Maintaining equilibrium is primarily a subconscious process. However, impending loss of equilibrium can be consciously prevented.

Upright gait and coordinated, targeted motion require complicated tonicity and balancing regulation. The cerebrum or the subcortical motor areas are relieved of these tasks. They are performed instead by the cerebellum and the vestibular system.[24,28]

The cerebellum modulates motor sequences that have been initiated by the cerebrum and turns them into targeted, well-coordinated motions. To do so, it receives information about the excitation state of muscles, the spatial position of the body, and information from the cortical and subcortical motor areas. The cerebellum receives information from the muscle spindles via the spinocerebellar tract. Vestibular nuclei provide information about the position and motions of the body in space. In parallel to the pyramidal and the parapyramidal tracts, fibers run to the cerebellum that informs it about motion patterns that have been preprogrammed by the cortex and the subcortical nuclei.

The impact of the cerebellum on motoricity is indirect. While the "rough" implementation plan for the motion pattern is supplied by the cortex, the cerebellum refines the motions by modulating the sensibility and motor areas. It regulates muscle activity by sending efferents to the thalamus, red nucleus, vestibular nuclei, and the olive. Performing this task requires the cerebellum to function soundly. This presupposes a healthy supply to the equilibrium apparatus as well as correct information from the posture receptors.

Practical Relevance

Somatic dysfunctions (blockages, muscle injuries, etc.) can direct misinformation to the cerebellum. Blockages in the spine are interference factors for forwarding all afferent and efferent stimuli. Eye motoricity and vestibular organ dysfunctions negatively impact the vestibular system.

The vascular supply for the cerebellum, inner ear, and brain stem is provided by the vertebral artery. Blockages in the upper thoracic spine (via the sympathetic nervous system) and especially in the cervical spine can negatively impact those vessels. This leads to vascular dysfunctions and, therefore, dysfunctions of the nuclei supplied by these vessels. From this perspective, the suboccipital region plays a special role. The vertebral artery is especially vulnerable in that region because it travels in a double arch and across the arch of the atlas before entering the head. Muscle tensions can easily impede blood flow through these vessels. The sympathicotonic condition present in case of blockages likely plays a much more important role because it leads to vasoconstriction.

The large number of afferents that reach the upper cervical segments (via the trigeminal nerve, vagus nerve, cervical plexus, and spinal cord) possibly explains the frequency of OAA joint dysfunctions. It also possibly explains the positive effect of normalizing the atlas.

Posture Receptors

The equilibrium is regulated by subconscious reflex arcs controlled by the central nervous system. Muscles are the implementing organ and posture (position sense) receptors are the sources of information. The following receptors are especially important for maintaining equilibrium.

■ Foot, Joint, and Muscle Proprioceptors

Proprioception from the muscle, joint, and tendon receptors provides information from the locomotor system for maintaining balance. Muscle spindles provide information about muscle length, while Golgi receptors in the tendons measure tensions. Pacini corpuscles are acceleration detectors that are present in skin, tendons, muscles, and joint capsules. They register the acceleration of motions. Merkel cells in the skin of the sole of the foot provide information about pressure shifts on the foot.[2,3,16,25]

■ Vestibular System

The vestibular system plays an important role in maintaining balance. Its sensory cells are in the inner ear. The information received there is transmitted via the vestibulocochlear nerve to the brain where they control balance together with other cerebral centers that are responsible for sensomotoricity.[8,24,25,28]

The vestibular system, together with the cochlea, resides in the bony labyrinth of the petrous part of temporal bone. It is surrounded by the perilymph fluid and essentially consists of:
- Three semicircular canals at the end of which are extensions called membranous ampullae.
- Two bladders, the utricle (utriculus vestibularis) and the saccule (sacculus vestibularis).

The canals, ampullae, and both bladders are also filled with endolymph fluid.

The ampullae, the utricle, and the saccule contain cilia that are the sensory organs of the vestibular system (statoconia and statoliths in the utricle and saccule). The canals are at a right angle to each other and are tilted by 45 degrees relative to the respective spatial planes.

When the head moves, the endolymph begins to oscillate, which stimulates the sensory cells. The cilia in the ampullae respond to rotational motions in three spatial planes, while the statoliths in the utricle and saccule only respond to linear motion and, therefore, the impact of gravity.

The vestibulocochlear nerve transmits these stimuli to the four vestibular nuclei at the bottom of the rhomboid fossa in the brain stem. These, in turn, project primarily to three regions in the brain:

- The cerebellum: vestibulocerebellum.
- The motor nuclei of the extrinsic (extraocular) eye muscles.
- The spinal cord.

■ Eyes

Eye movements must be coordinated with movements of the trunk and neck. This is necessary for maintaining level forward vision, maintaining focus on an object when the trunk moves, or following an observed object while in motion. This is possible via circuits that coordinate the visual area with the motor and equilibrium areas.

Proprioceptors in the sole of the foot, joints, and muscles as well as the vestibular system and the eyes can be viewed as primary organs of equilibrium. In addition, other structures are significant for posture because they support the muscles that maintain the body upright or they can have negative impacts in case of functional disorders.

- Cavity pressure.
- Masticatory apparatus.
- Suboccipital muscles.
- Lumbosacral junction.

■ Cavity Pressure

Cavity pressure in the thorax and in the abdomen helps erect the trunk. Therefore, one needs to consider that pressure changes in these cavities can cause posture adaptions.[5,23]

The sensible supply of the serosa and the attachment of organs (ligaments and mesos) reach the spinal cord segments. Stimuli, especially nociceptive stimuli (even subliminal or subconscious), are reported to the spinal cord and can contribute toward changing muscle tone of the paravertebral muscles in the respective segments.

Cavity pressure, however, is also very significant for another, perhaps more important, mechanism that also impacts posture indirectly. Thoracic respiration is the main pump for venolymphatic circulation. The respirator muscles and especially the diaphragm have the same function for the veins and lymph vessels of the trunk and the head as the muscle pump has for the veins and lymph channels in the extremities.

Veins of the head, trunk, and spine have no or very few functional venous valves. Venous return and lymph flow toward the heart is achieved through constant differences in pressure between the thoracic and abdominal cavities. Pressure in the thorax is lower than in the abdominal cavity. The inferior motion of the diaphragm during inspiration increases abdominal pressure and decreases thoracic pressure. This makes it possible to inhale air, but at the same time, blood and lymph (the cisterna chyli is located right below the peripheral parts of the diaphragm) is pumped toward the heart. The volume of blood and lymph are pumped in the direction of the heart correlates with the volume of inhaled air. The more the diaphragm and thorax expand during inspiration, the more blood and lymph pumped to the heart.

The attachment of the pericardium at the spine, sternum, and diaphragm as well as the fascial attachments of the veins in the superior thorax aperture is such that the heart is prepared to receive the blood pumped during inspiration. Without the supporting function of the thoracic venolymphatic pump, the human heart would experience overload within a short time.

The pressure gradient between the thorax and the abdomen can be changed by physiologic and pathologic conditions. The first structure to attempt to reestablish the physiologic pressure gradient is the diaphragm. If the pressure in the abdominal cavity increases, the diaphragm immediately shifts upward and functions in an expiration position. This presents as shallow breathing, especially inspiration, and a faster heartbeat. After a short time, the accessory muscles of respiration are increasingly recruited, which neutralizes the circulatory changes again. If that happens, the thorax is placed in the inspiration position, which influences posture.

Persistent changes in pressure that can happen because of organic pathologies, postsurgery or with inflammatory process that can create organ adhesions, can place continuous strain on the accessory muscles of respiration. This will lead to posture adaptations. Increased abdominal pressure causes extension of the spine (straightening of the spine with external rotation and abduction of the extremities). A decrease in abdominal pressure causes the opposite posture (kypholordosis of the spine with internal rotation and adduction of the extremities).

■ Masticatory Apparatus

The masticatory apparatus is not part of the primary organs of equilibrium. Nevertheless, the position of the jaw plays a significant role for cervical spine posture and especially the OAA. Pronation creates extension of the cervical spine and flexion position of the occiput over the atlas. Retrognathia creates the opposite position.[13]

The position of the OAA and the shape of the spinal curves harmonize with each other. Extension of the cervical spine results in a straightening of the entire spine, in the same way that lordosis increases the three spinal curves.

Malocclusion is a frequent cause of temporomandibular joint problems with head or neck pain. The roots of the teeth are highly sensible and they register even the smallest irregularities. The muscles of mastication respond by adjusting the bite, which can lead to temporomandibular joint dysfunctions in the long term.

One frequent malocclusion is cross-bite, where the upper and lower jaws are not correctly aligned above each other. Since teeth need contact for chewing and for their own stability, they "grow" or, better said, they reorient to reestablish contact. This leads to irregularities and occlusion problems. The real problem, however, is not aesthetics, but uneven strain on the muscles of mastication and problems with the kinematic behavior of the temporomandibular joints.

Dysfunctions in the masticatory apparatus can lead to posture problems or can aggravate existing spine dysfunctions. There is a neurologic explanation for this process:

- The trigeminal nerve sensibly supplies the entire cranium, except for the occiput and parts of the pharynx.
- The maxilla and mandible are sensibly supplied by their corresponding branches (V2 and V3).
- The nuclei of the trigeminal nerve are in the medulla oblongata and reach down to C3.
- Interneurons connect these nuclei with the remaining nuclei of the first three cervical segments as well as with the motor nuclei of these segments.
- Impulses from the spinal nucleus of trigeminal nerve can influence the other nuclei of the upper cervical segments and contribute to muscle imbalances and malpositions of the OAA joints.

The following muscles are entirely or partially supplied by these segments:

- Rectus capitis posterior major and minor.
- Rectus capitis lateralis and anterior.
- Long muscle of head.
- Superior and inferior oblique muscle of head.
- Semispinal muscle of head.
- Longissimus muscle of head.
- Sternocleidomastoid (SCM).
- Trapezius.
- Anterior and posterior scalene muscles.

Dysfunctions of the masticatory apparatus can influence these muscles and can lead to hypertonicity and mobility limitations of the OAA joints. Dysfunctions of the temporomandibular joints regularly present together with mobility limitations of the OAA joints on the side of the affected temporomandibular joint.

The connection between the masticatory system and the pelvis should also be noted. As we shall see later in the discussion of the Meersman test, we find increased muscle tonicity of the external hip rotators and the side of the dysfunctional temporomandibular joint.

■ Upper Cervical Spine and "Posture Muscles" of the Head

Microscopic studies have shown that the short neck muscles contain about nine times as many muscle spindles as the gluteal muscles. The short neck muscles are responsible for spatial positioning of the head. The upper cervical segments that supply these muscles are connected to the vestibular nuclei via neurons. The vestibular nuclei connect with the vestibular organs of the inner ear as well as with the nuclei that govern motor control for the eyes (oculomotor nerve, trochlear nerve, abducent nerve). This is of considerable functional importance:

- Besides the vestibular system, the eyes are the second most important organ for posture.
- Both provide "horizontality" for the head via vestibulocervical reflexes.
- The vestibular system uses positional reflexes to attempt to place the head into a position where both the eyes and the vestibular system can function optimally.

In our opinion, the suboccipital region is exceptionally important for posture, because dysfunctions in this area change the functionality of the entire postural system. The following important systems or structures relate to the upper cervical part of spinal cord:

- Meninges, sinuses, and masticatory apparatus via the trigeminal nerve.
- Thorax and abdominal organs and posterior cranial fossa via the vagus nerve, which has a connection to C2.
- Hyoid muscles via the ansa cervicalis (loop of hypoglossal nerve).

In addition to these nerve connections, there are myofascial connections to the entire locomotor system. Pathogenic stimuli from structures supplied by these nerves can impact the functionality of the upper cervical segments via interneurons. Tensions in the neck fasciae can change the position of the OAA joints.

Lumbosacral Junction and Sacroiliac Joints

The sacrum is the base of the spine. Malpositions of the base of the sacrum will inevitably impact the spine and the lower extremities. These changes immediately cause adaptations in the OAA joints (and vice versa). The explanation cranial osteopaths give for this process is the connection provided by the dura mater of spinal cord between the sacrum, C2, and the occiput. Villeneuve, a French posturologist, refers to a neurologic connection without providing details. Littlejohn, the great English osteopath, said that the atlas is to the occiput and the cervical spine what the sacrum is to the ilia. Whatever the explanations, these connections are regularly found in clinical practice.

It is interesting to note that there is a bone in each of the three cardinal areas of OAA, lumbosacral junction, and ankle joints, the behavior of which is barely or not at all determined by muscles, but rather by the forces that impact it: atlas, sacrum, and talus are dependent on gravity in upright posture. For this reason, they are valuable indicators for posture problems.

Summary: Maintaining Equilibrium

Like all body systems, the system of equilibrium consists of receptors, neural pathways and centers, and implementing organs and structures.

While myofascial structures are the implementing organ, the vestibular system—with its connections to the cortex, cerebellum, reticular formation, certain nuclei of the mesencephalon, and spinal cord—is the regulating organ that can provide an inhibiting or stimulating response. Receptors are found in the entire organism. The visceral as well as the cranial area can negatively impact the system of equilibrium.

The spine plays a central role because all information from the entire body arrives there. It has been shown that pathological and especially nociceptive influences impact normal functioning of the spinal segments.

The cervico-occipital junction, the lumbosacral junction, and the ankle joints are key areas for posture because this is where the central line of gravity of the body is directed to a different plane. For this reason, these areas are especially valuable for diagnosis and treatment.

9.5 Examination

The first step when examining a patient is to discover where the main interference factor is located. In other words: Which region of the body contains the dominant dysfunction? One should also examine the condition of the myofascial structure and the locomotor system in general:

- Are there indications about a chronic condition that could result in fascial contractions and adhesions? If that is the case, treating the dominant dysfunction is often not sufficient. The contracted or adhered structures must also be treated. Physical therapy and homework for the patient (positioning, stretching, etc.) are advisable.
- Is the condition acute? There are frequently muscle contractions or trigger points that need to be treated in addition to the cause.
- In many cases, acute problems occur against a chronic background. If so, pain needs to be alleviated before the chronic problem, which is often the cause of the pain symptoms, is addressed.

In every case, therapists should remember that the spine is always involved in the process and requires treatment. There are two reasons for this:

- Persistent pathogenic stimuli sooner or later lead to the phenomenon of sensitizing the spinal cord segments. This creates chronic spine dysfunctions.
- Dysfunctions and malpositions of the spine influence the head and the extremities via muscle chains. This changes posture and leads to dysfunctions of the posture receptors in the long term.

At this point, we would like our readers to note that the tests we are about to describe are employed in our clinical practice. There are certainly many other testing methods available that will achieve the same goals, but are not presented here. All these manual tests have one thing in common: they are rarely reproducible and therefore hardly statistically relevant. However, for the practitioner who is experienced in using these tests, they have diagnostic value.

Method

■ Impacted Area

Identification of the dominant area where the key lesion is located: cranial, visceral or parietal.

■ Searching for the Key Lesion

The key lesion is the dysfunction that causes the entire pathologic pattern, including so-called secondary dysfunctions. Frequently, but not always, the patient no longer perceives the key lesion as painful, because it is most often compensated by secondary dysfunctions. In most cases, pain results from compensatory secondary dysfunctions. The key lesion is usually the most functionally impacted dysfunction. In most cases, the key lesion presents as a considerable mobility limitation, but sometimes it presents as posttraumatic hypermobility.

From a posturology point of view, it is important to remember that over the course of a lifetime, the arches of the foot lose tension and yield. There are multiple possible reasons for this process (microtraumas, poor shoes, posture imbalances). This loss of tension can become an interference field and contribute toward the patient experiencing pain and dysfunctions in other areas.

With some older patients, the myofascial structures can no longer recover. This requires orthotics to externally correct (support) the arches and to "artificially" compensate the posture imbalance that originates in the fallen arches (pes planus). In many cases, however, dynamic proprioceptive orthotics and physical therapy following the correction of mobility limitations of the entire locomotor system are enough to correct the arches of the foot.

■ Differential Diagnostics

The therapist should ask the following questions:
- As a manual therapist, physical therapist, or osteopath, can I help this patient?
- Can I help this patient in cooperation with a specialist (ophthalmologist, orthodontist, neurologist, psychologist, or posturologist)?
- Is this a case that requires a specialist (surgeon, neurologist, or internist)?

A thorough anamnesis and clinical examination will help answer these questions.

In the following section, we introduce several clinical indicators and tests that provide information about dysfunctions of the postural system.

Posture Analysis

■ Examination While Standing

How do the individual motor units respond in relation to the line of gravity in the sagittal and frontal plane? In most cases, the motor unit that is the most imbalanced in both planes is the one that contains the key lesion.

Which of the following parts of the body is the most conspicuous in the frontal plane (▶ **Fig. 9.4**)?
- Foot position: calcaneus, tubercle of navicular bone of foot, forefoot.
- Pelvis: pelvic shift, pelvic torque.
- Shoulder girdle asymmetry: shoulder height, shoulder blade position, clavicle.
- Head position: sidebending, rotation.

Which of the following parts of the body is the most conspicuous in the sagittal plane (▶ **Figs. 9.5–9.7**)?
- Knee: flexed knee, hyperextension of the knee (genu recurvatum).
- Position of the pelvis: anteversion or retroversion? Normally, the posterior superior iliac spine (PSIS) and the anterior superior iliac spine (ASIS) are at the

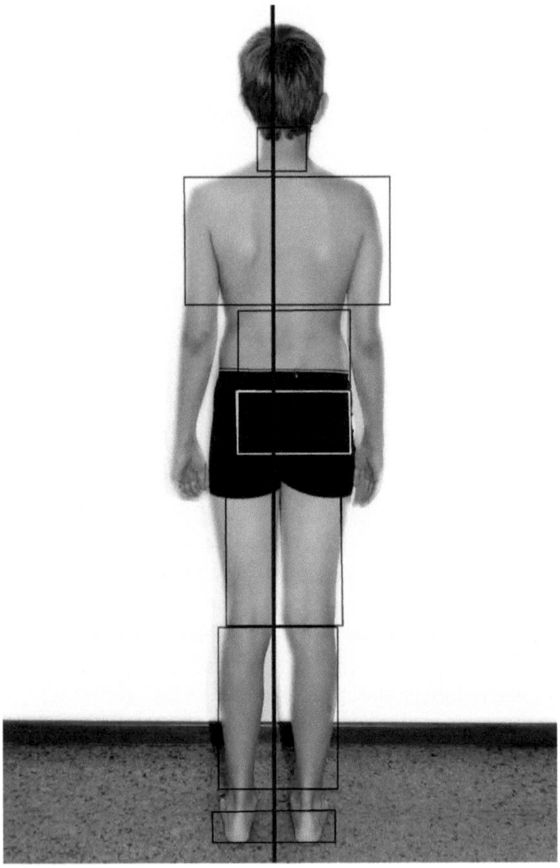

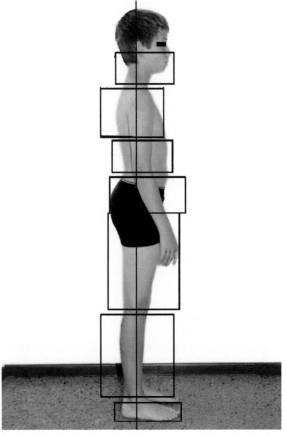

▶ **Fig. 9.4** Evaluation of individual motor units and vertical line in the frontal plane.

▶ **Fig. 9.5** Evaluation of individual motor units and vertical line in the sagittal plane.

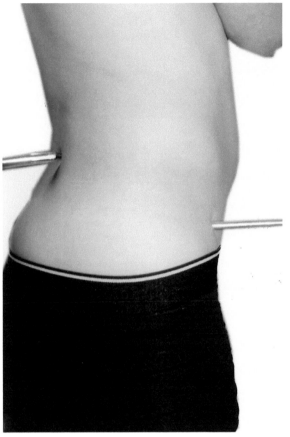

▶ **Fig. 9.6**   Comparison of the posterior superior iliac spine (PSIS) and anterior superior iliac spine (ASIS) positions (in this case, indicators for anterior rotation of ilium or anteversion of pelvis).

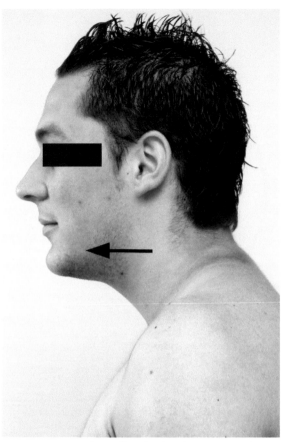

▶ **Fig. 9.7**   Antepulsion of head and neck in patient with temporomandibular joint dysfunction and cervical spine problems.

same level and the ASIS is on the same line as the pubic bone.
- How are the curves of the spine? Where are the vertices of the curves?
- Are the shoulders protracted? Is there a visible rotation of the shoulder girdle?
- Is the head protracted or retracted? A protracted head can indicate malocclusion. This head position is also often observable in the context of tensed or contracted anterior fasciae, which is frequently found to result from visceral dysfunctions.

The following are indicators of organ prolapse (ptosis; ▶ **Fig. 9.8**):
- Flat thorax, especially the upper part.
- Retraction between the shoulder blades.
- Tilt angle of the ribs in relation to the vertical line is less than 45 degrees.

- Small epigastric angle or wide, but flat lower thorax.
- Retraction of the abdominal wall below rib arches.
- Protrusion of the abdomen below the navel.
- Asthenic type.
- Frequently, anteversion of the pelvis and protraction of the head.

■ Comparison of Pelvic and Shoulder Girdle

Is the pelvic or shoulder girdle clearly asymmetric? As a rule, the dominant dysfunction is found in the area exhibiting the most pronounced asymmetry.
- Shoulder girdle: indication for cervical spine, head, upper extremities, upper to middle thoracic spine.
- Pelvic girdle: indication for lower extremities, pelvis, lower thoracic spine, and lumbar spine (▶ **Fig. 9.9**).

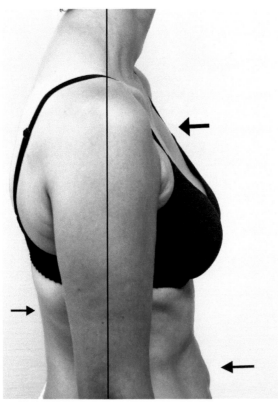

▶ **Fig. 9.8** Visible signs of organ prolapse: flat thorax, retraction below rib arches, and tilt angle of ribs.

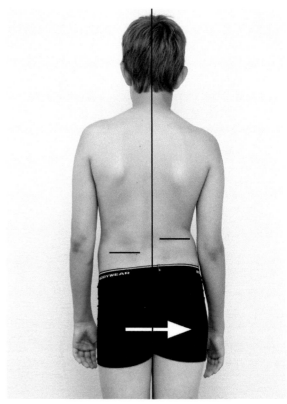

▶ **Fig. 9.9** Leg length difference and pelvic shift toward long leg, differences in iliac crest height, and changes in lumbar triangle.

Differentiation: Parietal–Visceral–Cranial

■ Examination

- Pronounced asymmetry in head posture is an indicator of possible cranial dominance.
- If the pelvis position is more clearly imbalanced than the shoulder girdle, the main problem is likely to be found in the lower half of the body.

■ Listening Test

The patient is relaxed and standing, with eyes closed. Therapist instructions:
- Stand next to the patient and, without exerting pressure, place one hand on the patient's head and the other hand on the sacrum.

This test allows you to feel in which direction the patient is being pulled by fascial tension.

■ Traction Test at Occiput and Sacrum

The patient is supine.
Therapist instructions:

- Place both hands under the occiput or one hand below the sacrum.
- Apply progressively more traction to feel the height of the restriction. The height of the restriction provides an indication about the area of spinal dysfunction.
- If the dominant problem is in the lower extremities or in the pelvis, you will quickly feel a restriction on the affected side when pulling on the sacrum. If the problem is cranial or cervical, you can feel this restriction immediately or very quickly when pulling on the occiput.

This test allows you to quickly delineate the region of the body where restrictions are most pronounced.

Modification 1

A modified version of this test allows therapists to determine the visceral influence on the restriction. Therapist instructions:
- Place one hand under the occiput and the other hand on the sternum of the patient (▶ **Fig. 9.10a, b**).
- Gently pull the head of the patient toward cranial to feel if the tension is in the direction of the spine or in the direction of the sternum. If the dominance is visceral, the anterior fasciae will be tense.

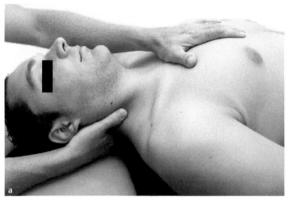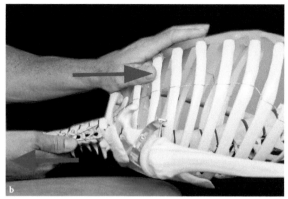

▶ **Fig. 9.10 (a)**   Examination of neck fasciae tension. **(b)** Traction test on cervical spine to differentiate visceral and parietal tensions.

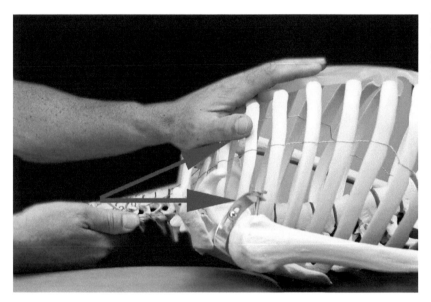

▶ **Fig. 9.11**   Traction test on head: tension toward anterior indicates dominant visceral component; tension toward posterior indicates parietal component.

- If you then attempt to push the sternum toward inferior, you will immediately feel traction at the hand that is placed on the occiput. If the anterior fasciae are relaxed, you can move the sternum toward inferior without palpable traction on the occiput (▶**Fig. 9.11**).

Modification 2

Therapist instructions:
- Place one hand under the sacrum. Place the other hand spread wide on the patient's abdomen, with the fingers pointing cranially (▶**Fig. 9.12**).
- With the hand on the abdomen, exert slight pressure and conduct a star-shaped test of the abdominal fasciae tension.
- Then pull the sacrum toward inferior until you feel a restriction on one side.

- With the abdominal hand, now reduce abdominal fascial tension and feel how the spine responds. If tension decreases, this indicates that the visceral tensions exert significant influence on spine mobility.

Examination of Posture Receptors

Once the therapist has determined the most vulnerable body region, the region needs to be examined in more detail:
- Cranial: eyes, temporomandibular joint, vestibular system.
- Visceral: cavity pressure, organ attachment.
- Parietal: spine, foot.

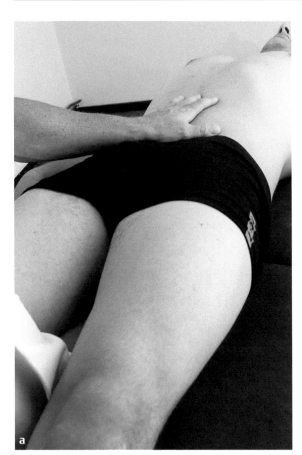
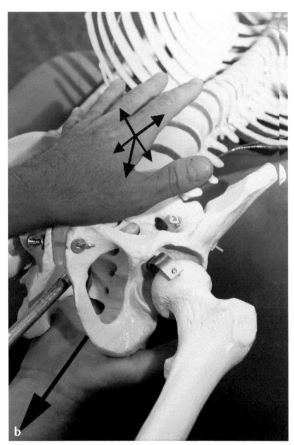

▶ **Fig. 9.12 (a, b)** Differentiation of visceral and parietal causes for pelvis or spine dysfunctions by traction on sacrum.

■ Examining the Eyes

Convergence Test

The patient is seated or supine.
Therapist instructions:
- Hold up a pencil with a light or colored tip in front of the patient's face and ask the patient to focus both eyes on the tip of the pencil.
- Move the pencil in all directions and observe if both eyes can follow the movement of the pencil at the same speed.
- Now move the tip of the pencil toward the root of the nose of the patient and observe if both pupils follow the pencil (▶ **Fig. 9.13**). If the extrinsic muscles of one eye are weaker, that eye usually cannot track the movement as quickly as the other eye. If there is a convergence problem, the pupil of the affected eye can no longer track the tip of the pencil as of a certain point when the pencil is moved close to the nose. Sometimes the pupil will visibly make a lateral evasive motion or the patient's eyes will blink.

Cover Test

The patient is seated.
Therapist instructions:
- Cover one eye of the patient and hold one of your fingers about one arm's length in front of the patient's face. Ask the patient to focus on your finger with the uncovered eye.
- Now uncover the other eye and observe the pupil of that eye. If you see a movement of this pupil, it indicates a motoricity dysfunction of that eye.

> If the eye examination shows suspicious results, an eye specialist should be consulted.

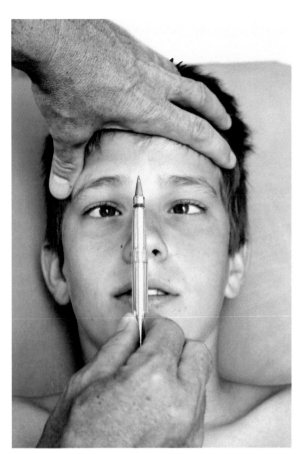

▶ **Fig. 9.13**   Convergence test of eyes.

▪ Examining the Masticatory Apparatus

Therapist instructions:
- Place your index fingers on the temporomandibular joints in front of the acoustic meatus and below the zygomatic process of temporal bone.
- Palpate the behavior of the jaw as the patient opens and closes their mouth.

In its physiologic state, both condyles perform identical rolling and gliding motions and the point of the chin does not make an evasive motion. The patient's mouth should open wide enough for the patient to place three middle fingers sideways between lower and upper jaws. Dysfunctional gliding motions or insufficient opening of the mouth indicate dysfunctions of the masticatory apparatus that should be examined further. The following tests may be performed to determine if these dysfunctions impact the locomotor system.

OAA Translation Test

The patient is supine.
Therapist instructions:
- Take the patient's head between both hands, with the fingertips placed on the transverse processes of the atlas.

- Perform a left and right translation and compare the amplitudes (▶ **Fig. 9.14a**). If there is a dominant cranial dysfunction, the translation will be restricted in one direction.

In a second phase, the same test is repeated.
Therapist instructions:
- This time, the patient holds two dental cotton rolls between their teeth (▶ **Fig. 9.14b**).
- After the patient has swallowed three times, repeat the translation test as described earlier and compare the amplitudes. If the temporomandibular joint dysfunction plays an important role for a spinal dysfunction, the translation will improve significantly because the dental cotton rolls inhibit the impulses issued by the masticatory apparatus (spinal nucleus of trigeminal nerve).

Hip Rotation Test (Meersman's Test)

The patient is supine.
Therapist instructions:
- Test the internal rotation of the hips first without and then with the dental cotton rolls, as for the OAA translation test discussed earlier.

If the result of this test is positive, the internal rotation will significantly improve on the side of the dysfunction when the dental cotton rolls are used. If this is the case, the temporomandibular joint dysfunction is an important factor in the pelvic dysfunction.

▪ Examining Cavity Pressure

The patient is standing upright and relaxed.
Therapist instructions:
- Palpate the paravertebral muscle tone using one hand.
- Place the other hand on the patient's abdomen, exert slight pressure, and feel if this decreases the paravertebral muscle tension. If tension does not decrease, the muscular tensions are not caused by visceral dysfunctions.

▪ Examining Plantar Receptors

Malalignment or deformities of the feet impact the position of the pelvis. For this reason, visual examination of the pelvis in addition to examination of the feet is of interest. Generally, the following applies:
- Fallen arches (pes planus) can cause anteversion of the ipsilateral pelvis.
- High arches (pes cavus, talipes cavus) can cause retroversion of the ipsilateral pelvis.
- Leg length differences cause fallen arches on the side of the long leg.

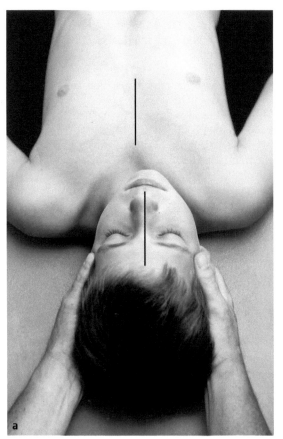 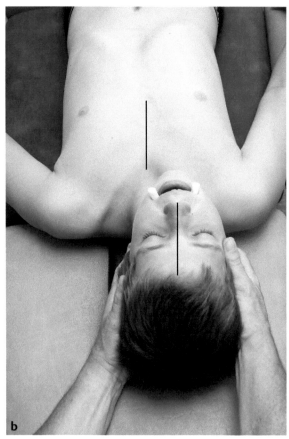

▶ **Fig. 9.14** Translation test on occiput without **(a)** and with small dental cotton rolls **(b)**.

- Leg length differences result in translation and rotation of the pelvis toward the side of the longer leg.
- Fallen arches (pes planus) lead to internal rotation of the leg and internal rotation of the ankle fork.
- High arches (pes cavus, talipes cavus) lead to external rotation of the leg and external rotation of the ankle fork.

Three conditions of the feet need to be differentiated:
- Change in the arches of the foot resulting from blockages of the foot: therapy consists of manipulation.
- Change in the arches of the foot resulting from structural changes in the aponeuroses and ligaments (support system, frequently seen in older patients): therapy consists of supportive orthotics.
- Change in the arch of the foot resulting from muscle insufficiency: therapy involves dynamic orthotics and muscle rehabilitation.

Visual examination provides initial indications for possible disturbances in the foot area. Another indicator is conspicuous posture imbalances of the pelvis. This is referred to as an ascending chain. Foot dysfunction leads to pelvis malpositions via the muscle chains. If a foot problem plays a significant role in pathogenesis, it is responsible for a pelvic dysfunction, which can be identified through motion tests such as the ones described next.

Hip Drop Test

This test can identify lumbosacral junction dysfunctions.
The patient is standing with feet about 30 cm apart.
Therapist instructions:
- Stand behind the patient and observe the behavior of the pelvis and the lower lumbar spine.
- Ask the patient to flex one knee without lifting the foot and to allow the pelvis to drop. The pelvis drops toward the side of the flexed knee and rotates slightly toward anterior. The lower lumbar spine sidebends to the other side.

In case of lower lumbar spine or sacroiliac joint dysfunctions, comparing both sides will indicate imbalances.

One-Legged Stance

The patient is standing.
Therapist instructions:
* Stand behind the patient and observe the behavior of the stance leg while the patient raises the other leg (± 90° hip and knee flexion).

Foot dysfunctions involve proprioception disturbances of the affected leg. This presents as instability at the beginning of the one-legged stance.

Rotation Test of Lower Extremity in Supine Position

The patient is supine.
Therapist instructions:
* Test the internal and external rotation of both legs to identify any differences. Note the most prominent rotation limitation.

Traction Test of Lower Extremity with Rotation Limitation

The patient is supine.
Therapist instructions:
* Rotate both legs of the patient toward the previously identified rotation dysfunction.
* From this position, apply progressive traction toward inferior. Pronounced resistance indicates dysfunction.
This test can be used to identify the height of dysfunction (foot, knee, hip, or sacroiliac joint).

Examination of Feet for Motion Limitation

It is interesting to observe the feet while the patient is standing, seated, and supine. If the shape of the feet changes when the patient is supine or seated compared to while standing, the problem is often muscular. If that is the case, the supine position can provide indicators for hypertonic or contracted muscle groups.

Conclusion

In addition to traumatic, cranial, and visceral causes, posture imbalances are a frequent cause of pain symptoms and dysfunctions of the locomotor system. They are also a frequent reason for treatment failures if they are not addressed. This is due to dysfunctions of the equilibrium system and especially of the receptors.

Structured examination of the patient enables therapists to quickly identify the source of the disturbance. Even if therapists are not always able to solve the problem on their own and require the help of an ophthalmologist, posturologist, or other kind of expert, they should never ignore the role of muscles.

Traumatic, visceral, postural, and emotional disturbances impact all muscles. Persistent disturbances can lead to structural changes of myofascial tissue. This causes trigger points and contractions. The resulting circulatory problems—first venolymphatic and neurologic, then arterial—eventually impact the health of the entire organism.

9.6 Leg Length Differences

True leg length differences are common:
* Ten percent of all people have leg length differences of more than 1 cm.[27]
* Friberg [in[27]] conducted a radiological examination of 359 asymptomatic soldiers and found the following:
  - Fifty-six percent had leg length differences of 0 to 4 mm.
  - Thirty percent had leg length differences of 5 and 9 mm.
  - Fourteen percent had leg length differences of 1 cm.
* Two of three patients presenting with chronic lumbago have radiologically verified leg length differences.

Leg length differences lead to a tilted base of sacrum with compensation of the entire spine (rotoscoliosis). On the other hand, a tilted base of sacrum, regardless of its cause, always results in ilium rotation, which changes leg length. This is referred to as functional leg length difference.

Before equalizing leg length using orthotics, it needs to be determined if the difference is structural or functional. The only reliable method to make this determination is through radiology imaging after treating somatic dysfunctions in the entire organism. This is important because ilium rotations cause changes in leg position, which can change leg length by up to 1 cm.[7] The pelvis and both legs need to be X-rayed in the standing posture. The error rate with X-ray measurements varies from 1 to 5 mm.[12]

Leg Length Differences and Posture Changes of Pelvis and Spine

* The ilium on the side of the long leg rotates toward posterior and the ilium on the side of the shorter leg rotates toward anterior.
* The iliac crest on the side of the long leg is higher.

- The entire pelvis tilts toward the short leg and rotates toward the long leg.
- The base of the sacrum tilts toward the short leg.
- The entire pelvis is anteriorized.
- Lordosis of the lumbar spine is increased in most cases, especially in the lumbosacral junction.
- The lumbar spine, as a rule, performs an NSR with rotation toward the short leg. The thoracic spine performs an NSR toward the long leg and the cervical spine performs a translation toward the side of the short leg.
- The shoulder is lower on the side of the long leg except in cases in which the leg length difference is more than 1.5 to 2 mm.
- The head is tilted toward the side of the shorter leg.
- The pelvis performs a translation toward the long leg, which increases the size of the lumbar triangle on the side of the short leg.

Notes:
- In 80% of all cases, the lumbar spine sidebends toward the long leg with increase in lordosis. In the remaining cases, it does not sidebend at all or sidebends toward the short leg. This happens when structural damage prevents it from sidebending toward the long leg.
- Shoulder height is of course influenced by muscle tension in the trapezius and levator muscle of scapula. Problems in the upper cervical spine can change the position of the shoulder.
- Ilium dysfunction changes leg length (functional leg length difference), position of the iliac crest, and position of the PSIS and ASIS in the standing position.
  - With true leg length differences, the iliac crest is positioned higher and the PSIS lower (depending on length difference) and posterior. The ASIS is higher and posterior (posterior rotation of the ilium).
  - With ilium anterior dysfunction, the iliac crest is higher, but the PSIS is higher than on the other side. The ASIS is lower and anterior in comparison to the other side.
- In the initial stage, the spine adapts by adopting a C-shaped scoliosis with sidebending toward the long leg. However, the entire musculoskeletal system responds very quickly and establishes an S-curve. This distributes stress and levels the eyes and vestibular system horizontally.

Symptoms of Leg Length Differences and Impact on Musculoskeletal System

Most leg length differences remain asymptomatic until a trauma or excessive strain lead to pain symptoms. Even then, in most cases only substantial differences are registered. Some patients report that they noticed their pelvis was "lopsided" or that they were told by a doctor when they were young that their spine is curved.

Uncorrected leg length differences lead to myofascial tensions in the entire locomotor system. Pain usually manifests first in the lumbosacral junction region, then the spine is impacted all the way up to the head. Myofascial tissue is contracted in the concavities and stretched in the convexities.

Depending on the type of additional stress impacting a body region, pain develops in those regions when the adaption mechanisms are exhausted. In the lumbosacral junction, the iliolumbar ligaments on the convex side (short leg) are stretched. This causes localized pain that radiates along the iliac crest and into the groin to the inner side of the thigh. A local pressure pain point is often found at the insertion of ligaments along the iliac crest or in the transverse processes of L4 or L5. The iliosacral ligaments on the same side are also frequently stressed. In addition to local pain, they can produce pain on the lateral side of the thigh. Often, there are painful trigger points of the quadratus lumborum on the side of the lumbar spine concavity. According to Lewit[86], the scalene muscles on the same side are also hypertonic.

Frequently found dysfunctions in the lumbosacral junction include unilateral dysfunction of the sacrum on the side of the short leg, forward torsion of the sacrum with rotation toward the long leg as well as an extension–rotation–sidebending (ERS) dysfunction of L4 or L5.

With a sacrum torsion towards posterior, the base of the sacrum is usually posterior on the side of the long leg. Of the lower extremities, the long leg is usually the most stressed mechanically. Hip arthrosis, gonarthrosis (lateral tibial plateau), and muscle strain of the adductors, psoas, and gluteal muscles frequently present in this area. Sciatic pain syndrome is also more frequently found on the side of the long leg (60%).

Leg length differences normally present with pronation of the hindfoot valgus and external leg rotation of the long leg. Supination of the foot is more frequent on the short leg. This explains why patients wear down the heel of their shoes on the outside more quickly on the side of the short leg.

These phenomena have been documented by various studies (all in[27]):
- Taillard and Morscher (1965): Increased electromyographic (EMG) activity in the erector muscle of spine (erector spinae), gluteus maximus, and triceps muscle of calf (triceps surae) on the side of the short leg.
- Strong (1966) found increased EMG activity in the muscles of the concavity with scoliosis caused by leg length differences as well as in the postural muscles of the long leg.
- Bopp (1971) describes pain at the greater trochanter, lesser trochanter, transverse processes of the lumbar

vertebrae, and on the pubic bone on the side of the long leg.

- Mahar et al (1985) found in a radiology study that artificial lengthening of one leg causes substantial pelvic shift toward the side of the long leg.
- Wiburg (1983, 1984) describes the influence of a long leg on the hip joint. The pelvic shift toward the long leg decreases the pressure area on the hip joint, which leads to increased pressure on the bones.
- Gofton and Trueman (1971) discovered in their study that 81% of patients who suffered from hip arthrosis also had different leg lengths, and that the long leg was the one impacted.

Diagnosing Leg Length Differences

A confirmed diagnosis of leg length differences with iliac crest height differences of below 1.5 cm requires radiology imaging. It is advisable to treat the patient osteopathically beforehand to normalize motion limitations and to adequately treat myofascial structures. This prevents those dysfunctions from distorting the image. There still remains a significant error rate.

Kuchera and Kuchera[12] therefore recommend subtracting 25% from the measured difference. Palpation and visual examination can still provide clear indicators for leg length differences.

The following clinical findings indicate leg length differences if they occur together:

- Iliac crest and greater trochanter are higher on the same side.
- PSIS and ASIS are higher on the side of the higher iliac crest.
- PSIS is anterior and ASIS is superior and anterior on the side of the higher iliac crest.
- With feet side by side, translation to the side of the long leg is found.
- Horizontal gluteal fold is higher on the side of the long leg.
- Lumbar triangle is larger on the side of the short leg.
- Shoulder is higher on the side of the short leg. It is advisable to palpate the lower shoulder blade angle.
- Pronation position of the foot on the long leg and supination position on the short leg.
- Relaxed posture with leg length differences presents as weight shifted to short leg, with slight abduction and knee flexion of the long leg. Often, persons stand with their legs apart.
- With maximum forward bend, the inferior lateral angle (ILA) is higher on the side of the long leg.

The following indicators can also be found when examining the patient in supine position:

- In supine position with flexed knees, the knee is higher on the side of the long leg.

- In prone position with flexed knees, the thigh is longer (the knee is further inferior) and/or the lower leg is longer (heel is higher) on the side of the long leg.

If these indicators are mostly present and the iliac crest heights differ by 1 cm, then it can be assumed that there is a leg length difference. This supposition can be confirmed if the patient is asked to walk and it can be observed that on the side of the supposed longer leg the pelvis is raised during the swing phase and the hip flexion is more pronounced than on the other side.

Should Leg Length Differences be Corrected?

Kuchera and Kuchera[12] write that newer studies show that a sacral tilt of 1.5 mm changes the tonicity of the lumbar spine muscles and causes lumbago. Klein et al[76] conducted an interesting study: In 7 of 11 children between the ages of 1.5 and 15 years, leg length differences normalized completely within 3 to 7 months following shoe equalization. Leg length differences ranged from 1.3 to 1.9 cm. Irvin[29] writes that complete equalization of leg length differences until the base of the sacrum is horizontal normalizes so-called idiopathic scoliosis by one-third.

These indications confirm the advisability of orthotics for true leg length differences (congenital or acquired). This should be accompanied by manual therapy to help the organism adapt.

Differences of less than 3 mm are not normalized as a rule. Larger differences are equalized progressively. Irvin recommends the first raise to be a maximum of 3 mm. This is followed 2 weeks later by a raise of 2 mm. From then on, leg length is corrected by 2 mm every 2 weeks until the measured tilt of the base of the sacrum is completely equalized. At the end of this entire procedure, another radiological image of the pelvis is obtained and more corrections are applied, if necessary. Pain symptoms disappear progressively towards cranial, starting at the pelvis.

If the difference to be equalized is greater than 8 mm, the sole of the shoe on the long leg should be lowered. Too much one-sided equalization can change gait too much and cause complications.

Kuchera and Kuchera[12] recommend correcting leg length differences of 5 mm or more by using orthotics. With larger differences, 50 to 75% of the radiologically measured difference should be equalized using orthotics or raised shoes (because one can assume a measuring error of about 25%). The general condition of the patient and duration of the imbalance should be taken into consideration.

- Patients with arthrosis or osteoporotic bones or unstable patients should be started with an increase of 2 mm, with 2 mm added every 2 weeks.
- Patients whose musculoskeletal condition is not very affected can be started on a rise of 4 mm, with 2 mm added every 2 weeks.
- Leg length differences arising from trauma or surgery (prosthesis) should be equalized all at once.

Orthotics should be no thicker than 0.5 cm or they will feel uncomfortable in the shoe. If a larger rise is necessary, the sole of the shoe can be raised or the sole of the shoe on the long leg can be lowered.

Since raising only the heel causes a pelvic rotation to the other side, it is advisable to raise the entire sole of the shoe if a rise of 1.2 cm or more is required. Raising only the heel or only the forefoot influences pelvic rotation. Leg length differences with tilt of the base of the sacrum are often accompanied by pelvic rotation (usually toward the long leg) and it is often necessary to address this aspect when fitting raised shoes. The reason is obvious: pelvic rotation increases scoliosis of the spine.

- Raising the heel rotates the pelvis to the other side.
- Raising the forefoot rotates the pelvis to the same side.
- Evenly raising the entire sole of the foot rotates the pelvis to the same side because raising the forefoot has a larger impact than raising the heel.

For leg length differences with pelvic rotation, the following rules of thumb apply if the goal is to level the sacral base:

- Pelvic rotation of less than 5 mm: Traditional increase in shoe height according to the principles described above.
- Pelvic rotation of between 5 and 10 mm: Begin with an increase of 3 mm under the forefoot and then add of 3 mm every 2 weeks under the heel.
- Pelvic rotation greater than 10 mm: First correct the pelvic rotation using orthotics, afterwards increase both forefoot and heel 3 mm each in 2 week intervals.

With children, it is advisable to correct leg length differences using orthotics, because it increases pressure on the short leg. This stimulates growth of bone length.

Children should wear orthotics until the leg length is equalized. Adults should wear orthotics as regularly as possible.

The procedures described are generally applicable and can be adapted as needed.

Conclusion

True leg length differences are very common. Medical literature states that about 50 to 70% of the population has unequal leg lengths. Studies of patients with chronic lumbago show that leg length differences are even more frequent in this population. Above all, these are leg length differences of 5 mm or more.

Newer studies seem to show that tilts in sacral base of 1.5 mm change the muscle tone in the lumbar region and can trigger lumbago. An improvement of symptoms by up to 80% after correcting leg length differences, as described by Kuchera and Kuchera,[12] speaks for itself.

These facts underscore the importance of posture in the presence of back pain. Blockages and traumas lead to malpositions of the base of sacrum, with predictable impact on the entire locomotor system. Rapid adaptation of the myofascial tissue leads relatively quickly to structural changes that disturb the function of the entire organism. Systematic osteopathic treatment must address this process and treat myofascial tissue accordingly. Therapists who understand the physiology and pathophysiology of myofascial tissue and muscle chains can apply targeted treatment. They can also give precise instructions to the patient about which muscle groups to stretch or strengthen, with priority given to stretching of contracted muscles over strengthening of their antagonists.

10 Diagnostics

Before a patient can be treated, the therapist needs to conduct a thorough anamnesis and examination.

10.1 Anamnesis

Anamnesis helps arrive at a differential diagnosis and should provide information to the therapist that is useful for treatment. It should include questions about traumas, surgeries, illnesses, and previous treatments as well as questions about the type, duration, and development history of the patient's symptoms. The therapist needs to gain an understanding of the neurovegetative condition of the patient.

10.2 Examination

The examination includes:
- Observation.
- Palpation.
- Motion test.
- Differentiation test (see Chapter 9.5).

Observation

The patient's **posture** is observed both in standing and supine positions. Observation includes noting posture asymmetries, muscle tensions, and tissue changes. In the standing position, various motion tests can be performed for the individual regions of the body and anomalies can be assessed.

It is interesting to observe how the patient stands naturally and then to note the patient's posture when both feet are positioned close together. By reducing their base of equilibrium, patients are compelled to demonstrate their posture patterns.

When the patient is supine, gravity is excluded. Motion patterns visible in this position are manifestations of muscle imbalances caused by dysfunctions (or structural changes).

Note: We are not big proponents of comprehensive gait analysis. Often, the therapist's office is not suitable because of limited size or the limited information provided by gait analysis does not justify the time required.

We prefer to analyze gait by using the hip drop test, one-legged stance, and shoulder motions.

Palpation

Palpitation provides information to the therapist about the position of structures and the condition of tissue. In addition to observing the patient's posture while standing and supine, palpation can identify dominant muscle chains and the position of joint partners. It also enables differentiation between chronic and acute processes. These results are further confirmed by motion tests.

Motion Tests

Global motion tests are designed to identify the region of the body with the most pronounced mobility limitation. During forward bending and sidebending (▶ **Fig. 10.1**), the therapist looks for harmonious motion sequences. Discontinuities and evasive motions are then examined in more detail.

The affected region is examined using segmental tests and palpation for muscular or segmental restrictions. By using differentiation tests, the therapist then attempts to find out whether the visceral, cranial, or parietal component of the problem dominates with

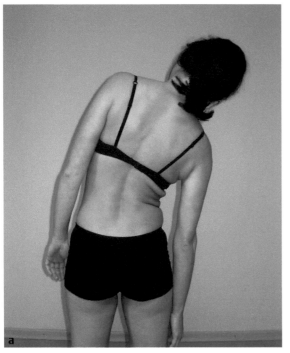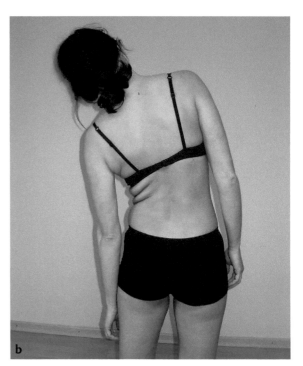

▶ **Fig. 10.1 (a, b)** Sidebending test for lumbar spine.

this patient. The part of the body region assessed to be dominant during the examination is then targeted for treatment using appropriate techniques.

We would now like to introduce a different but very rational examination approach. It is based on Zink patterns and traction tests on the head, pelvis, and legs.

After we briefly observe the patient while standing and noting rough deviations, we ask the patient to bend forward (▶ **Fig. 10.2**) and perform the hip drop test or a translation test on the pelvis. This provides indications for the position and mobility of the sacrum and lumbar spine and possibly for dominant muscle chains.

If we note problems in the lower extremities, we ask the patient to perform a one-legged stance. This allows us to observe the behavior of the pelvis, knees, and feet. Neuromuscular disturbances of the leg muscles present as posture asymmetries because of the muscular imbalances and the different behavior of receptors due to segmental facilitation.

A flexion test can indicate a dominant chain on the leg and in the spine. The hip drop test and the translation test provide information about the position of the sacrum and the lower lumbar spine.

While the patient is supine, we observe rotation of the legs (▶ **Fig. 10.3**), pelvis (▶ **Fig. 10.4**), inferior thorax aperture (▶ **Fig. 10.5**), and superior thorax aperture (▶ **Fig. 10.6**) before we test the Zink patterns. We then perform a traction test on the head and on the pelvis (or on the legs). This enables us to identify the dominant side and helps us to locate the main restriction and to differentiate between an ascending or descending

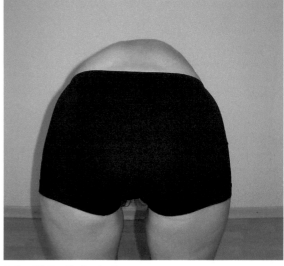

▶ **Fig. 10.2** Flexion test.

chain. The sooner the resistance to traction is encountered, the closer the restriction is to the hand applying traction.[137,148]

When testing the Zink patterns, we not only test for torsions at the junctions to determine where they do not alternate, but also, primarily, try to find out at which junction the rotation pattern is the most pronounced, i.e., where right rotation is most clearly differentiated from left rotation. This is followed by a differentiation that determines if the muscles causing the torsion pattern are posterior or anterior (▶ **Figs. 10.4–10.7**).

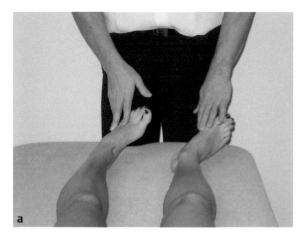

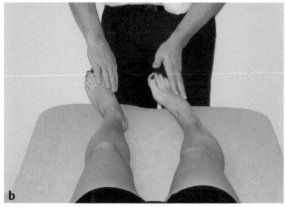

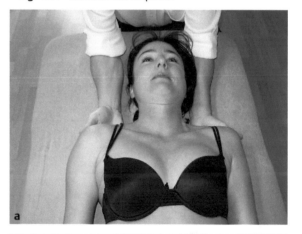

▶ **Fig. 10.3 (a, b)**   Rotation test of hip, comparing both sides.

▶ **Fig. 10.4**   Rotation test for pelvis.

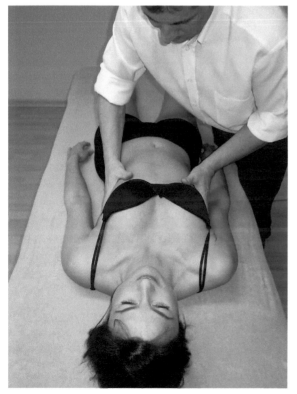

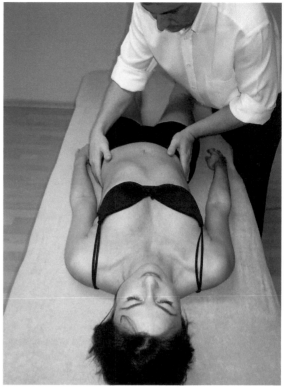

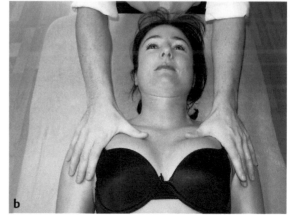

▶ **Fig. 10.5**   Rotation test for inferior thorax aperture.

▶ **Fig. 10.6 (a)**   Rotation test for superior thorax aperture. **(b)** Variation.

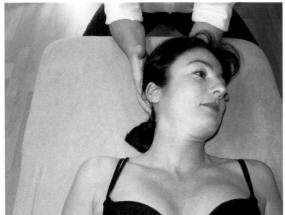

► **Fig. 10.7** Rotation test of occipitoatlantoaxial joints.

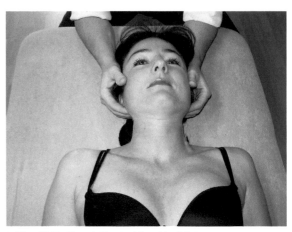

► **Fig. 10.8** Translation test for atlas joint.

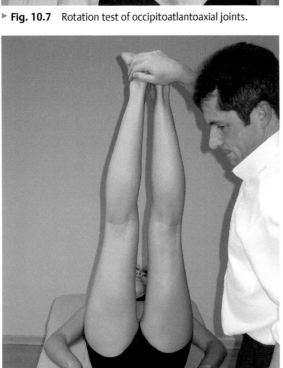

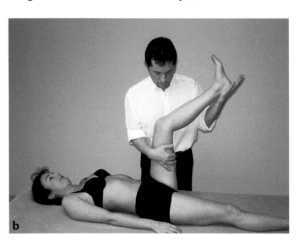

► **Fig. 10.9 (a)** Test of ischiocrural muscles (hamstrings). On the left, the ischiocrural muscles are contracted; this raises the ischial tuberosity. **(b)** Variation.

Each junction represents a specific region of the body, as we described in the previous chapters. This is illustrated by anatomical muscles and neurologic connections (► **Figs. 10.8–10.11**).

Here, we provide another brief overview.

Occipitoatlantoaxial Complex

Suboccipital muscles:
• Segments C1–C3.

Superior Thoracic Aperture

Sibson fascia:
• Segments C4–T4.

Inferior Thoracic Aperture

Diaphragm, abdominal muscles, and 6th to 12th ribs:
• Segments T5–T12.

Pelvis

Psoas, pelvic floor:
• Segments L1–S4.

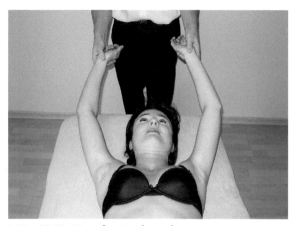

▶ **Fig. 10.10**   Test of pectoral muscle.

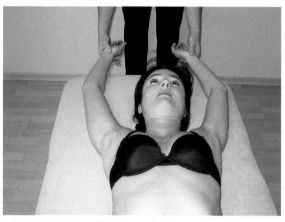

▶ **Fig. 10.11**   Test of latissimus dorsi.

11 Therapy

Once we have identified a dominant pattern, we need to examine all structures that have a segmental (neural) connection with this pattern in more detail to target treatment as closely as possible. The guiding principle is: "Find it, fix it, and leave it alone."

From our osteopathic perspective, myofascial structures play an important role:

- In acute, painful cases, we regularly find active trigger points. These frequently cause so-called pseudoneuralgias.

Example: Trigger points in the scalene muscles imitate neuralgia of the median nerve. Trigger points in the gluteus minimus present with the same symptoms as L4 sciatica.

- So-called silent trigger points change the normal behavior of muscles and cause muscle imbalances.
- Retractions and muscle fibrosis frequently contribute to relapses.

The likelihood of fast pain reduction will be quite high and the risk of relapse will be reduced once the therapist has:

- Identified and treated the dominant dysfunction (visceral, parietal, or cranial).
- In acute cases, also treated the trigger points.
- In chronic cases, normalized the contracted muscles in the affected muscle chain.

11.1 Muscle Energy Techniques

Muscle energy techniques (METs) are very popular with manual therapists. Physical therapists, chiropractors, osteopaths, and manual therapists all use MET or variations of this technique to detonify or tonify muscles, mobilize joints, or stretch fasciae. One reason for the popularity of METs may be the fact that they are low risk and often successful even if not precisely applied. It is possible that Kabat was the first therapist to use muscle techniques to treat spasms and muscle contractions.

Osteopaths attribute the development of muscle techniques for the treatment of joint dysfunctions to Fred Mitchell, Sr. He caught the attention of the osteopathy world after writing two notable articles (1948, 1958) about manipulative treatment of mechanical pelvic dysfunctions using METs. Mitchell was influenced in the development of his method by the work of other osteopaths (T.J. Ruddy, 1874–1964, and Carl Kettler). He also referred to Still himself who said that "the attempt to restore joint integrity before smoothingly restoring muscle and ligamentous normality was putting the cart before the horse."

Since then, METs have been substantially refined. Studies have tested their effectiveness and the neurophysiologic characteristics of myofascial structures have been incorporated.

It is safe to assume that other professions (physical therapists, chiropractors) have been conducting parallel developments in the field of muscle techniques. It is notable that there are now active exchanges of information and meetings between experts in the various fields of therapy. This includes Fred Mitchell, Jr., Stiles, Greenman, Liebenson, Lewit, Janda, Grieve, and Norris, to name just a few. This may explain the scientific progress in the MET field.

Definition

METs are defined as a type of osteopathic treatment that requires patients to tense muscles from a precisely controlled position in a specific direction, against the precise resistance provided by the therapist.

METs are used for:

- Treatment of joint mobility restrictions.
- Stretching of tense muscles and fasciae.
- Stimulating localized circulation.
- Changing muscle tone via neuromuscular mechanisms.

METs require patient cooperation to tense muscles, breathe in or out, or move joint partners in a specific direction. For these reasons, this type of therapy cannot be used for comatose, uncooperative patients, or patients who are unable to follow the therapist's direction.

Indications and Contraindications

Indications and contraindications can be derived from the definition mentioned earlier.

▪ Indications

There are many indications for this type of treatment. Here is a nonprioritized list:
- Inhibit hypertonic, spastic muscles.
- Tonify hypotonic, weak muscles.
- Stretch contractions and fibrosis.
- Loosen adhesions.
- Normalize joint dysfunctions.
- Stimulate localized, venolymphatic circulation.
- Alleviate pain.
- Positively influence motion and posture patterns.
- Break through a pain-induced "vicious circle."

▪ Contraindications

In addition to the classic contraindications for osteopathic treatment, the following contraindications apply for muscle techniques:
- Communication and coordination problems between therapist and patient.
- Bone or muscle injuries that have not yet healed in the segments to be treated.

Prerequisites for Optimal Muscle Energy Technique Application

- One of the most important prerequisites is to obtain a **precise diagnosis**. The therapist should be able to determine what is causing the pain, limiting mobility, or is the reason for imbalance or faulty motion pattern.

Examples:
- Pain in the shoulder and neck region can have many causes, but they all result in muscle changes:
  - Joint blockage of the cervical spine.
  - Trigger points.
  - Intervertebral disk problems.
  - Reflected pain.
  - Ligament pain following trauma.
  - Hypertonicity or spasms in response to excess posture or functional strain due to contraction of other muscle groups.

Treatment focus and choice of MET varies, depending on the cause.
- Hip extension limitations can result from:
  - Hip joints (beginning or advanced arthrosis).
  - Chronically contracted iliopsoas.
  - Spastically contracted iliopsoas (with lumbar spine complaints).

Careful diagnosis enables the therapist to identify the main problem—muscles, fasciae, or joints—and which of these three is the dominating component, since frequently, all three are present.

Optimally effective treatment requires focused impact on the element that is causing the pathologic mechanism. This is true for the examination techniques used as well as for treatment.
- Precise assessment of the **neurovegetative condition** of the patient is important. Typical examples include fibromyalgia patients, patients presenting with depression, or patients with acute pain symptoms. The right diagnosis at the right moment in the right body region is key for treatment success.
- **Choice of treatment technique** is significant. The technique must be able to precisely impact the lesion mechanism. It needs to be appropriate for the neurovegetative condition of the patient. It must not be painful and should ideally achieve instant, measurable success.
- **Precise intervention.** Meeting the requirements listed earlier necessitates a treatment technique that provides the precise degree of impact on the joint to be treated, the hypertonic or spastic muscle fibers to be relaxed, or the contracted fascia to be stretched in the right direction.

Technical Prerequisites and Enhancers for Muscle Energy Techniques

Therapists are required to have a good sense of touch and the ability to differentiate between chronic and acute dysfunctions. They must be able to feel the affected muscle fibers in a hypertonic muscle. They need to be able to sense the direction in which a muscle needs to be stretched and when the muscle fibers respond to the stretch.

When METs are used to treat joints, it is important for the therapist to sense the limits of motion in three planes and to correctly position the joint partners without stretching the muscles to be treated (avoidance of stretch reflex). It is important to sense muscle limits. Muscle limits are reached before joint limits and before fascial limits.

In general, joint blockages are removed before treating muscles or fasciae. This applies to cases where the joint blockage triggers muscle hypertonicity. In other cases, however, muscles need to be detonified before joints can be treated.

Patients must be able to follow the therapist's instructions. They must, above all, be able to relax and feel the difference between tension and relaxation. Patients should be able to apply the requested amount of tension.

Treatment enhancers for MET include respiration, eye movement, and visualization.

■ Respiration

- Inspiration facilitates tension, while expiration dampens it.
- It is helpful if the patient "breathes into" the area of treatment.
- Inspiration should be slow and progressive.
- Patients should tense muscles before breathing in.

■ Eye Movement

- Eye movement is especially important for treating the cervical spine.
- In general, patients should look in the direction they are applying tension.

■ Visualization

Mental visualization of motions helps patients with tensioning and relaxation.

Muscle Energy Technique Variants

Before describing different forms of MET, we would like to briefly explain a few terms.

■ Isometric Contraction

The distance between origin and insertion of muscles does not change when the muscle is tensed. The forces of the therapist and the patient neutralize each other.

■ Isotonic Concentric Contraction

Muscles shorten during contraction. The patient overcomes the therapist's resistance.

■ Isotonic Eccentric Contraction

Muscles lengthen despite contraction. Muscle fibers are stretched.

Physiologic Principles

The following physiologic principles apply.

■ Postisometric Relaxation

Muscles relax more easily after they have been contracted. During the relaxation phase, it is easier to stretch the previously contracted fibers. The relaxation phase is not the same as latent period, which is much shorter.

The current thinking is that postisometric relaxation (PIR) involves activation of the Golgi tendon organ, leading to a 10- to 15-second inhibition. During this relaxation phase, the muscle group is stretched just to the point where renewed tension occurs.

■ Reciprocal Innervation or Inhibition of Antagonists

Tensioning the agonist relaxes the antagonist (for this motion pattern).

This provides the basis for the different MET variants.

■ Muscle Strengthening

Isokinetic contractions of ± 4 seconds in a range of motion that correspond as closely as possible to the motion pattern. Contraction should be close to maximum.

Treatment involves concentric as well as eccentric contractions. Brief series of contractions are preferable to frequent repetitions.

■ Isolytic Muscle Energy Technique

This type of MET is used to stretch muscles or to loosen adhesions. It involves isotonic, eccentric contraction.

To optimally break down the fibrosis in as many muscle fibers as possible, muscle contractions must be sufficiently strong. The therapists require significant strength for this, because they need to stretch the contracting muscle. To reduce the strength required by the therapist, we recommend prestretching the muscle until the tension is felt in the fibers to be treated and then asking the patient to contract the muscles.

■ Muscle Energy Technique for Resolving Spasms and Hypertonicity

Isometric contractions are best suited for this application. PIR and antagonist inhibition can be used. These two methods can also be combined. It is important to only stretch the muscle or the muscle group to its muscle limit. The contraction the patient is asked to make should not exceed 20% of the maximum contraction.

Optimal contraction should be just palpable in the hypertonic fibers. Hypertonic fibers are the first to contract in a tensed muscle. The decision whether to use PIR or antagonist inhibition depends on the degree of pain in the hypertonic muscle. If the antagonist inhibition principle is used, contraction can be stronger. The decisive effect of this treatment results from passive stretching. It must be absolutely pain free.

■ Joint Normalization and Muscle Energy Technique

Both PIR and antagonist inhibition may also be used for this application. While ilium lesions are primarily treated using antagonist inhibition, vertebrae dysfunctions are primarily corrected using PIR. Isometric contractions are preferable in all cases.

Since the intent is to inhibit primarily postural (type I) muscle fibers, light contractions that are held a little longer (5–7 seconds) are advisable.

MET treatments can cause a slight sensation of numbness in the treated areas for ± 24 hours. This seems to be caused by the release of waste products in the tissue.

Muscle imbalances require stretching of hypertonic muscles or muscles that are too short before the weak, hypotonic muscles can be strengthened. Janda explains this is due to the principle of antagonist inhibition.

11.2 Myofascial Release Techniques

Paula Sciarti and Dennis J. Dowling refer to myofascial release techniques as "myofascial–tendon–ligament–osseous–viscera techniques." This gives an indication of the interrelations between the various systems provided by connective tissue.

From Still's writing, we know that he viewed connective tissue as very important. He appears to also have used myofascial relaxation techniques. Still's techniques taught by van Buskirk are the best proof. The goal of myofascial release techniques is to relax connective tissue. If we consider that connective tissue consists of muscles, skin, fasciae, tendons, ligaments, capsules, serosa, mesos, etc., then treatment takes on a holistic nature.

Terms like "loose–tight" and "direct–indirect" as well as three-dimensionality are also important for diagnosis and treatment.

■ Loose–Tight

These terms describe the two extreme tissue conditions. Both are pathologic and contribute to imbalance. If a muscle or muscle group is hypertonic and contracted, it is tight. Their antagonists, as a rule, then are hypotonic and loose (flaccid).

The goal of myofascial release technique is to reestablish balance via neuromuscular reflexes to support physiologic functions.

■ Direct–Indirect

These terms are important in treatment. Direct treatment applies a little more contraction to already tight tissue. This activates receptors in the tissue that produce relaxation. The other method is to bring tight tissue closer together. This reduces tensions and calms receptors.

Both methods require a good sense of touch. The tissue in most fasciae is aligned multidirectionally rather than unidirectionally.

Direct treatment involves continuous palpation to determine the direction in which tension manifests. With indirect treatment, the therapist follows the "relaxations" during treatment.

■ Three-Dimensional

Diagnosis and treatment involve testing the movability of tissue in all three planes. Depending on the treatment variant, this is followed by "stacking" of "ease" or "bind." The therapist actively uses both hands for palpation and treatment.

The following enhancers are recommended for treatment:
- Respiration.
- Movements of the extremities.
- Eye movements.
- Combinations of these three enhancers.

Depending on the treatment variant used, the enhancers are selected to support either direct or indirect therapy methods.

■ Clinical Practice

The patient is seated, supine, or prostrate.
Therapist instructions:
- Contact the region to be treated with both hands. Test tissue movability using both hands and test tension between hands in all planes. If tension is felt, a decision needs to be made about the treatment variant to be used.
- If indirect treatment is used, move the hands in the directions of unrestricted movement to bring the tissue closer together.
- During treatment, the direction of movement changes. Follow the respective new direction. If fasciae are to be treated directly, create tension between both hands by palpating the fascial tracks in the three planes of motion with both hands.

- Maintain tension on the tissue until you feel a harmonious cranial-inferior movement or until you clearly sense respiration below your hands. Inspiration and movement of the extremities can help increase tension. It is interesting to invite the patient to "breathe into" the region being treated. If the patient moves the extremities, you need to inform the patient which tension to increase or to reduce and then allow the patient to perform the motion accordingly.

Several other treatment methods are also based on the same principles as myofascial release technique. We list these here without describing them further:
- Strain–counterstrain.
- Facilitated positional release.
- Functional techniques.
- Balanced ligamentous release.
- Unwinding.
- Cranial osteopathy.

11.3 Neuromuscular Technique

Neuromuscular technique (NMT) is another interesting myofascial treatment method. NMT involves deep tissue massage performed with one or more fingers or the side of the hand. This technique was developed in the 1940s by Stanley Lief while trying to develop a method of preparing tissue for treatment.

Lief was a chiropractor and osteopath. He was convinced that joint problems were only partly the cause of illness, neuralgia, and circulation disorders, as chiropractors believed at the time. He also realized that spine blockages often resulted from indurations in paravertebral tissue. He therefore began to sensitively massage tissue using progressively deeper pressure. He paid attention to knots, retractions, swelling, and resistance in tissue movability.

He was surprised to find that this neuromuscular treatment, as he called it, not only resolved mobility limitations, but also affected distant regions. He called his technique neuromuscular treatment because it allowed him to treat not only the muscles, but also to reflectively treat other disorders via the nervous system.

Indeed, treatment success for this method does seem to be primarily of a reflective nature. This method allows successful treatment of trigger points, Chapman's reflex points, and other reflex points. On the other hand,

therapists can use deep massage to target and influence connective tissue, stimulate localized circulation, and activate the metabolism. This treatment can be used on the entire body or only in specific regions.

■ Clinical Practice

The patient is seated or lying down as comfortably as possible.
Therapist instructions:
- Push a finger into the tissue without causing pain until you feel a slight resistance.
- Then move the finger forward at a rate of ±2 to 3 cm/s.
  - If you encounter indurations, knots, or resistance, move the finger more slowly without decreasing pressure.
  - Generally, draw lines of about 5 to 10 cm in length.
  - In regions containing indurations, draw several lines until the tissue softens.
  - For knots, you can apply friction or intermittent pressure.
  - Lines can be drawn across or parallel to muscle fibers.
  - Trigger points generally need to be treated separately (see Part B, Trigger Points: Diagnosis and Treatment).

11.4 Myofascial Release Technique with Ischemic Compression

This method is interesting for treating muscle indurations and trigger points.

■ Clinical Practice

Therapist instructions:
- The patient is seated or lying down comfortably.
- Search for muscle indurations, tensed fibers, or trigger points.

- Once a painful (when pressed too hard) point is located, compress this point using the elbow or one of the knuckles of the hand.
- Ask the patient to perform a motion that moves the muscle fibers being treated below your elbow or knuckle.
- Maintain contact until the pain is significantly reduced.
- Stretch the treated muscle or muscle group a few times.

B

Trigger Points: Diagnosis and Treatment

Eric Hebgen

12 Definition

A **trigger point (TP)** is a strongly irritated region within a taut (hypertonic) band of skeletal muscle or muscle fascia. Trigger points are painful when palpated. Each trigger point can trigger reactions that are specific to that point:

- Referred pain.
- Muscle tension (also in other muscles).
- Vegetative reactions.

Trigger points are also found in other tissues, for example, skin, adipose tissue, tendons, ligaments, joint capsules, or the periosteum. Unlike myofascial trigger points, however, these trigger points are not as consistent or predictably located. They also do not cause referred pain.

13 Classification of Trigger Points

Active and Latent Trigger Points

Trigger points can be active or latent. Active trigger points cause pain at rest as well as during muscle activity. Latent trigger points, on the other hand, may present all the diagnostic indicators of active trigger points (see below), but they only generate pain when palpated.

Active trigger points may convert to latent trigger points, especially if factors that have been perpetuating the active trigger point are no longer present or when the muscle containing the active trigger point has been sufficiently stretched by normal daily activity.

Conversely, latent trigger points can persist silently in muscles for years and then be transformed into active trigger points. Factors that promote this conversion are muscle strain dysfunctions in the most general sense, for example, excessive stretching or excessive use of a muscle.

Symptoms

The following symptoms indicate active or latent trigger points:
- Limited active and/or passive mobility when a muscle is stretched or contracted. The patient experiences a feeling of stiffness.
- Weakness in the muscle containing the trigger point(s).
- Referred pain exhibiting characteristic patterns that are defined for each muscle. With active trigger points, referred pain is present during activity, rest, or palpation of the trigger point. Latent trigger points generate the characteristic referred pain pattern only during diagnostic palpation.

Muscle stiffness and weakness appear especially after longer periods of rest or generally following inactivity.

Typical examples include morning stiffness or "startup" pain when resuming motion after longer periods of sitting.

The level of symptoms and sensitivity to palpation of active trigger points can change within hours or from day to day. Trigger point symptoms often endure well beyond the presence of the trigger point cause.

Other symptoms that may be caused by trigger points include:
- Vegetative changes in the zone of referred pain, for example, local vasoconstriction, perspiration, lacrimation, increased nasal secretion, and increased pilomotor activity (goose bumps).
- Deep sensibility dysfunctions.
- Vertigo and dizziness.
- Changes in motor neuron activity with increased irritability.
- Impaired muscle coordination.

Factors Contributing to Trigger Points

The following factors are conducive to the development of trigger points:
- Acute excessive muscle strain.
- Chronic excessive muscle strain or excessive muscle fatigue.
- Direct trauma.
- Hypothermia (muscle activity without prior warm-up).
- Other trigger points.
- Internal organ disorders.
- Arthritic joints.
- Segmental reflectory dysfunction (see Chapter 18).
- Distress.

14 Pathophysiology of Trigger Points

■ Local Tension Increase in Trigger Points: Referred Pain

The local increase of tension in the trigger point is attributed to changed or increased irritability of group 3 and 4 nerve fibers. In muscles, these nerves are the nociceptors in the form of free (nonencapsulated) nerve endings. If such a nerve fiber is hyperirritable, even small stimuli—in this case, pain stimuli—can trigger an amplified response in the body. This response can develop into increased pain perception (lowered pain threshold) or a more pronounced vegetative response. In general, the stronger response of afferent nociceptive nerve fibers to stimuli can trigger responses from efferent nerve fibers that normally would not react. The information processing for this phenomenon takes place in spinal cord segments.

Substances known to increase the excitability of group 3 and 4 fibers are, for example, bradykinin, serotonin, prostaglandins, or histamine. Afferent impulses from group 3 and 4 nociceptor fibers can also be responsible for the brain's "misinterpretation" of these impulses and for responding to them as referred pain or increased tension. The mechanisms responsible for this process are described in the following sections.

■ Convergence: Projection

The spinal cord contains two possible different mechanisms for coupling afferents with efferent neurons (▶ Fig. 14.1):

- An afferent nociceptive impulse from the skin, a muscle, or an inner organ is switched in the spinal cord to an interneuron that is responsible for both

afferents before this neuron is switched back to efferent for responding to the impulse.

- Skin, muscle, and visceral afferents share an end path before the stimulus is conducted to the efferent.

Afferent information is not only conducted to the efferent to respond to stimuli, but also via the anterior and lateral spinothalamic tract to the central nervous system (CNS). The afferent impulse flow arrives in the CNS. With both mechanisms, it is not possible for the CNS to determine whether the nociceptive impulse arrives from the skin/muscle or from an inner organ. Since our body/CNS has learned over time that nociceptive or damaging stimuli generally impact the body from the outside, they are interpreted as impulses arriving from the skin or from a muscle. A pain impulse conducted via the anterior and lateral spinothalamic tracts for conscious perception is noticed as referred pain in the section of skin that is associated with the respective segment.

The CNS treats afferent impulse activity arising from a trigger point like nociceptive afferents from an inner organ. The pain is perceived in the skin, which is the reference zone segmentally associated with the trigger point.

■ Convergence: Facilitation

Many afferent nerves display some background activity. It could be said that these nerves generate a kind of ambient noise of impulse activity that is not generated by external (or internal) stimuli. Its neurophysiological cause is a lowering of the impulse threshold via changes in the ion channel that makes it easier to

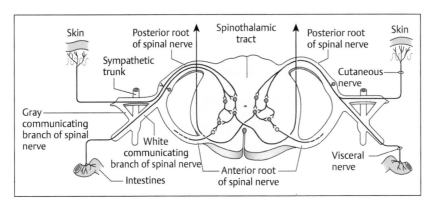

▶ **Fig. 14.1** Development of referred pain. (From Schmidt RF, Thews G, eds. Physiologie des Menschen. 29th ed. Berlin: Springer; 2004.)

generate action potentials. This may be a protective mechanism vis-à-vis nociceptive impulses, because it allows these impulses to be recognized and responded to more quickly.

If this background activity is amplified in an area of the skin by a series of afferent nociceptive impulses from an inner organ or from a trigger point (convergent facilitated) and conducted on *one* neuron of the spinothalamic tract to the CNS (see previous section on "Convergence: Projection"), the pain will be felt very strongly in that skin area.

■ Axon Reflex

The dendrites of afferent nerves bifurcate into many branches and one nerve can sensibly supply many different regions of the body. This can result in the CNS misinterpreting the afferent impulse flow: as of the axon hillock, the individual areas of the body can no longer be differentiated. Instead, the pain is registered as coming from the entire innervation area of the neuron.

■ Sympathetic Nerves (Hyperexcitability)

It is possible that these nerves help sustain referred pain by releasing substances that further increase the sensitization of nociceptive afferents in the pain region and lower their impulse threshold. It is also possible that because of sympathetic innervation, the blood supply of afferents from the pain zone is reduced.

■ Metabolic Derailment

Trigger point regions are areas in a muscle characterized by metabolic derailment. These areas present with a combination of increased energy requirement with simultaneous lack of oxygen and energy, likely caused by reduced blood circulation in that area. This sets off a vicious circle that results in the development of trigger points in the area experiencing a decreased supply of energy. Existing trigger points may be sustained by this metabolic derailment.

■ Muscle Stretching Influences Muscle Metabolism

Stretching contracted sarcomere to their maximum length has immediate effects on the muscle (▶**Fig. 14.2**): it reduces adenosine triphosphate (ATP) consumption, normalizes metabolism, and decreases muscle tension.

If metabolic derailment caused substances to be released in the muscle (e.g., prostaglandins) that can trigger different pathological mechanisms of relevance to trigger points, restoring metabolism to normal reduces the concentration of these substances. It is also believed that balancing the metabolism normalizes the excitability of afferent nociceptive nerve fibers.

■ Hypertonic Palpable Muscle Strands (Taut Bands)

Hypertonic palpable muscle strands are taut bands of muscle fibers surrounding a trigger point. They measure about 1 to 4 mm in thickness and, when palpated, are noticeably firmer than their surroundings. These taut bands stand out because they exhibit hyperesthesia or even pronounced painfulness. The easiest way to palpate taut bands is to slightly stretch the taut muscle fibers while the remaining muscle fibers stay relaxed.

Stretching or strong contraction of taut bands or pressure on a trigger point within the taut band can trigger localized pain and, following a certain latency period, also referred pain.

Sarcomeres within muscle fibers in normal muscles are of equal length. Muscle fibers are arranged lengthwise to enable maximum development of muscle strength. This muscle strength requires actin and myosin filaments to overlap by a specific ratio. If they overlap too much or too little, muscle strength is reduced.

Muscle fibers in taut muscle bands look histologically different. Sarcomere length within taut bands varies. If sarcomeres are shortened around a trigger point without exhibiting electromyography activity, they are **contracted** (▶**Fig. 14.4**). These contracted fibers are compensated by lengthened sarcomeres at the end of the taut band near the muscle–tendon junction.

This unique feature explains why muscles with hypertonic, palpable muscle bands exhibit decreased elasticity (contracted sarcomeres) as well as reduced strength (contracted and lengthened sarcomeres: sarcomeres outside the optimal length range; ▶**Fig. 14.3**).

■ Muscle Weakness and Rapid Fatigue

Patients with trigger points likely present with both these symptoms because of reduced circulation and the resulting hypoxia in the affected muscle.

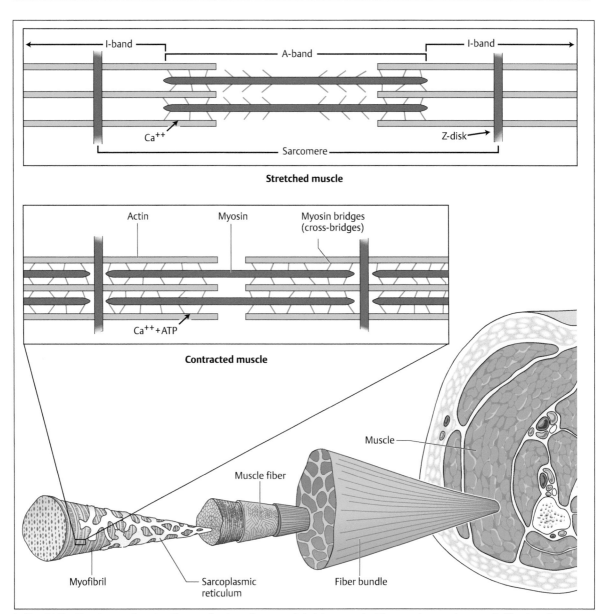

▶ **Fig. 14.2** Structure and contraction mechanism of a normal skeleton muscle. The muscle contains muscle fiber bundles consisting of fasciated, striated muscle cells or muscle fibers. A single fiber generally contains about 1,000 myofibrils. Each myofibril is surrounded by a sarcoplasmic reticulum, a sacklike webbed structure.
Zoom: Adenosine triphosphate and free calcium (Ca^{2+}) activate the myosin cross-bridges, which causes them to pull on the actin filaments. This traction brings the Z-lines closer together and contracts the sarcomere (contracting unit), which shortens the muscle. The actin filament sections that do not contain myosin filaments in both sides of a Z-disk make up the I-band. The A-band corresponds to the length of the myosin filaments. If there is only an A-band and no I-band, maximum contraction has been reached (according to Travell and Simons 1999).

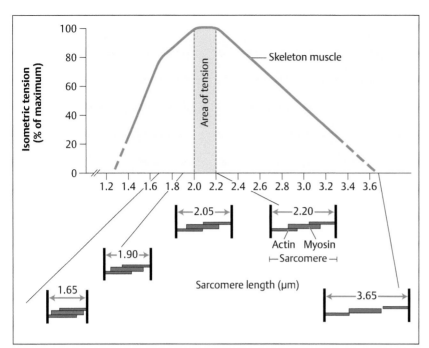

▸ **Fig. 14.3** Isometric muscle tension determined by length of sarcomeres. (From Silbernagl S, Despopoulos A. Taschenatlas Physiologie. 7th ed. Stuttgart: Thieme; 2007:67.)

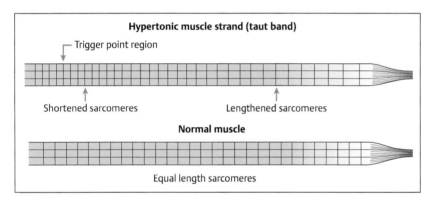

▸ **Fig. 14.4** Comparison: sarcomeres of equal length in normal muscle and sarcomeres of varying length in a muscle with trigger points. Shortened sarcomeres in the trigger point region increase tension in hypertonic muscle strands and reduce muscle elasticity. (From Simons D. Myofascial pain syndrome due to trigger points. In: Goodgold J, ed. Rehabilitation Medicine. St. Louis, MO: Mosby Year Book; 1988:686–723.)

15 Diagnosing Trigger Points

Trigger points are most effectively diagnosed using the following step-by-step process.

■ Precise Anamnesis

Identifying the muscles that developed trigger points and that led to the current symptoms requires a precise anamnesis:

- Were the symptoms caused by trauma? Did the pain appear, for example, after significant exertion or after a fall?
- In which position or during which motion did the pain first appear?
- Are there segmental dysfunctions (for example, joint blockages or herniations of intervertebral disks) that could have facilitated the entire segment?
- Are there visceral dysfunctions that have promoted the development of trigger points via hypertonic facilitation of muscles that share the same segmental innervation, in the sense of a viscerosomatic reflex?

■ Charting Pain Patterns

It can be helpful to chart pain patterns onto a diagram of the patient's body to recognize typical patterns assigned to individual muscles. Patterns should be classified historically by when they appeared. Frequently, patterns will overlap. The following questions should be addressed:

- Is it possible to determine the sequence in which pain appeared despite overlapping patterns? Is it possible to isolate muscle-specific regions?
- Do the overlapping patterns share commonalities, for example, segmental innervation, that would point to structural or visceral dysfunctions?

Pain (and increased tension) caused by a trigger point is generally projected and perceived some distance from the location of the trigger point. It is important to note that symptoms may vary widely depending on the posture or muscle activity causing the pain. Therefore, symptoms may fluctuate during the day as well as from one day to the next.

Pain that occurs not only during motion but also at rest indicates more pronounced impairment by trigger points.

In addition to pain, trigger points can also cause paresthesia of surface and deep sensibility in muscle-specific areas of the skin. Concomitant vegetative symptoms may also present in these areas, for example, increased vasomotor activity with pale skin during trigger point stimulation, reflectory hyperemia following stimulation, goose bumps (cutis anserina), as well as increased lacrimal and nasal secretions.

■ Examining Muscle Activity

The muscles identified during previous tests are now examined while active. The goal is to observe the muscle during its entire active range of motion to identify postures and/or motion areas that cause pain. The muscle is also tested actively and passively to its maximum stretched length. The therapist looks for local pain in the trigger point area as well as referred pain.

The following findings are possible if trigger points are present:

- Maximum strength of the affected muscle is reduced during active resistance testing, without presenting with atrophy.
- Typical pain patterns occur or are amplified if the muscle is exercised isometrically or eccentrically.
- Active and passive stretching causes referred pain.
- Active and passive muscle elasticity is impaired.

■ Searching for Trigger Points

The next step is to search for trigger points in the previously identified muscles (▶Fig. 15.1). This examination is conducted in a neutral posture—the affected muscle fibers should not be stretched or approximated. The therapist palpates the muscle tissue using the tip of a finger. Superficial muscles are palpated vertically to their long axis (**flat palpation**). Hypertonic muscle strands that likely contain the expected trigger point will present as a bandlike area of significantly increased tension (taut band; ▶Fig.15.1). Within this band, the therapist now searches for the most sensitive spot—this will be the trigger point. Applying pressure to the trigger point elicits local pain and persistent pressure elicits referred pain. Local pain can present so strongly, sharply, and spontaneously that patients exhibit a **jump sign**: they wince, produce a pain-related vocalization, or pull the muscle away from the therapist.

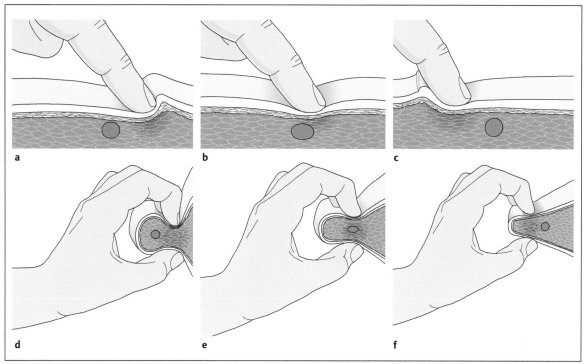

▶ **Fig. 15.1 (a–c)** Cross-section showing flat palpation of a taut muscle fiber band (black circle) and its trigger point. **Flat palpation** is used for muscles that can only be accessed from one side, for example, the infraspinous muscle. **(a)** Start palpation by pushing skin away. **(b)** Slide fingertip across the muscle fibers. A taut band of fibers is recognized by its ropelike structure. **(c)** Then push the skin away to the other side. This motion is also called **snapping palpation** if it is performed more quickly. **(d–f)** Cross-section showing **pincer palpation** of a taut muscle fiber band (*black circle*) at a trigger point. Pincer palpation is suitable for muscles that can be gripped with fingers, for example, sternocleidomastoid, greater pectoral muscle, and latissimus dorsi. **(d)** Muscle fibers held in **pincer grip** using thumb and fingers. **(e)** Firmness of taut fiber band is clearly palpable when rolled between fingers. Changing the position of the finger end joints creates a swinging motion that allows more details to be observed. **(f)** Palpable margin of taut fiber band is clearly distinguishable when it slides out between finger tips. Often accompanied by a simultaneous **local twitch response** (according to Travell and Simons 1999).

Searching for hypertonic taut muscle bands in deeper muscles can be more difficult or impossible because of the overlaying structures. In these deeper tissue areas, the therapist uses direct **deep palpation** to locate trigger points.

Using **pincer palpation** can be helpful for finding trigger points in muscles that can be held between two fingers (e.g., trapezius). The therapist rolls the area of the muscle belly back and forth between thumb and index finger to search for the hypertonic taut band. The same grip is then used to search for the trigger point within the taut band.

When a muscle is palpated near a trigger point, a brief contraction of the muscle fibers can often be observed. The therapist feels or observes this muscle reaction as a twitch. This **local twitch response** (LTR) is characteristic for trigger points (▶**Fig.15.2**). The localized muscle contraction is most pronounced when the muscle is palpated perpendicular to the long axis of the muscle band **using snapping palpation**: the band is plucked and stretched horizontally and then released, like a guitar string.

As a final confirmation of the trigger point location, palpation is repeated: active trigger points present reproducible results.

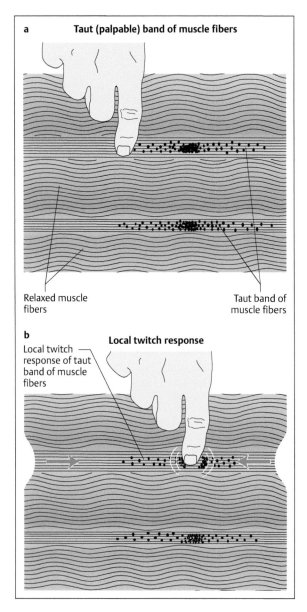

a   **Taut (palpable) band of muscle fibers**

Relaxed muscle
fibers

Taut band of
muscle fibers

b

Local twitch
response of taut
band of muscle
fibers

Local twitch response

▶ **Fig. 15.2** Taut fiber band, myofascial trigger points, and local twitch response in longitudinal cross-section of muscle. **(a)** Palpation of taut fiber band (*straight lines*) surrounded by flaccid, relaxed muscle fibers (*wavy lines*). Density of dots reflects degree of pressure sensitivity of the taut fiber band. The trigger point is the most pressure-sensitive location in the fiber band. **(b)** Quickly rolling the fiber band below finger tips (snapping palpation) frequently elicits a local twitch response. Most clearly visible as skin movement between trigger point and insertion location of muscle fibers (after Travell and Simons 1999).

Note: Pain originating from muscles must be distinguished from other types of pain:
- Neurologic.
- Rheumatic.
- Tumorous.
- Psychogenic.
- Inflammatory.
- Vascular.

Muscle-induced pain typically comes and goes as the affected muscle is activated by motion or by certain malpostures.

16 Trigger Point Therapy

In addition to the many techniques for treating trigger points, two factors are very important for therapy success:

- Even if the treatment of trigger points is initially successful, factors that perpetuate trigger points will quickly and predictably reactivate trigger points and their associated symptoms. Therefore, eliminating these factors is as important as treating the muscles.
- Patients need to be included in their treatment. It is about their own body and they need to participate in the process. This includes making patients aware of problems with their posture or motion patterns as well as providing patients with a program they can perform on their own to stretch affected muscles or muscle groups.

■ Spray and Stretch Technique

The goal of this technique is to deactivate trigger points by stretching the muscle to its maximum without triggering reflectory countertension or appreciable pain.

Applying Cooling Spray

The treatment objective is for the cooling spray to irritate the skin and trigger a flow of "distracting" afferent impulses that blocks the reflectory hypertonicity/spasm of the muscle being treated at the level of the spinal cord.

Instructions for therapists:

- Apply the cooling spray to the skin in parallel lines in locations where the muscle to be treated projects to the body's surface. Icing up or freezing of the skin must be avoided.
- Apply the spray at a rate of 10 cm/s along the entire length of the muscle from a distance of about 45 cm and at an angle of 30 degrees to the skin surface.
- Include the referred pain region in the treatment. Treat the extremities from proximal to distal and the trunk from superior to inferior.

Passive Stretching

Instructions for therapists:

- After applying the first two to three sprays, begin to passively stretch the muscle. Slowly, and while

observing tension barriers along the way, stretch the muscle to its maximum length.
- Continue spraying while stretching the muscle. To further support reflectory relaxation, you can ask the patient to slowly exhale and look down while stretching the muscle.

The cooling spray decreases reflectory muscle tonicity and allows the muscle to be easily stretched without pain.

> *Important:* Application of the cooling spray serves as a distraction at the level of the spinal cord. Stretching is the treatment.

Active Stretching

Actively exercise the range of motion achieved by the spray and stretch application with the patient.

■ Postisometric Relaxation/Muscle Energy Techniques/Myofascial Release

Instructions for therapists:

1. Stretch the muscle to be treated until muscle tension prevents further stretching of the muscle.
2. Ask the patient to contract the muscle against your resistance while applying three-dimensional resistance (at about 25% of maximum strength) in the direction of muscle contraction without allowing movement (isometric contraction). Hold this resistance for 3 to 7 seconds.
3. Ask the patient to relax while you continue to passively stretch the muscle to a new tension barrier. During this relaxation phase, the effectiveness of this technique can be enhanced by asking the patient to slowly exhale and look down.
4. Repeat the contraction exercise in step 2.
5. Once normal muscle length is reached, actively exercise the newly achieved range of motion with the patient.

■ Ischemic Compression/Manual Inhibition

Instructions for therapists:
- Apply manual compression to the trigger point. The pain elicited by this treatment must be well tolerable and reflects treatment progress.
- Once the pain disappears (15 seconds to 1 minute), increase pressure to the next pain barrier. Repeat this compression until the trigger point is no longer painful.
- Actively exercise the newly achieved range of motion with the patient.

■ Deep Friction Massage

Instructions for therapists:
- Apply manual, crosswise stretching along the taut, hypertonic muscle band containing the trigger point. Work at a constant speed along the entire muscle band. Initially, this technique is painful and the level of pain must be well tolerable for the patient. Continue to stretch until the pain disappears (2–3 minutes).
- Actively exercise the newly achieved range of motion with the patient.

■ Stretching Exercises

Successful treatment requires therapists to motivate patients to share the responsibility for and be integrated into treatment. For this purpose, the following chapters on trigger points contain various stretching exercises that can be taught to patients for performing on their own. The objective of these exercises is to stretch either individual muscles or, more frequently, whole muscle groups. Our choice of muscles is based on clinical relevance in our daily practice. All stretching exercises have been tested numerous times in clinical practice, are easy to teach and to learn, and can be performed by lay persons with little effort. We believe that these factors achieve manifold increases in patient compliance with exercise programs.

Each exercise is designed to be practiced about 15 to 20 times a day. These repetitions do not have to be achieved in one session, but can be spread throughout the day and integrated into the patient's lifestyle. This is another important aspect for enhancing patient acceptance of the exercise and thereby increasing treatment effectiveness.

These exercises are designed for static stretching. They can quickly lengthen muscle structures and range of motion. This prevents trigger point relapses and significantly decreases trigger point activity. In some cases, the trigger point is no longer palpable in patients after they have consistently exercised for 1 to 2 weeks on their own.

17 Trigger Point Perpetuating Factors

Treatment of trigger points may lead to only temporary freedom from symptoms if there are factors that perpetuate trigger points. Long-term freedom from pain can only be achieved if these factors are recognized and eliminated.

It is possible that a trigger point develops in a muscle after a fall or short-term strain. If this trigger point is eliminated as soon as possible following the trauma, the body can quickly be restored to its original condition (restitutio ad integrum). This type of treatment success can generally be observed with professional athletes who are cared for by therapists on an ongoing basis.

However, if treatment does not occur immediately following a trauma, the body has time to develop protective postures and evasive motions to protect the injured muscle against further strain. These evasive mechanisms in turn can strain other ligaments, joints, etc., and cause new symptoms. The initial trauma then recedes into the background and the weakest link in the protective chain emerges. If only the original trigger point is clinically diagnosed and treated without also treating the protective mechanisms that developed later, treatment success would be temporary and not satisfactory.

The following is a partial list of factors that perpetuate trigger points.

■ Mechanical Factors

- Leg length differences.
- Malpostures while sitting or standing.
- Spinal curvatures.
- Torticollis (wryneck).
- Winged scapula (alar scapula).
- Pelvic tilt (ilium or sacrum dysfunctions).
- Malpositions of coccygeal bone.
- Arm length differences.

■ Systemic Factors

Systemic factors include everything that can negatively impact the energy metabolism of muscles. Reduced energy supply in muscles promotes the development and perpetuation of trigger points. Systemic factors include:
- Vitamin B deficiency.
- Electrolyte imbalances (e.g., calcium, copper, magnesium, iron).
- Gout.
- Anemia.
- Hypoglycemia.
- Chronic infections.
- Lowered immunity.
- Psychological stress.

18 Facilitated Segments

Innervation of spinal segments is multifaceted. The somatic (cerebrospinal) and the autonomic nervous systems both originate there. Afferent nerve fibers travel via the posterior horn of the spinal cord into the spinal cord. Efferents leave the spinal cord segment via the anterior horn of the spinal cord. In between, we find a multitude of synapsis of these two nerve types in the spinal cord itself. Transmission of afferent impulses onto interneurons provides a range of modulation opportunities for the original nerve impulse. Stimuli can be not only amplified, but also inhibited. The mechanisms responsible for this modulation are partly found at the segmental level. In addition, excitation or inhibition signals sent by the cranial centers, for example, via the extrapyramidal system, also influence this modulation.

If we now take a closer look at afferents, we find that we can divide the spinal cord segment into various compartments. We find afferent nerves from the **sclerotome**. We refer to the nerve supply not only of bones, but also of joints (including cartilage), joint capsules, fasciae, synovia, and ligaments. Sclerotome neurons also handle the perception of deep sensibility and pain.

Muscles also exhibit segmental innervation via the **myotome**. Muscles and their associated fiber and tendon sensors also provide information about deep sensibility and pain.

Individual skin areas are exclusively innervated by a spinal cord segment, the **dermatome**. This is where surface sensibility is perceived via afferents.

The last innervation area of a segment is the **viscerotome**. It transmits afferent information about pain and generally damaging agents to the spinal cord.

The information about afferents also applies to efferents. The efferents for each innervation area also originate in the spinal cord and motorically supply fasciae or muscles in the skin, inner organs, or skeleton muscles.

Altogether, this could be called the segmental "hardware." The "software" is what we refer to as the **facilitated segment**. Afferent stimuli are largely processed and modulated at the level of the spinal cord and responded to as an efferent impulse. Processing can include all innervation areas of a segment and the efferent response can also be multifaceted.

Example: A person is suffering from duodenal ulcers. The information about damage to the mucous membrane is transmitted to the spinal cord via visceral afferents. Responding to this information now challenges the entire segment. The viscerotome may respond: smooth muscles become hypertonic, resulting in a spasm in the intestinal wall. The dermatome may respond via spinal cord synapses: segmental abdominal skin areas could exhibit hyperesthesia, circulatory changes (paleness or redness), or pilomotor activity. The sclerotome responds by fascial contraction of the damaged region, resulting in immobilization of the inflamed intestinal sections or development of segmental joint blockages in the physiologic motor pattern. And finally, trigger points may develop in the myotome, that is, the abdominal muscles.

This complex segmental response serves regeneration or the body's self-healing. All parts of the body work on removing the ulcer in the duodenum.

Once healing has occurred, two response areas may continue their immobilization work even though it is no longer needed: fasciae and muscles.

Concerning muscles, it can be said that trigger point activity should be eliminated by therapy. Otherwise, mobility limitations can persist that could in turn trigger new pathologies. The same applies for fascial tension.

> *Important:* For each muscle discussed in this book, we list the associated organs, because the reaction chain can also be traced in reverse. If a trigger point is found in a muscle, the segmentally associated organs should also be examined and treated for dysfunctions. If only the trigger points are eliminated and visceral dysfunctions are overlooked, then either it is not possible to achieve a pain-free state for muscles or there will be relapses.

Facilitated segments challenge therapists again and again to shed one-dimensional thinking, engage neuroanatomy, and place the symptom complex into a greater segmental context. No therapist should be satisfied with only treating a trigger point to eliminate, for example, painful shoulder motions. Our complex body deserves more. Therapists who commit to this more holistic approach will obtain a substantially higher rate of treatment success and much more long-lasting results.

19 Trigger Points

19.1 Head and Neck Pain: Related Muscles

The muscles listed in this chapter can cause pain in the head and neck area if they contain trigger points (TPs). This pain may be misdiagnosed as:
- Migraine.
- Temporomandibular joint arthrosis.
- Sinusitis.
- Pharyngitis.
- Laryngitis.
- Tooth disorders.
- Trigeminal neuralgia.

Trapezius Muscle (▶Figs. 19.1–19.4)

Origin

- Middle third of superior nuchal line.
- Nuchal ligament.
- Spinous processes and supraspinal ligaments up to thoracic vertebral body (TVB) 12.

Insertion

- Outer third of posterior border of clavicle.
- Medial section of acromion.
- Upper edge of spine of scapula.

Action

- External rotation in shoulder joint.
- Raises scapula.
- Retraction of scapula toward spine.
- With fixed scapula: extension and lateral flexion of the cervical spinal column (CSC).

Innervation

- Accessory nerve.
- Proprioceptive fibers from C3/C4.

Trigger Point Location

Trapezius TPs are found in the entire muscle.
- TP1: Palpable in free border of the descending part as hypertonic taut bands.
- TP2: Posterior to TP1 and above the spine of the scapula, roughly in the center of the spine of the scapula.
- TP3: In the area of lateral border of the ascending part, near the medial border of the scapula.
- TP4: In the ascending part, directly below the spine of the scapula, near the medial border of the scapula.
- TP5: In the horizontal part, about 1 cm medial of insertion of the levator scapula muscle at the scapula.
- TP6: In the supraspinous fossa of scapula, near the acromion.

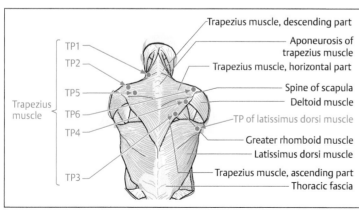

▶ **Fig. 19.1**

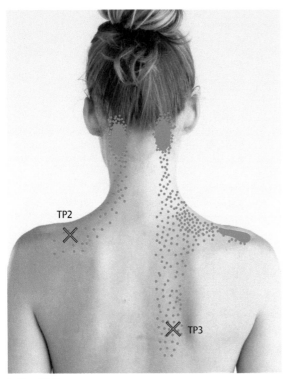

▶ **Fig. 19.2**

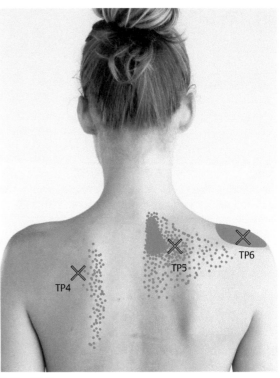

▶ **Fig. 19.3**

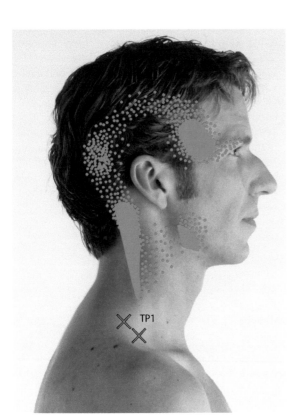

▶ **Fig. 19.4**

Referred Pain Areas

- TP1: Posterolateral in the cervical and nuchal area to the mastoid process and lateral on the head, especially in the temple area and eye socket (orbit), and angles of mandible.
- TP2: Mastoid process and the upper CSC (posterolateral).
- TP3: Mastoid process and the upper CSC (posterolateral) and in the area of the acromion.
- TP4: Along the medial border of the scapula.
- TP5: Paravertebral between CVB 7 and TP5.
- TP6: Acromion.

Associated Inner Organs

- Liver.
- Gallbladder.
- Stomach.

Sternocleidomastoid Muscle (▸Figs. 19.5–19.7)

Origin

- Anterosuperior at the manubrium of the sternum.
- Upper border of the medial third of clavicle.

Insertion

- Exterior surface of the mastoid process.
- Lateral half of the superior nuchal line.

Action

- Ipsilateral lateral flexion and contralateral rotation of the CSC.
- Bilateral contraction: extension of the CSC with anterior translation.

Innervation

- Accessory nerve.

Trigger Point Location

- TPs are found in the sternal and clavicular part throughout the entire length of the muscle.

Trigger Points in Sternal Part

- Manubrium of the sternum.
- Supraorbital and in the orbit.
- Cheek.
- Outer acoustic meatus.
- Temporomandibular joint region.
- Pharynx and tongue.
- Occiput, posterior of the mastoid process.

Trigger Points in Clavicular Part

- Forehead, sometimes also bilaterally.
- Outer acoustic meatus.
- Immediately behind the ear.

Referred Pain Areas

TPs of the sternocleidomastoid can cause facial pain that can easily be misdiagnosed as trigeminal neuralgia.

Associated Inner Organs

- Liver.
- Gallbladder.
- Stomach.

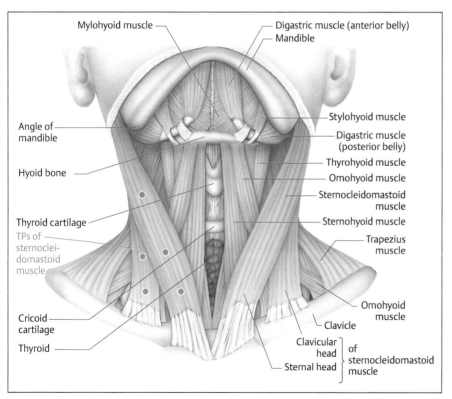

▸ **Fig. 19.5**

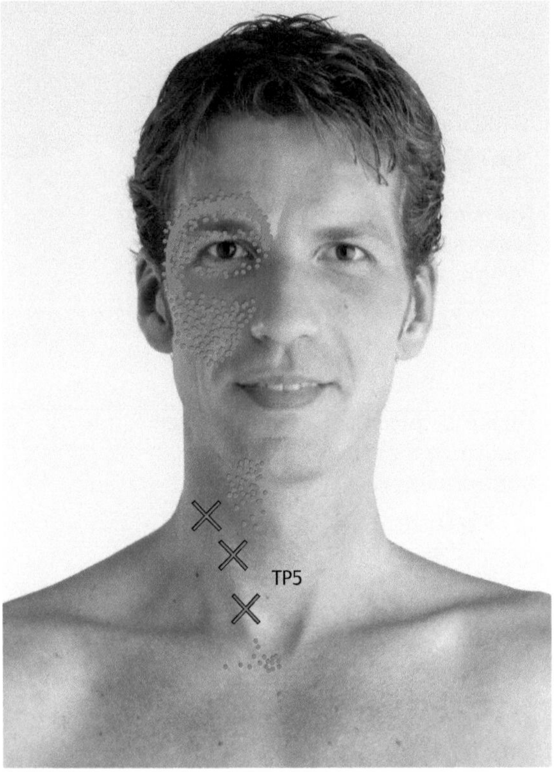

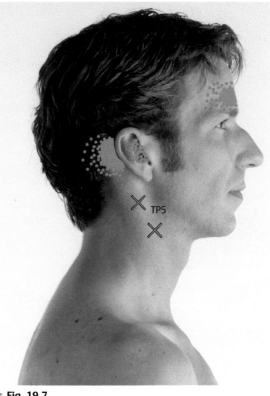

► Fig. 19.6

► Fig. 19.7

Masseter Muscle (►Figs. 19.8, 19.9)

Origin

- Anterior two-thirds of the zygomatic arch.
- Zygomatic process of the maxilla.

Insertion

- Exterior surface of the angle of the mandible.
- Lower section of the ramus of the mandible.

Action

Raises mandible (closes mouth).

Innervation

Mandibular nerve (from the trigeminal nerve).

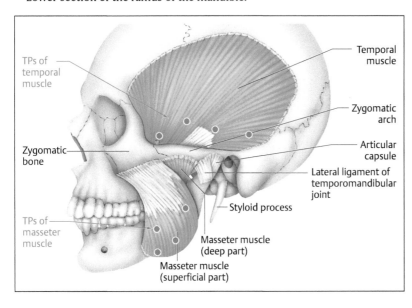

► Fig. 19.8

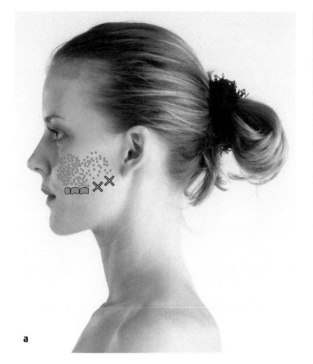

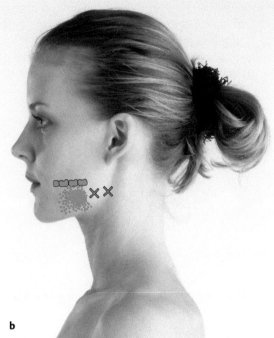

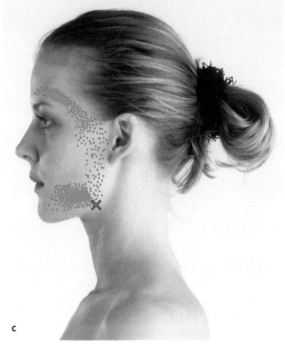

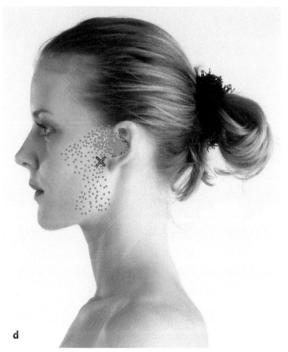

▶ **Fig. 19.9 (a–d)**

Trigger Point Location

TPs are found distributed throughout the entire muscle.

Referred Pain Areas

- Maxilla and upper molars.
- Mandible and lower molars.

- From the temple to above the eyebrows.
- Temporomandibular joint.
- Outer acoustic meatus.

Sometimes, TPs in the masseter muscle cause tinnitus.

Associated Inner Organs

None.

Temporal Muscle (▶ Figs. 19.8, 19.10)

Origin

Temporal fossa between the inferior temporal line of the parietal bone and the infratemporal crest.

Insertion

Medial and anterior section of the coronoid process of the mandible.

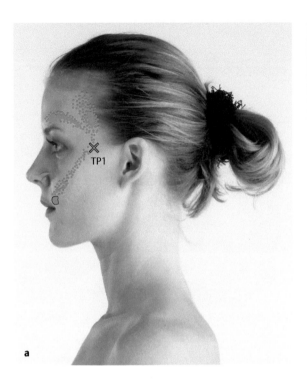

a

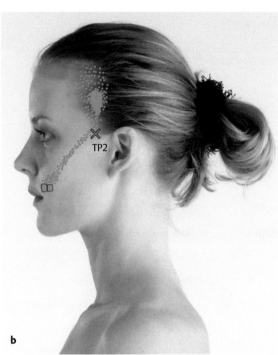

b

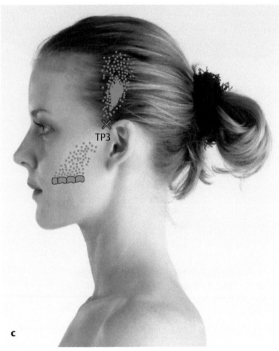

c

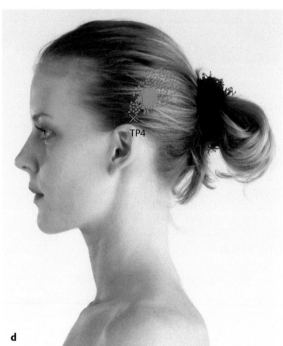

d

▶ **Fig. 19.10 (a–d)**

Action

Raises and guides back the mandible.

Innervation

Mandibular nerve (from trigeminal nerve).

Trigger Point Location

* TP1–TP3: Above the zygomatic process.
* TP4: Above the ear.

Referred Pain Areas

* Radiating from the temple toward the parietal.
* Above the eyebrows.
* Upper row of the teeth.
* Behind the eye.

Associated Inner Organs

None.

Lateral Pterygoid Muscle (▶Figs. 19.11, 19.12)

Origin

* Lower surface of the greater wing of the sphenoid bone.
* Exterior surface of the lateral pterygoid plate.

Insertion

* Pterygoid fossa below the condylar process of the mandible.
* Mandibles.
* Articular disk of the temporomandibular joint.

Action

Opens mouth (draws the mandible with the articular disk forward).

Innervation

Lateral pterygoid nerve from the mandibular nerve (from the trigeminal nerve).

Trigger Point Location

TPs of this short muscle are found by intraoral palpation approximately in the middle of the muscle belly.

Referred Pain Areas

* Temporomandibular joint.
* Maxilla.

Associated Inner Organs

None.

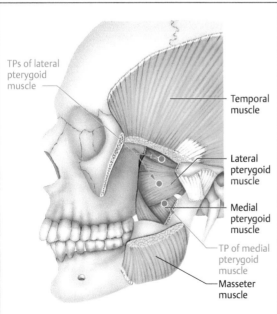

▶ **Fig. 19.11**

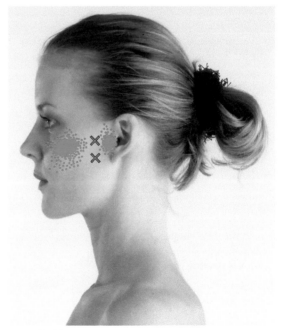

▶ **Fig. 19.12**

Medial Pterygoid Muscle (▶Figs. 19.11, 19.13)

Origin

- Interior surface of the lateral pterygoid plate.
- Pterygoid fossa.
- Maxillary tuberosity.
- Pyramidal process of the palatine bone.

Insertion

Inner side of the angle of the mandible.

Action

Moves mandible forward, upward, and laterally (chewing).

Innervation

Medial pterygoid nerve from the mandibular nerve (from the trigeminal nerve).

Trigger Point Location

TPs of this short muscle are found by intraoral palpation approximately in the middle of the muscle belly.

Referred Pain Areas

- Tongue.
- Pharynx.

Digastric Muscle (▶Figs. 19.14, 19.15)

Origin

- Anterior head: digastric fossa at the posterior surface of the mandibular symphysis.
- Posterior head: mastoid notch at the mastoid process.

Insertion

At the intermediate tendon that inserts laterally at the hyoid bone.

Action

- Raises the hyoid bone.
- Draws the mandible forward.
- Supports swallowing.

Innervation

- Anterior head: mandibular nerve (from the trigeminal nerve).

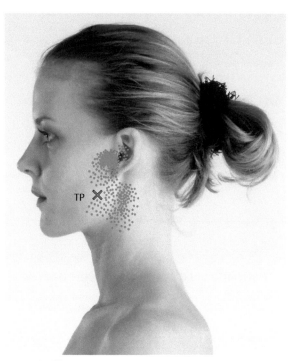

▶ **Fig. 19.13**

- Larynx.
- Temporomandibular joint.

Associated Inner Organs

None.

- Posterior head: facial nerve.

Trigger Point Location

TPs are palpated along the muscle as hypersensible points medial of the sternocleidomastoid.

Referred Pain Areas

Posterior head:
- Into upper area of the sternocleidomastoid muscle.
- Occiput.
- Neck area, near the mandible.

Anterior head: lower incisors and the mandible below.

Associated Inner Organs

None.

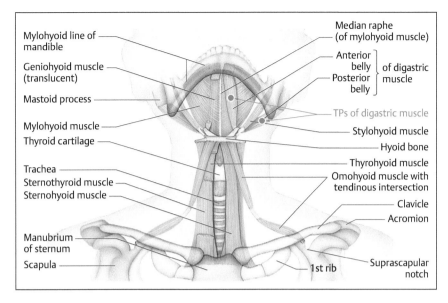

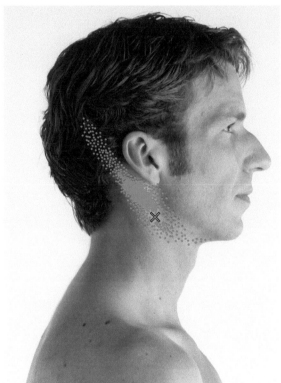

▶ **Fig. 19.15**

Orbicular Muscle of Eye, Greater Zygomatic Muscle, Platysma Muscle (▶Fig. 19.16)

▪ Orbicular Muscle of Eye

Origin

Medial border of the orbit, wall of lacrimal sac.

Insertion

Palpebral ligament.

Action

Eyelid closure, supports lacrimation.

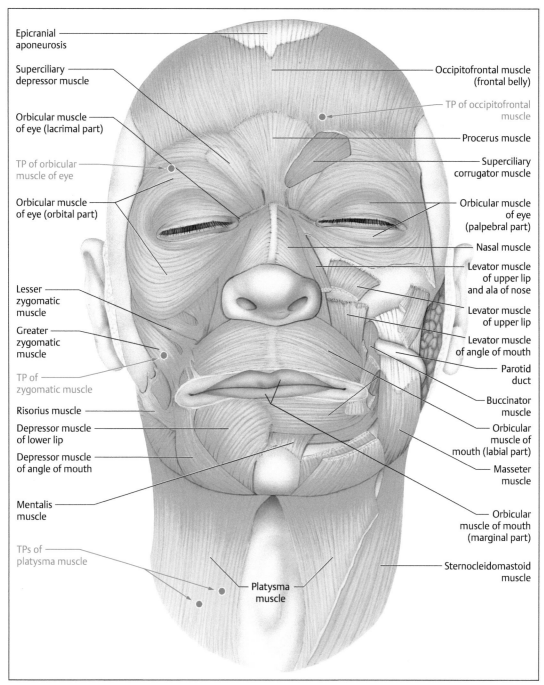

Epicranial aponeurosis

Superciliary depressor muscle

Orbicular muscle of eye (lacrimal part)

TP of orbicular muscle of eye

Orbicular muscle of eye (orbital part)

Lesser zygomatic muscle

Greater zygomatic muscle

TP of zygomatic muscle

Risorius muscle

Depressor muscle of lower lip

Depressor muscle of angle of mouth

Mentalis muscle

TPs of platysma muscle

Platysma muscle

Occipitofrontal muscle (frontal belly)

TP of occipitofrontal muscle

Procerus muscle

Superciliary corrugator muscle

Orbicular muscle of eye (palpebral part)

Nasal muscle

Levator muscle of upper lip and ala of nose

Levator muscle of upper lip

Levator muscle of angle of mouth

Parotid duct

Buccinator muscle

Orbicular muscle of mouth (labial part)

Masseter muscle

Orbicular muscle of mouth (marginal part)

Sternocleidomastoid muscle

▶ **Fig. 19.16**

■ Greater Zygomatic Muscle

Origin

Anterior surface of the zygomatic bone.

Insertion

Lateral of the angle of the mouth.

Action

Draws the angle of the mouth backward and upward.

▪ Platysma Muscle

Origin

Skin in the lower cervical region and upper outer thorax region.

Insertion

Lower edge of the mandible, skin in the lower facial region, angle of the mouth.

Action

Draws skin of the lower facial and mouth regions and the mandible downward.

Innervation

Facial nerve.

Trigger Point Location

Orbicular Muscle of Eye
Above the eyelid, immediately below the eyebrow.

Occipitofrontal Muscle (▶Figs. 19.16–19.18)

Origin

- Highest nuchal line, mastoid process.
- Radiates into the fibers of the upper facial muscles.

Greater Zygomatic Muscle
In the area of the muscle close to the insertion—superolateral to the angle of the mouth.

Platysma Muscle
About 2 cm above the clavicle, at the crossing with the sternocleidomastoid muscle.

Referred Pain Areas

Orbicular Muscle of Eye
- Dorsum of nose.
- Upper lip.

Greater Zygomatic Muscle
Starting at the TP running lateral to the nose and medial to the eye to the forehead (median).

Platysma Muscle
- Mandible.
- Cheek.
- Chin.

Associated Inner Organs

None.

Insertion

Epicranial aponeurosis (galea aponeurotica).

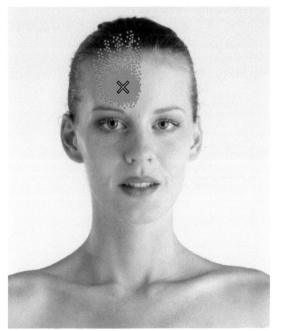

▶ **Fig. 19.17**

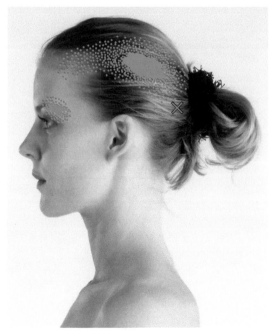

▶ **Fig. 19.18**

Action

- Fixation of epicranial aponeurosis.
- Frowning.

Innervation

Facial nerve.

Trigger Point Location

- Frontal: above the medial end of the eyebrow.

- Occipital: above the superior nuchal line and about 4 cm lateral of the median line.

Referred Pain Areas

Radiates along the muscle from the orbit via the ipsilateral half of the cranium.

Associated Inner Organs

None.

Splenius Muscle of Head and Splenius Muscle of Neck (▶Figs. 19.19, 19.20)

Origin

- Splenius muscle of head: nuchal ligaments and spinous processes and supraspinal ligaments of the TVB 1 to 3.

- Splenius muscle of neck: spinous processes and supraspinal ligaments of TVB 3 to 6.

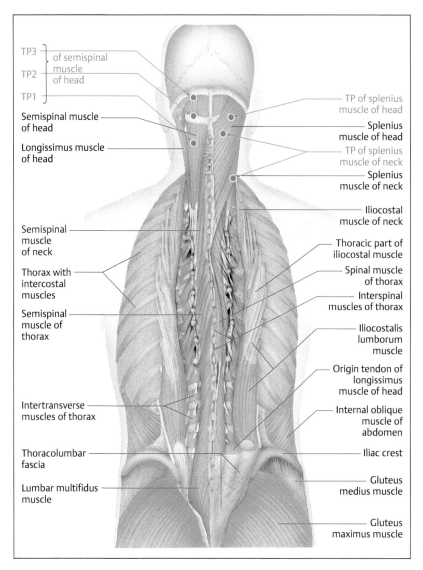

TP3 ⎱ of semispinal muscle
TP2 ⎰ of head
TP1
Semispinal muscle of head
Longissimus muscle of head
Semispinal muscle of neck
Thorax with intercostal muscles
Semispinal muscle of thorax
Intertransverse muscles of thorax
Thoracolumbar fascia
Lumbar multifidus muscle

TP of splenius muscle of head
Splenius muscle of head
TP of splenius muscle of neck
Splenius muscle of neck
Iliocostal muscle of neck
Thoracic part of iliocostal muscle
Spinal muscle of thorax
Interspinal muscles of thorax
Iliocostalis lumborum muscle
Origin tendon of longissimus muscle of head
Internal oblique muscle of abdomen
Iliac crest
Gluteus medius muscle
Gluteus maximus muscle

▶ **Fig. 19.19**

► **Fig. 19.20 (a–c)**

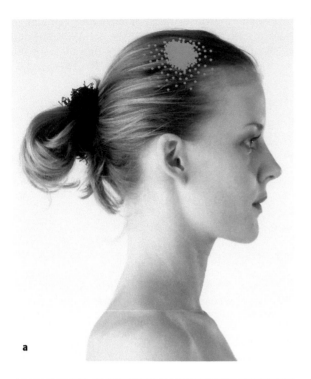

a

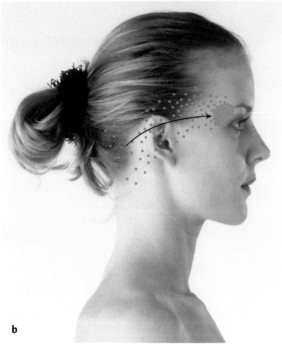

b

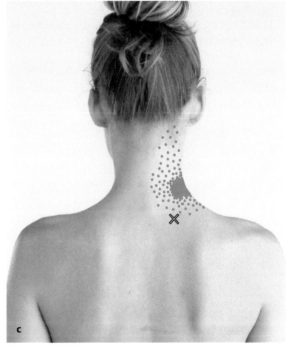

c

Insertion

- Splenius muscle of head: between the superior and inferior nuchal ligaments (lateral at occiput).
- Splenius muscle of neck: posterior tubercles of the atlas, CVB 1 to 3.

Action

Extension and ipsilateral rotation of the CSC.

Innervation

- Splenius muscle of head: spinal nerves C3/C4 (posterior branches).
- Splenius muscle of neck: spinal nerves C5/C6 (posterior branches).

Trigger Point Location

- Splenius muscle of head: in the muscle belly at about the level of the spinous process of the axis.

- Splenius muscle of neck: at the level of the transition from shoulder to neck and slightly further above that, a second TP near the muscle insertion at the level of CVB 2 to 3.

To palpate these TPs, slide the palpation finger between the trapezius muscle and the levator muscle of scapula.

Referred Pain Areas

Splenius muscle of head: into the vertex of the cranium—ipsilateral.

Splenius muscle of neck: through the cranium to back of eye; sometimes also at the occiput, transition of shoulder to neck, and ipsilaterally upward along the neck.

Associated Inner Organs

- Liver.
- Gallbladder.

Semispinal Muscle of Head, Semispinal Muscle of Neck, Multifidus Muscles (▶Figs. 19.19, 19.21, 19.22)

Origin

- Semispinal muscles: transverse processes.
- Multifidus muscles: lamina of vertebral arch.

Insertion

- Semispinal muscles: spinous processes (about six vertebrae superior to the origin).
- Multifidus muscles: spinous processes (about two to three vertebrae superior to the origin).

These muscles run approximately from TVB 6 to the superior/inferior nuchal line.

Action

Extension and lateral flexion ipsilateral to the spine.

Innervation

Posterior branches of the segmental spinal nerves.

Trigger Point Location

- TP1: At the base of the neck, at the level of CVB 4 to 5.
- TP2: 2 to 4 cm below the occiput.
- TP3: Immediately below the superior nuchal line.

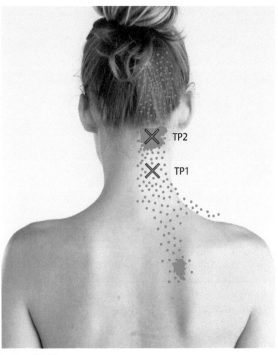

▶ **Fig. 19.21**

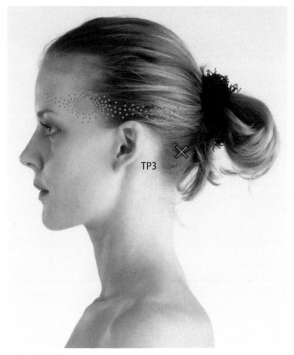

▶ **Fig. 19.22**

Referred Pain Areas

- TP1: Along the neck into the suboccipital region and toward the inferior to medial border of the scapula.
- TP2: From the occiput toward the vertex.
- TP3: Painful horizontal band along the cranium to the temple area.

Associated Inner Organs

- Heart.
- Lungs/bronchia.

Rectus Capitis Posterior Major and Minor Muscles, Inferior and Superior Oblique Muscles of Head (▶Figs. 19.23, 19.24)

Origin

- Rectus capitis posterior major: spinous process of CVB 2.
- Rectus capitis posterior minor: posterior tubercle of the atlas.
- Inferior oblique muscle of head: spinous process of CVB 2.
- Superior oblique muscle of head: lateral mass of the atlas.

Insertion

- Rectus capitis posterior major: outer half of the inferior nuchal line.
- Rectus capitis posterior minor: medial half of the inferior nuchal line.
- Inferior oblique muscle of head: lateral mass of the atlas.
- Superior oblique muscle of head: lateral half of the inferior nuchal line.

Action

- Rectus capitis posterior major: extension of the head and ipsilateral rotation in the occipitoatlantoaxial (OAA) joint.
- Rectus capitis posterior minor: extension of the head.
- Inferior oblique muscle of head: ipsilateral rotation in the OAA joint.
- Superior oblique muscle of head: sidebending of the head.

Innervation

Suboccipital nerve (posterior branch from C1).

Trigger Point Location

No definable, palpable TP; only general tension in the muscle belly.

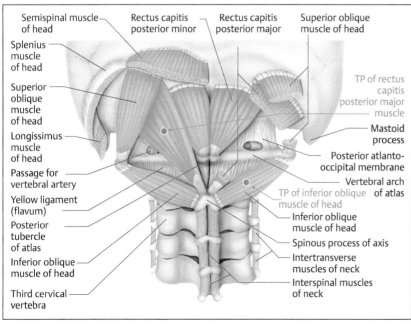

Semispinal muscle of head — Rectus capitis posterior minor — Rectus capitis posterior major — Superior oblique muscle of head

Splenius muscle of head

Superior oblique muscle of head

Longissimus muscle of head

Passage for vertebral artery

Yellow ligament (flavum)

Posterior tubercle of atlas

Inferior oblique muscle of head

Third cervical vertebra

TP of rectus capitis posterior major muscle

Mastoid process

Posterior atlanto-occipital membrane

Vertebral arch of atlas

TP of inferior oblique muscle of head

Inferior oblique muscle of head

Spinous process of axis

Intertransverse muscles of neck

Interspinal muscles of neck

▶ **Fig. 19.23**

Referred Pain Areas

From the occiput via the temple region to the orbit and forehead (ipsilateral). Pain cannot be clearly and precisely located.

Associated Inner Organs

None.

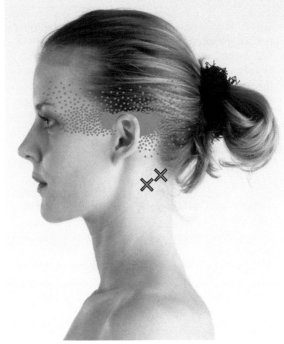

▶ **Fig. 19.24**

Stretching the Lateral Cervical and Nuchal Muscles (▶Fig. 19.25)

Starting Posture

The patient is seated upright on a chair.

Procedure

1. The patient grasps the edge of the chair with the hand on the side to be stretched (in this example, right).
2. The patient turns the head to the opposite side (in this example, left) and looks down to the floor along the outside of the knee. This creates a stretch in the lateral cervical and nuchal area.
3. The patient holds the stretch for 30 seconds.

Slight shifts in the head posture, for example, turning or tilting more sideways, can shift the location of the stretch. If the stretch is felt in the lateral area of the neck, it is performed correctly.

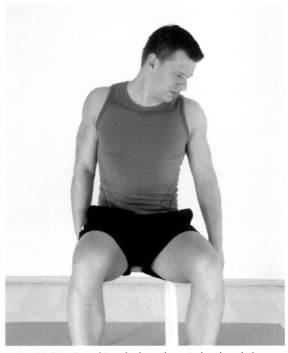

▶ **Fig. 19.25** Stretching the lateral cervical and nuchal muscles.

19.2   Upper Thorax, Shoulder, and Arm Pain: Related Muscles

Levator Muscle of Scapula (▶Figs. 19.26a, 19.27)

Origin

Posterior tubercles of the CVB 1 to 4.

Insertion

Medial border of the scapula (superior).

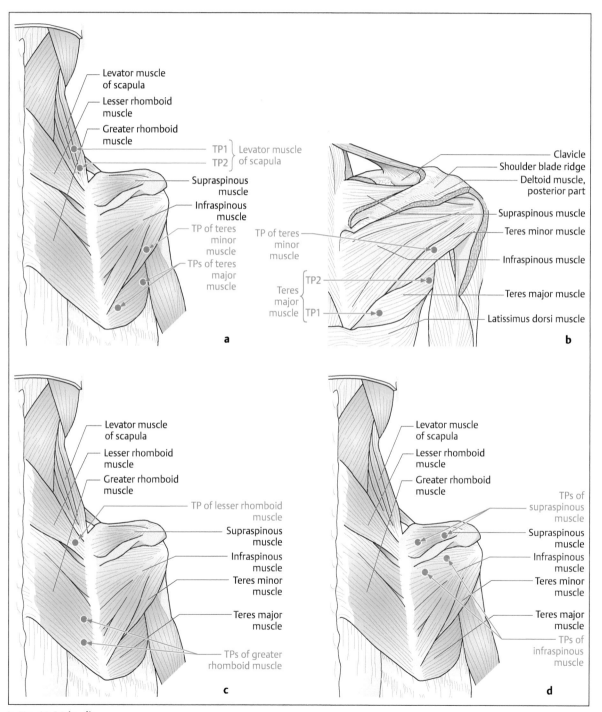

▶ **Fig. 19.26 (a–d)**

Action

- Rotates the inferior angle of the scapula toward medial and raises the superior angle of the scapula toward superomedial.
- Extension (bilateral contraction) and ipsilateral rotation of the CSC.

Innervation

Dorsal scapular nerve (C5) and anterior branches of the spinal nerves C3–C4.

Trigger Point Location

- TP1: Transition from shoulder to neck, palpable by displacing the trapezius muscle backward.
- TP2: About 1.3 cm above the superior angle of the scapula.

Referred Pain Areas

- Transition from shoulder to neck.
- Medial border of the scapula.
- Posterior shoulder area.

Associated Inner Organs

- Liver.
- Gallbladder.
- Stomach.
- Heart.

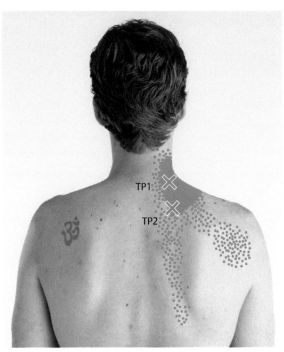

▶ **Fig. 19.27**

Scalene Muscles (▶Figs. 19.28–19.30)

Origin

- Anterior scalene muscle: anterior tubercles of CVB 3 to 6.
- Middle scalene muscle: posterior tubercles of CVB 2 to 7.
- Posterior scalene muscle: posterior tubercles of CVB 4 to 6.
- Smallest scalene muscle: anterior tubercle of CVB 7.

Insertion

- Anterior scalene muscle: scalene tubercle of the first rib.
- Middle scalene muscle: upper border of the first rib (near neck of rib).
- Posterior scalene muscle: lateral posterior exterior surface of the second rib.
- Smallest scalene muscle: suprapleural membrane.

Action

- Muscles of inspiration.
- Anterior scalene muscle: also supports sidebending of the CSC with the fixed rib.
- Smallest scalene muscle: braces cupola (dome) of the pleura.

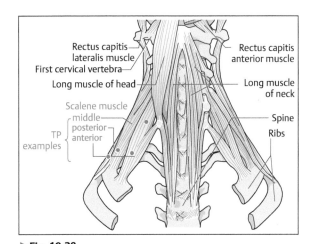

▶ **Fig. 19.28**

Innervation

Anterior branches of the spinal nerves:
- Anterior scalene muscle: C5–C6.
- Middle scalene muscle: C3–C8.
- Posterior scalene muscle: C6–C8.
- Smallest scalene muscle: C7.

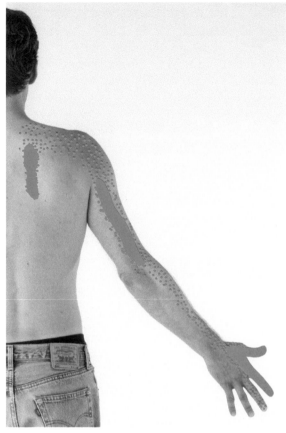

► **Fig. 19.29**

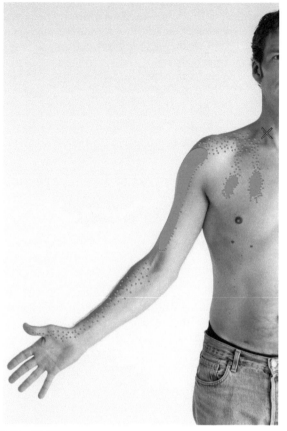

► **Fig. 19.30**

Trigger Point Location

The scalene muscles are searched for in the greater supraclavicular fossa and are partially compressed against the transverse processes of the cervical vertebrae. The TPs are distributed in the muscles at various levels.

Referred Pain Areas

- Chest area.
- Radial anterior and posterior upper arm and lower arm.

- From posterior, thumb and index finger (smallest scalene muscle: entire dorsum of hand).
- Medial border of the scapula.

> These referred pain areas may mimic the pain patterns of a cardiac infarction!

Associated Inner Organs

See teres major muscle.

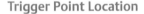

Supraspinous Muscle (►Figs. 19.26d, 19.31, 19.32)

Origin

- Supraspinous fossa (of scapula).
- Spine of the scapula.

Insertion

- Greater tubercle of the humerus (proximal facet).
- Shoulder joint capsule.

Action

- Abduction of the arm.
- Shoulder joint stabilizer.

Innervation

Suprascapular nerve (C5–C6).

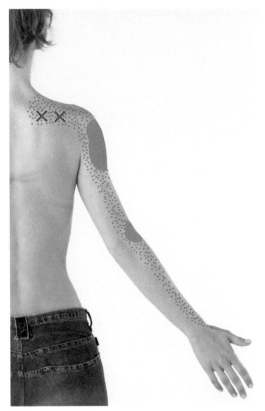

▶ **Fig. 19.31**

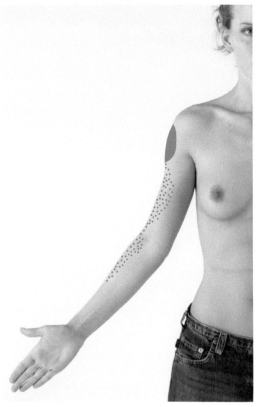

▶ **Fig. 19.32**

Trigger Point Location

Both TPs are easily palpable in the supraspinous fossa of the scapula.

Referred Pain Areas

* Lateral deltoid muscle area.
* Lateral epicondyle.

* Lateral upper and lower arms.
* Acromion.

Associated Inner Organs

See teres major muscle.

Infraspinous Muscle (▶ Figs. 19.26d, 19.33, 19.34)

Origin

Infraspinous fossa of scapula.

Insertion

* Greater tubercle of the humerus (middle facet).
* Shoulder joint capsule.

Action

* External rotation of the arm.
* Shoulder joint stabilizer.

Innervation

Suprascapular nerve (C5–C6).

Trigger Point Location

In the infraspinous fossa of scapula, immediately below the spine of the scapula. TP1 is located near the medial border of the scapula; TP2 is located slightly further lateral.

Referred Pain Areas

* Anterior shoulder area.
* Anterolateral upper and lower arm.
* Radial palm and dorsum of hand.

Associated Inner Organs

See teres major muscle.

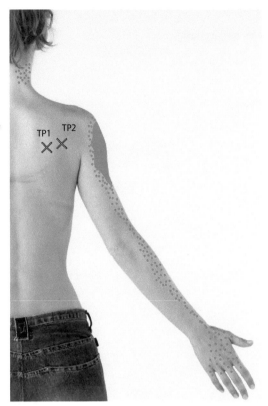

► **Fig. 19.33**

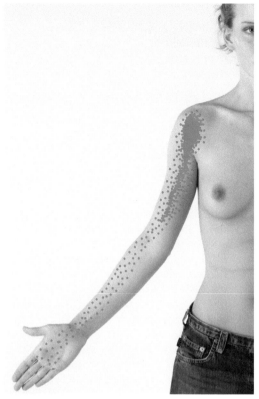

► **Fig. 19.34**

Teres Minor Muscle (►Figs. 19.26a, b, 19.35)

Origin

Lateral border of the scapula (middle third), above the teres major muscle.

Insertion

- Greater tubercle of the humerus (lower facet).
- Shoulder joint capsule.

Action

- External rotation of the arm.
- Shoulder joint stabilizer.

Innervation

Axillary nerve (C5–C6).

Trigger Point Location

Lateral of lateral border of the scapula between the infraspinous muscle and the teres major muscle.

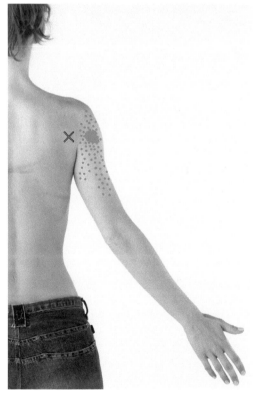

► **Fig. 19.35**

Referred Pain Areas

- Posterior deltoid muscle area, slightly above the insertion of the deltoid.
- Posterior upper arm.

Associated Inner Organs

See teres major muscle.

Stretching the External Shoulder Rotators (▸Fig. 19.36)

Starting Posture

The patient is seated on a chair.

Procedure

- The patient clasps both hands together behind the back, with the upper body slightly flexed.
- The patient extends the upper body while continuing to clasp the hands. This creates a stretch in the anterior shoulder area.
- The patient holds the stretch for 30 seconds.

If internal rotation and retroversion of the shoulders are very limited, patients may not be able to clasp their hands behind the back. If this is the case, patients can "hook" their thumbs into the waist bands of their clothing. Over time, if their shoulder range of motion improves, patients can clasp their hands behind their back.

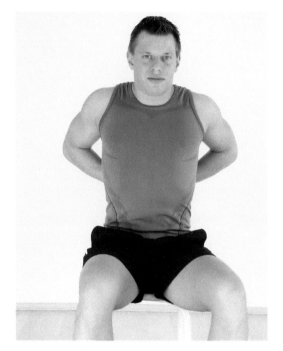

▸ **Fig. 19.36** Stretching the external shoulder rotators.

Teres Major Muscle (▸Figs. 19.26a, b, 19.37)

Origin

- Distal third of the lateral border of the scapula (below the teres minor muscle).
- Inferior angle of the scapula.

Insertion

Crest of the lesser tubercle of the humerus.

Action

- Internal rotation.
- Adduction.
- Shoulder joint stabilizer.

Innervation

Subscapular nerve (C5–C6).

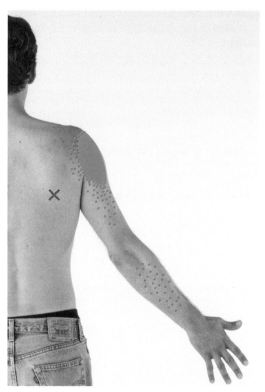

▸ **Fig. 19.37**

Trigger Point Location

- TP1: In area of lower angle of the scapula.
- TP2: Lateral in the muscle belly in the posterior axillary fold.

Referred Pain Areas

- Posterior deltoid muscle area.
- Along the long head of the triceps muscle of arm.
- Posterior lower arm.

Associated Inner Organs

- Herniations of cervical disks (C4/C5, C5/C6, C6/C7) frequently lead to development of TPs in the scalene, supraspinous, infraspinous, teres major/minor, and deltoid muscles.
- Heart.

Latissimus Dorsi Muscle (▶Figs. 19.1, 19.38)

Origin

- Spinous processes and supraspinal ligaments of all thoracic, lumbar, and sacral vertebrae from TVB 7 downward.
- Thoracolumbar fascia.

- Iliac crest (posterior third).
- Ribs 9 to 12.
- Inferior angle of the scapula.

Insertion

Crest of the lesser tubercle of the humerus.

Action

- Extension, internal rotation, and adduction of the arm.
- Deep inspiration and forced expiration.

Innervation

Thoracodorsal nerve (C6–C8).

Trigger Point Location

Free border of the posterior axillary fold, at about the level of the middle of the lateral border of the scapula.

Referred Pain Areas

- Lower angle of the scapula and in a circle around that area.
- Posterior shoulder area.
- Posteromedial upper and lower arm, including fingers 4 and 5.

Associated Inner Organs

None.

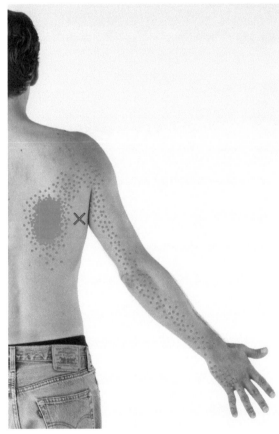

▶ **Fig. 19.38**

Stretching the Lateral Side of the Trunk (▶ Fig. 19.39)

Starting Posture

The patient is standing with feet apart.

Procedure

- *On* the side to be stretched, the patient raises the arm to maximum abduction, flexes the lower arm, and places the palm of the hand in approximately the center of the upper thoracic spine area.
- With the other hand, the patient holds the elbow on the side to be stretched and passively pulls the arm into additional abduction.
- At the same time, the patient sidebends the upper body to the contralateral side. This may create a stretch in the posterior upper arm and on the entire lateral side of the trunk.
- The patient holds the stretch for 30 seconds.

This exercise primarily stretches the triceps muscle of the arm and the teres major and latissimus dorsi muscles.

Subscapular Muscle (▶ Figs. 19.40, 19.41)

Origin

Subscapular fossa.

Insertion

- Lesser tubercle of the humerus.
- Crest of the lesser tubercle of the humerus (proximal).
- Shoulder joint capsule.

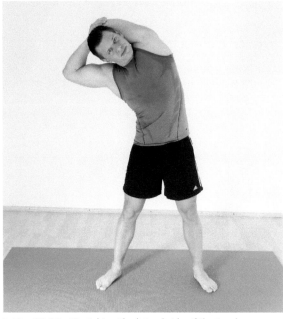

▶ **Fig. 19.39** Stretching the lateral side of the trunk.

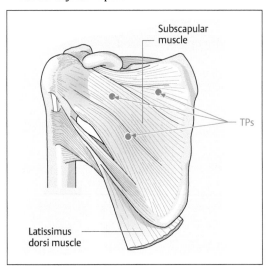

▶ **Fig. 19.40**

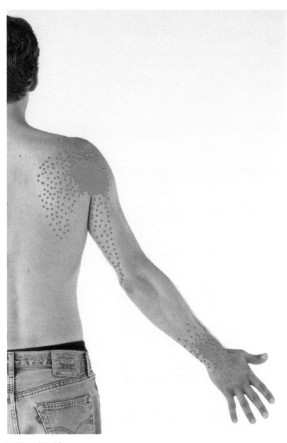

▶ **Fig. 19.41**

Action

- Internal rotation.
- Shoulder joint stabilizer.

Innervation

Subscapular nerve (C6–C7).

Trigger Point Location

- Near the lateral borders of the scapula in the subscapular fossa.

Rhomboid Muscles (▶Figs. 19.26c, 19.42)

Origin

- Nuchal ligament.
- Spinous processes and supraspinal ligaments of the CVB 7 to TVB 5.

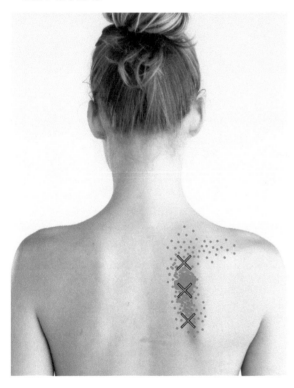

Deltoid Muscle (▶Figs. 19.43–19.45)

Origin

- Clavicle (lateral third).
- Acromion.
- Spine of the scapula.

Insertion

Deltoid tuberosity.

- Also in the subscapular fossa further medial, toward the upper angle of the scapula.

Referred Pain Areas

- Posterior shoulder area.
- Entire scapula area.
- Posterior upper arm up to the elbow.
- Wrist (posterior and palmar).

Associated Inner Organs

None.

Insertion

Medial border of the scapula.

Action

Retraction of the scapula.

Innervation

Dorsal scapular nerve (C5).

Trigger Point Location

Along and near the medial border of the scapula.

Referred Pain Areas

- Along the medial border of the scapula between the scapula and the paravertebral muscles.
- Supraspinous fossa of the scapula.

Associated Inner Organs

Heart.

▶ **Fig. 19.42**

Action

- Abduction of the arm.
- Anterior part: flexion, internal rotation.
- Posterior part: extension, external rotation.

Innervation

Axillary nerve (C5–C6).

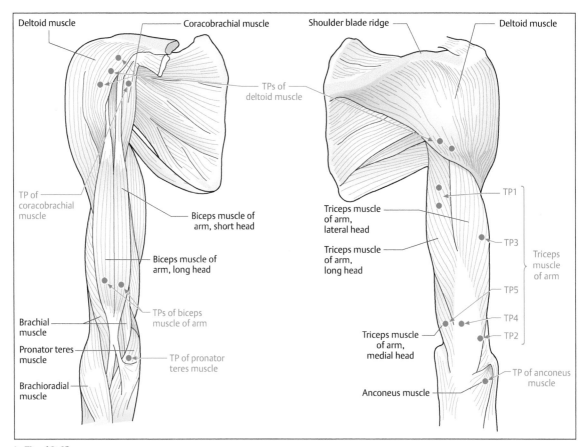

▶ **Fig. 19.43**

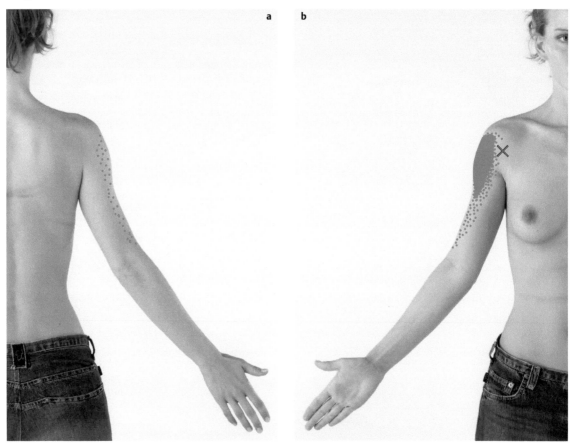

▶ **Fig. 19.44 (a, b)**

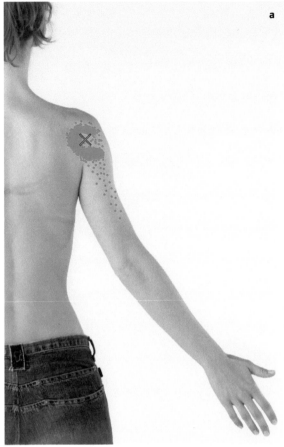 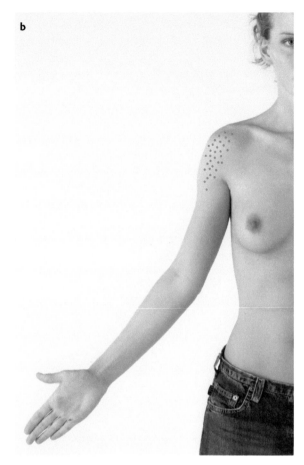

▶ **Fig. 19.45 (a, b)**

Trigger Point Location

- Anterior TPs: in the upper third of the muscle belly in front of the glenohumeral joint and near its anterior border.
- Posterior TPs: along the posterior margin of the muscle belly in its lower half.

Referred Pain Areas

- Anterior TPs: anterior and lateral deltoid muscle area and the upper arm.
- Posterior TPs: posterior and lateral deltoid muscle area and the upper arm.

Associated Inner Organs

See teres major muscle

Coracobrachial Muscle (▶Figs. 19.43, 19.46)

Origin

Coracoid process (of the scapula).

Insertion

Medial area of the humerus (proximal half).

Action

Flexion, adduction of the arm.

Innervation

Musculocutaneous nerve (C5–C7).

Trigger Point Location

Found by palpating the axilla between the deltoid and the greater pectoral muscles and pushing the superior part of the muscle against the humerus.

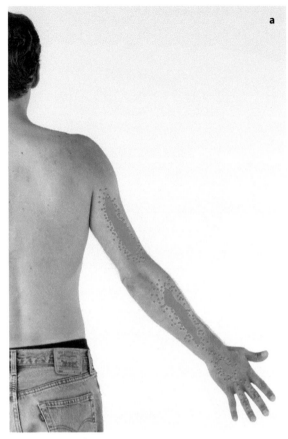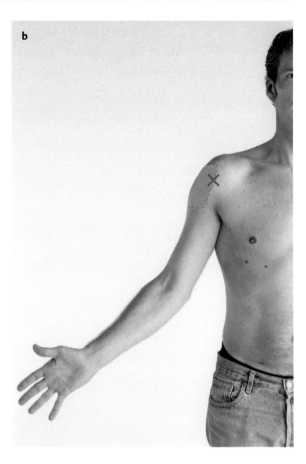

▶ **Fig. 19.46 (a, b)**

Referred Pain Areas

- Anterior aspect of the deltoid muscle.
- In a discontinuous line on parts of the upper arm, lower arm, and dorsum of the hand.

Associated Inner Organs

None.

Biceps Muscle of Arm (▶Figs. 19.43, 19.47)

Origin

- Long head: supraglenoid tubercle (of the scapula).
- Short head: coracoid process (of the scapula).

Insertion

- Radial tuberosity.
- Aponeurosis of biceps muscle of arm.

Action

- Flexion of the arm.
- Flexion of the elbow.
- Supination of the lower arm.

Innervation

Musculocutaneous nerve (C5–C6).

Trigger Point Location

In distal third of the muscle.

Referred Pain Areas

- Anterior deltoid muscle area.
- Anterior upper arm along the course of the muscle.
- Cubital fossa.
- Suprascapular region.

Associated Inner Organs

None.

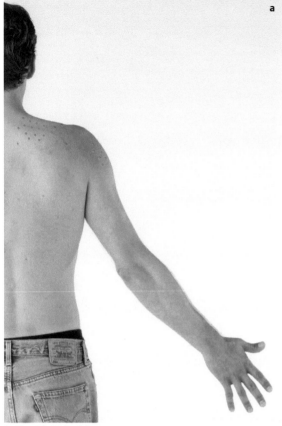

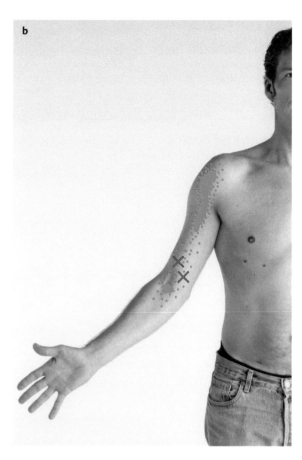

▶ **Fig. 19.47 (a, b)**

Stretching the Biceps Muscle of Arm
(▶Fig. 19.48)

Starting Posture

Patient is standing upright.

Procedure

- Patient places the dorsum of the hand on the side to be stretched inside a door frame or on the side of a cabinet, with the arm stretched and the elbow joint extended.
- Patient turns away from the arm to be stretched, placing the shoulder in retroversion. This creates a stretch in the anterior shoulder area and the upper arm, sometimes also in the cubital fossa.
- Patient holds the stretch for 30 seconds.

If the described stretch does not occur, it may be because the arm is placed too high or too low on the door frame.

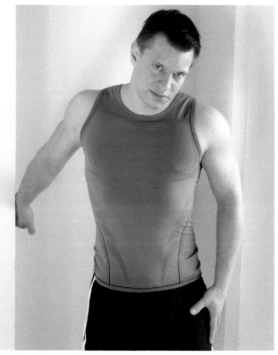

▶ **Fig. 19.48** Stretching the biceps muscle of the arm.

Brachial Muscle (▶Figs. 19.49, 19.50)

Origin

Anterior surface of the humerus (distal half).

Insertion

- Tuberosity of the ulna.
- Coronoid process of the ulna.

Action

Flexion in the elbow joint.

Innervation

- Musculocutaneous nerve (C5–C6).
- Radial nerve (C7).

Trigger Point Location

- TP1: A few centimeters above the cubital fossa.
- TP2: In the upper half of the muscle belly.

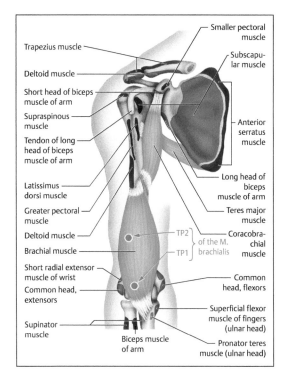

▶ **Fig. 19.49**

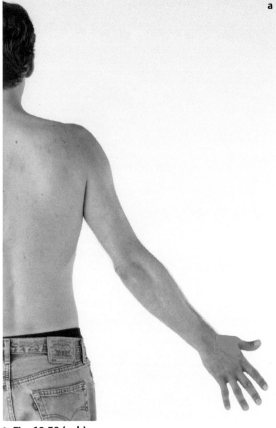

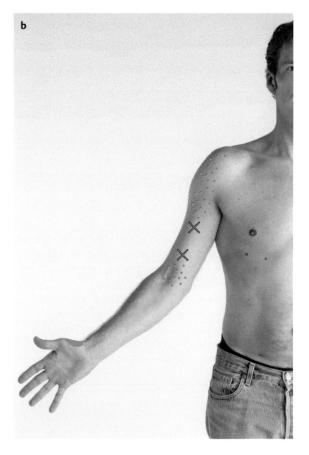

▶ **Fig. 19.50 (a, b)**

Referred Pain Areas

- Dorsum of the hand in the areas of the carpometacarpal joint 1 and the metacarpophalangeal joint of the thumb.
- Cubital fossa.
- Anterior upper arm and deltoid muscle area.

Associated Inner Organs

None.

Triceps Muscle of Arm (▶ Figs. 19.43, 19.51, 19.52)

Origin

- Long head: infraglenoid tubercle (of the scapula).
- Lateral head: posterior surface of the humerus (proximal half).
- Medial head: posterior surface of the humerus (distal half), inferomedial of the groove for the radial nerve.

Insertion

- Olecranon.
- Elbow joint capsule.

Action

- Extension in the elbow.
- Shoulder joint stabilizer.

Innervation

Radial nerve (C7–C8).

Trigger Point Location

- TP1: In the long head, a few centimeters distal to the location where the teres major muscle crosses the long head of triceps.
- TP2: In the medial head, about 4 to 6 cm above the lateral epicondyle of the humerus, at the lateral margin of the muscle.
- TP3: In the lateral head, at the lateral margin of the muscle, about the middle of the upper arm, at the level of palpation points of the radial nerve on the posterior upper arm.
- TP4: In the medial head, slightly above the olecranon.
- TP5: At the medial margin of the medial head, slightly above the medial epicondyle of the humerus.

Referred Pain Areas

- TP1:
  - Posterior upper arm.
  - Posterior shoulder area up to the neck.

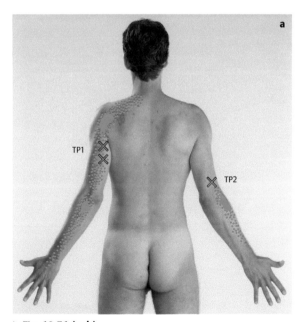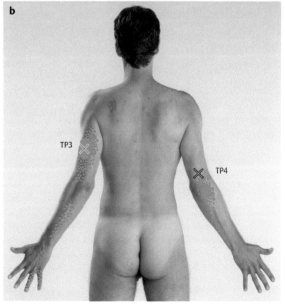

▶ **Fig. 19.51 (a, b)**

– Posterior lower arm to dorsum of the hand (skipping elbow).
- TP2:
  – Lateral epicondyle of the humerus.
  – Radial lower arm.
- TP3:
  – Posterior upper arm.
  – Posterior lower arm.
  – Fingers 4 and 5 (posterior).
- TP4:
  – Olecranon.
- TP5:
  – Medial epicondyle of the humerus.
  – Anteromedial lower arm.
  – Fingers 4 and 5 palmar.

Associated Inner Organs

None.

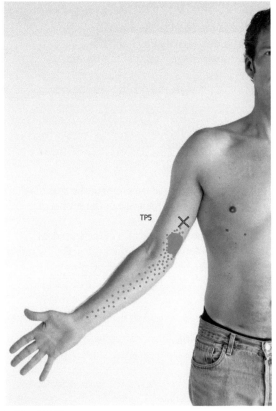

▶ **Fig. 19.52**

Anconeus Muscle (▶Figs. 19.43, 19.53)

Origin

Lateral epicondyle of the humerus (posterior surface).

Insertion

Elbow joint capsule.

Action

Tensor of joint capsule (prevents elbow joint capsule from being pinched during extension of the elbow).

Innervation

Radial nerve (C6–C8).

Trigger Point Location

Slightly distal of annular ligament of the radius.

Referred Pain Areas

Lateral epicondyle of the humerus.

Associated Inner Organs

None.

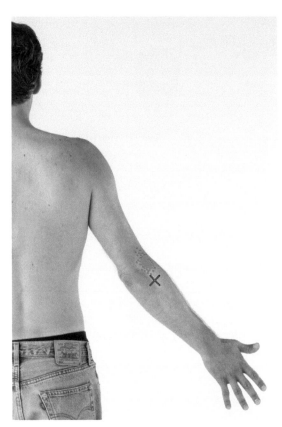

▶ **Fig. 19.53**

19.3   Elbow and Finger Pain: Related Muscles

Brachioradial Muscle (▶Figs. 19.54, 19.55)

Origin

* Lateral supraepicondylar ridge of the humerus (upper two-thirds).
* Lateral intermuscular septum of the arm.

Insertion

Styloid process of the radius.

Action

* Flexion in the elbow joint.
* Positions lower arm halfway between supination and pronation.

Innervation

Radial nerve (C5–C6).

Trigger Point Location

Radial head of the humerus 1 to 2 cm, distal, on the radial side of the lower arm, at about the middle of the muscle belly.

Referred Pain Areas

* Dorsum of the hand in the area between the carpometacarpal joint of the thumb and metacarpophalangeal joint of the index finger.
* Lateral epicondyle.
* Radial lower arm.

Associated Inner Organs

None.

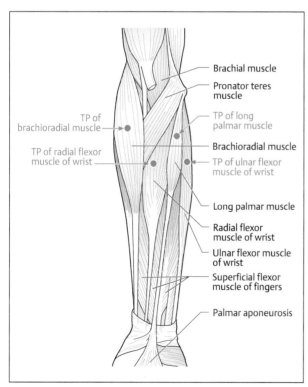

▶ **Fig. 19.54**

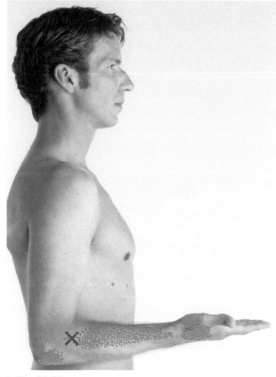

▶ **Fig. 19.55**

Long Radial Extensor Muscle of Wrist (▶Figs. 19.56, 19.57a)

Origin

- Lateral supraepicondylar ridge of the humerus (distal third).
- Lateral intermuscular septum of the arm.

Insertion

Base of second metacarpal bone (extension side).

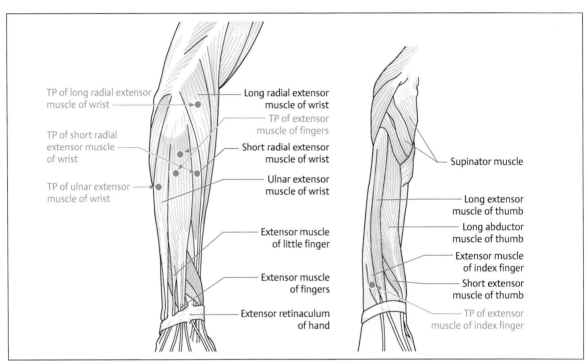

▶ **Fig. 19.56**

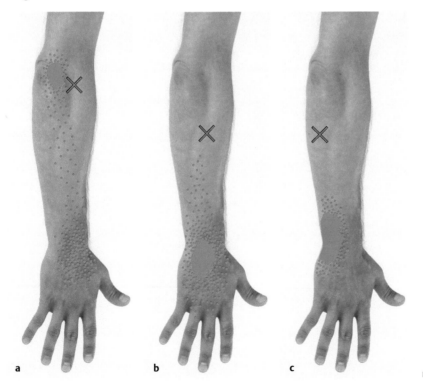

a   b   c

▶ **Fig. 19.57 (a–c)**

Action

Posterior extension and radial abduction in the wrist.

Innervation

Radial nerve (C6–C7).

Trigger Point Location

Radial head, 1 to 2 cm distal, at about the level of the TP of the brachioradial muscle, but further ulnar.

Referred Pain Areas

- Lateral epicondyle.
- Radial half of the wrist and dorsum of the hand, in the area of the metacarpal bones 1 to 3.

Associated Inner Organs

None.

Short Radial Extensor Muscle of Wrist (▶Figs. 19.56, 19.57b)

Origin

Lateral epicondyle of the humerus (anterior surface).

Insertion

Base of the third metacarpal bone (extension side).

Action

Posterior extension and radial abduction in the wrist.

Innervation

Radial nerve (C7–C8).

Trigger Point Location

About 5 to 6 cm distal of radial head (approximately in the middle of the muscle belly).

Referred Pain Areas

Middle area of the wrist and dorsum of the hand.

Associated Inner Organs

None.

Ulnar Extensor Muscle of Wrist (▶Figs. 19.56, 19.57c)

Origin

Lateral epicondyle of the humerus (anterior surface).

Insertion

Base of the fifth metacarpal bone.

Action

Posterior extension and ulnar abduction in the wrist.

Innervation

Radial nerve (C7–C8).

Trigger Point Location

About 7 to 8 cm distal to the lateral epicondyle.

Referred Pain Areas

Ulnar half of the wrist.

Associated Inner Organs

None.

Extensor Muscle of Fingers (▸Figs. 19.56, 19.58a–d)

Origin

Lateral epicondyle of the humerus (anterior surface).

Insertion

Middle and distal phalanges of fingers 2 to 5 (indirectly via radiation of the four muscle tendons into the posterior aponeurosis).

Action

Extension of the finger joints.

Innervation

Radial nerve (C7–C8).

Trigger Point Location

- TPs for the middle finger: 3 to 4 cm distal and slightly posterior to the radial head.

- TPs for ring finger and little finger: slightly distal to the TP for middle finger, deep in the muscle belly.

Referred Pain Areas

- Lateral epicondyle of the humerus (sometimes involved if ring finger or little finger is impacted).
- Posterior lower arm.
- Wrist.
- Dorsum of the hand.
- Fingers, except distal phalanx.

Depending on the TP location, pain radiation is sensed in a different finger.

Associated Inner Organs

None.

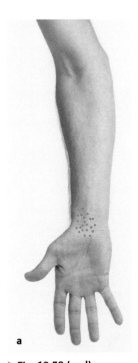 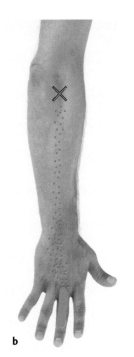 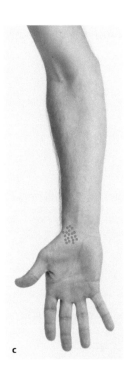 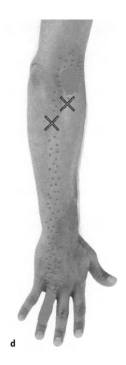

a　　　　b　　　　c　　　　d

▸ **Fig. 19.58 (a–d)**

Extensor Muscle of Index Finger (▸Figs. 19.56, 19.59)

Origin

- Posterior surface of the ulna (distal section).
- Interosseous membrane.

Insertion

Radiates into the extensor aponeurosis (dorsal digital expansion) of the index finger.

Action

Extension of the index finger.

Innervation

Radial nerve (C7–C8).

Trigger Point Location

In the distal half of the muscle, in the middle of the lower arm, between the radius and the ulna.

Referred Pain Areas

Radial side of the wrist and dorsum of the hand.

Associated Inner Organs

None.

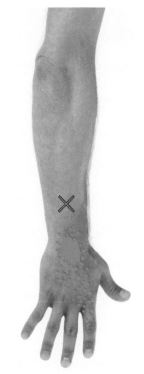

▶ **Fig. 19.59**

Supinator Muscle (▶ Figs. 19.60, 19.61)

Origin

- Supinator crest of the ulna.
- Lateral epicondyle.
- Radial collateral ligament.
- Annular ligament of the radius.

Insertion

Neck and body of the radius (between radial tuberosity and insertion of the pronator teres muscle).

Action

Supination of the lower arm.

Innervation

Radial nerve (C5–C6).

Trigger Point Location

Slightly lateral and distal to biceps tendon, in the superficial part of the muscle, on the anterior side of the radius.

Referred Pain Areas

- Lateral epicondyle of the humerus and into the lateral area of the elbow.
- Posterior dorsum of the hand, between the first and second metacarpal bones.
- Posterior proximal phalanx of the thumb.

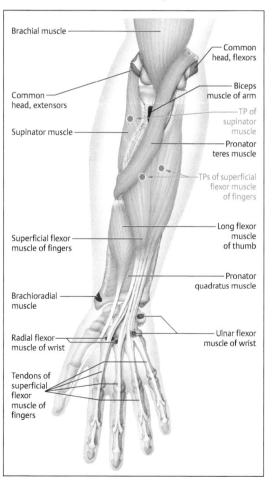

Brachial muscle

Common head, flexors

Biceps muscle of arm

Common head, extensors

TP of supinator muscle

Supinator muscle

Pronator teres muscle

TPs of superficial flexor muscle of fingers

Long flexor muscle of thumb

Superficial flexor muscle of fingers

Pronator quadratus muscle

Brachioradial muscle

Radial flexor muscle of wrist

Ulnar flexor muscle of wrist

Tendons of superficial flexor muscle of fingers

▶ **Fig. 19.60**

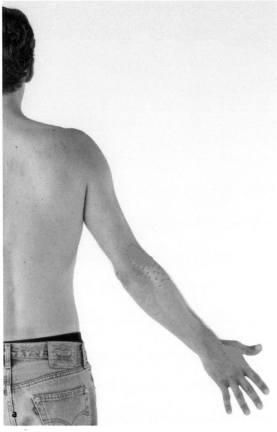

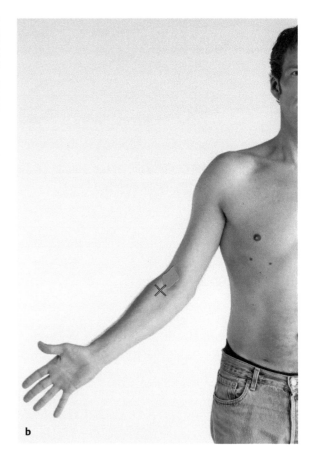

▶ **Fig. 19.61 (a, b)**

Associated Inner Organs

None.

Stretching the Lower Arm Extensors
(▶Fig. 19.62)

Starting Posture

Patient is seated.

Procedure

The following describes the stretching procedure for the right side:
- Patient places the right hand on the left upper leg, with the posterior side of thumb resting on the leg and the right shoulder in internal rotation.
- Patient uses the left hand to grasp the fingers of the right hand on their posterior side and fully extends the elbow joint of the right arm.
- Patient's left hand pulls the fingers of the right hand and right wrist into palmar flexion until a stretch is felt in the right posterior lower arm.
- Patient holds the stretch for 30 seconds.

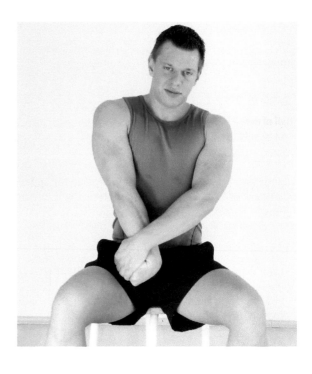

▶ **Fig. 19.62** Stretching the lower arm extensors.

Long Palmar Muscle (▸Figs. 19.54, 19.63)

Origin

Medial epicondyle of the humerus.

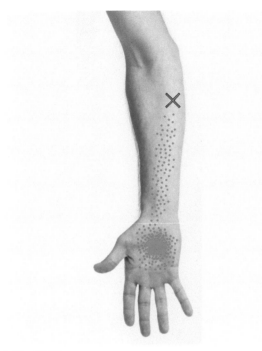

▸ **Fig. 19.63**

Insertion

- Flexor retinaculum of the hand.
- Palmar aponeurosis.

Action

Tensor of the palmar aponeurosis.

Innervation

Median nerve (C7–C8).

Trigger Point Location

At transition from proximal to middle third of the anterior lower arm.

Referred Pain Areas

- Palm of the hand.
- Distal half of the anterior lower arm.

Associated Inner Organs

None.

Radial Flexor Muscle of the Wrist (▸Figs. 19.54, 19.64a)

Origin

Medial epicondyle of the humerus.

Insertion

- Base of the second and third metacarpal bones.
- Scaphoid bone.

Action

- Palmar flexion.
- Radial abduction.

Innervation

Median nerve (C6–C7).

Trigger Point Location

In the middle of the muscle belly (middle of the anterior lower arm, proximal half).

Referred Pain Areas

- Anterior wrist area between the thenar and the hypothenar.
- Proximal half of the palm of the hand.
- Narrow band in the distal half of the lower arm.

Associated Inner Organs

None.

Ulnar Flexor Muscle of Wrist (▸Figs. 19.54, 19.64b)

Origin

- Medial epicondyle of the humerus.
- Olecranon.

- Posterior border of the ulna.
- Antebrachial fascia.

Insertion

- Pisiform bone.
- Hook of hamate bone.
- At the base of the fifth metacarpal bone via the pisohamate ligament and the pisometacarpal ligament.

Action

- Palmar flexion.
- Ulnar abduction.

Innervation

Ulnar nerve (C6–C7).

Trigger Point Location

In the middle of the muscle belly, at the ulnar border of the anterior lower arm (in proximal half).

Referred Pain Areas

- Anterior wrist in the area of the ulnar border of the hypothenar.
- Proximal half of the palm of the hand (hypothenar area).
- Narrow band in the distal half of the lower arm (hypothenar area).

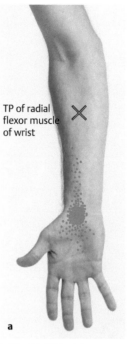
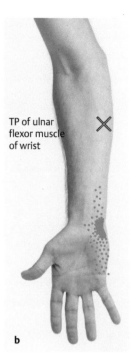

TP of radial flexor muscle of wrist

TP of ulnar flexor muscle of wrist

a

b

▶ **Fig. 19.64 (a, b)**

Associated Inner Organs

None.

Superficial Flexor Muscle of Fingers (▶Figs. 19.60, 19.65)

Origin

- Medial epicondyle of the humerus (up to the medial collateral ligaments of the elbow).
- Coronoid process of the ulna (medial border).
- Oblique cord of the elbow joint.
- Interior surface of the radius along the oblique line of the radius.

Insertion

Lateral at the middle phalanges of fingers 2 to 5.

Action

- Flexion of the proximal interphalangeal joints and the metacarpophalangeal joints of fingers 2 to 5.
- Flexion in the wrist.

Innervation

Median nerve (C7–C8).

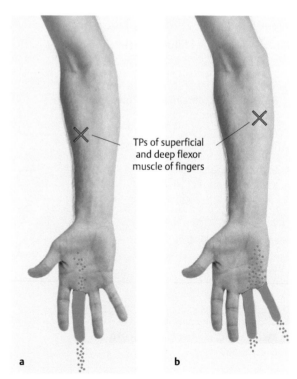

TPs of superficial and deep flexor muscle of fingers

a

b

▶ **Fig. 19.65 (a, b)**   Dots beyond fingers illustrate that pain can shoot explosively from fingers like a stroke of lightening.

Deep Flexor Muscle of Fingers (▶Figs. 19.65, 19.66)

Origin

- Olecranon (medial).
- Anterior and medial surface of the ulna.
- Interosseous membrane (of the lower arm).

Insertion

Distal phalanges of fingers 2 to 5.

Action

- Flexion of all the finger joints.
- Flexion of the wrist.

Innervation

- Median nerve (C6–C7).
- Ulnar nerve (C7–C8).

Trigger Point Location for Both Muscles

Anterior lower arm in the proximal half, on a line with TPs of the radial flexor muscle of the wrist and ulnar flexor muscle of the wrist.

Referred Pain Areas for Both Muscles

Plantar surfaces of fingers 3 to 5 (individual fingers can also exhibit pain).

Associated Inner Organs for Both Muscles

None.

Long Flexor Muscle of Thumb (▶Figs. 19.66, 19.67a)

Origin

- Anterior surface of the radius (distal to oblique line of the radius).
- Interosseous membrane of the lower arm.

Insertion

Base of distal phalanx of the thumb.

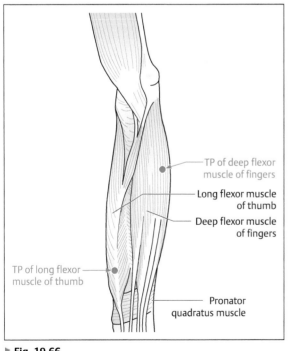

TP of deep flexor muscle of fingers

Long flexor muscle of thumb

Deep flexor muscle of fingers

TP of long flexor muscle of thumb

Pronator quadratus muscle

▶ **Fig. 19.66**

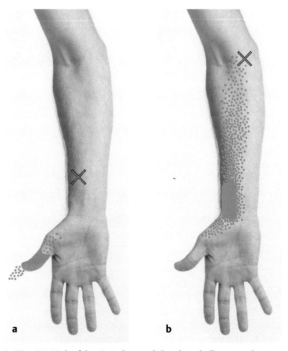

a   b

▶ **Fig. 19.67 (a, b)**   Dots beyond the thumb illustrate that pain can shoot explosively from the thumb like a stroke of lightening.

Action

Flexion of distal phalanx of the thumb.

Innervation

Median nerve (C7–C8).

Trigger Point Location

Slightly proximal to the wrist and radial to the median line of the lower arm.

Pronator Teres Muscle (▶Figs. 19.43, 19.67b)

Origin

- Medial epicondyle of the humerus.
- Medial intermuscular septum of the arm.
- Coronoid process of the ulna.

Insertion

Pronator tuberosity.

Action

- Pronation of the lower arm.
- Flexion in the elbow joint.

Referred Pain Areas

Anterior surface of the thumb.

Associated Inner Organs

None.

Innervation

Median nerve (C6–C7).

Trigger Point Location

Near cubital fossa, ulnar of the aponeurosis of the biceps muscle of arm.

Referred Pain Areas

- Anterior and radial area of the wrist.
- Radial, anterior half of the lower arm.

Associated Inner Organs

None.

Stretching the Lower Arm Flexors (▶Fig. 19.68)

Starting Posture

Patient is standing in the gait posture in front of a table.

Procedure

- Patient places palms of the hands on the table, with tips of fingers pointing back toward the patient and the edge of the table.
- Patient fully extends arms in the elbow joints. This creates a stretch in the anterior lower arm.
- Patient holds the stretch for 30 seconds.

The intensity of the stretch can be modified by moving the legs closer to or further away from the table. Patients who are not able to fully place their hands on the table due to insufficient posterior extension of the wrists can grasp the edge of the table instead (fingers below the table and thumbs above the table).

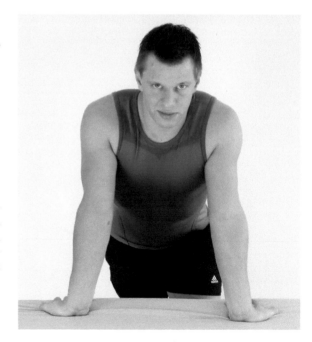

▶ **Fig. 19.68** Stretching the lower arm flexors.

Adductor Muscle of Thumb (▶Figs. 19.69, 19.70)

Origin

- Base of metacarpal bones 2–3.
- Trapezoid bone.
- Capitate bone.
- Body of the metacarpal bone 3.

Insertion

- Ulnar sesamoid bone.
- Proximal phalanx of the thumb (ulnar surface).
- Tendon of the long extensor muscle of the thumb.

Action

Adduction of the thumb.

Innervation

Ulnar nerve (T1).

Trigger Point Location

Near the cutaneous fold between the thumb and the index finger; easily palpable in the muscle belly using pincer palpation.

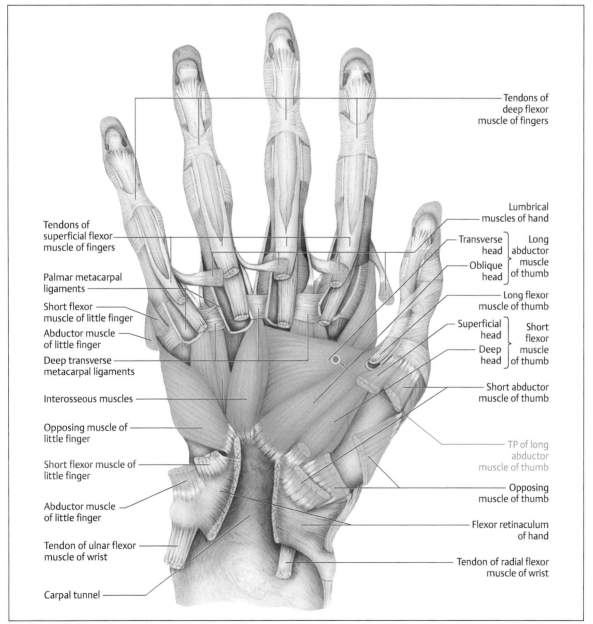

▶ **Fig. 19.69**

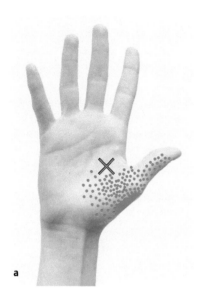
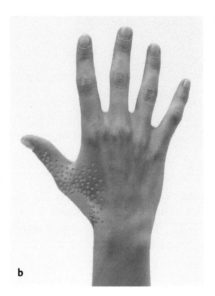

► **Fig. 19.70 (a, b)**

a   b

Referred Pain Areas

- Radial side of the metacarpophalangeal joint of the thumb to the carpometacarpal joint of the thumb.
- Thenar.
- Posterior dorsum of the hand in area of the thumb.

Associated Inner Organs

None.

Opposing Muscle of Thumb (►Figs. 19.71, 19.72)

Origin

- Flexor retinaculum of the hand.
- Tubercle of the trapezium bone.

Insertion

First metacarpal bone (radial).

Action

Opposition of the thumb.

Innervation

- Median nerve (C8–T1).
- Ulnar nerve (T1).

Trigger Point Location

In the muscle belly, near the wrist.

Referred Pain Areas

- Palmar surface of the thumb.
- Radial and plantar half of the wrist.

Associated Inner Organs

None.

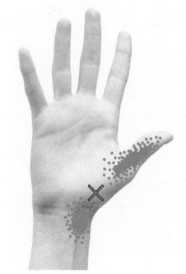

► **Fig. 19.71**

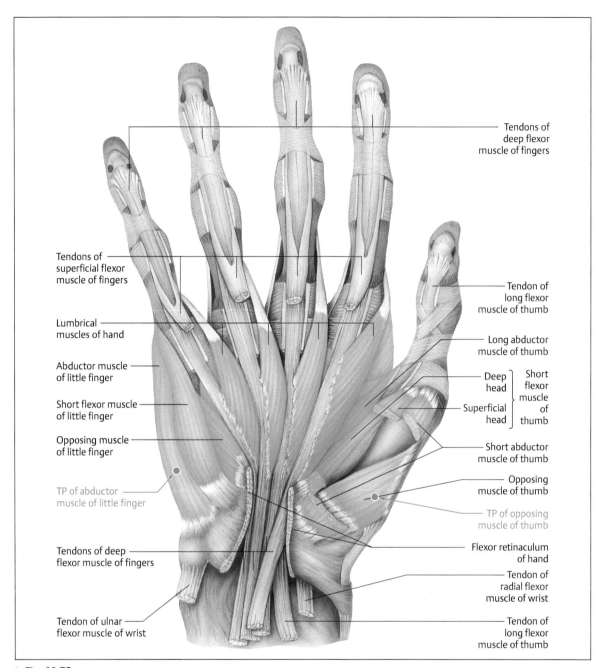

Tendons of
deep flexor
muscle of fingers

Tendons of
superficial flexor
muscle of fingers

Lumbrical
muscles of hand

Abductor muscle
of little finger

Short flexor muscle
of little finger

Opposing muscle
of little finger

TP of abductor
muscle of little finger

Tendons of deep
flexor muscle of fingers

Tendon of ulnar
flexor muscle of wrist

Tendon of
long flexor
muscle of thumb

Long abductor
muscle of thumb

Deep ⎱ Short
head ⎰ flexor
         muscle
Superficial ⎱ of
head ⎰ thumb

Short abductor
muscle of thumb

Opposing
muscle of thumb

TP of opposing
muscle of thumb

Flexor retinaculum
of hand

Tendon of
radial flexor
muscle of wrist

Tendon of
long flexor
muscle of thumb

▶ **Fig. 19.72**

Abductor Muscle of Little Finger (▶Figs. 19.72, 19.73)

Origin

Pisiform bone.

Insertion

Ulnar base of the proximal phalanx and the extensor aponeurosis (dorsal digital expansion) of finger 5.

Action

- Flexion and abduction in the metacarpophalangeal joint of the little finger.
- Extension in proximal and distal interphalangeal joint of the little finger.

Innervation

- Ulnar nerve (C8–T1).

Trigger Point Location

In the muscle belly near the base of metacarpal bone 5.

Referred Pain Areas

Ulnar side of the little finger.

Associated Inner Organs

None.

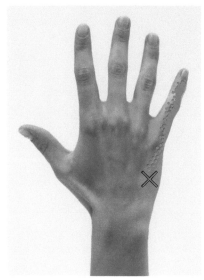

▸ **Fig. 19.73**

Interosseous Muscles of Hand (▸Figs. 19.74, 19.75)

■ Dorsal Interosseous Muscles of Hand

Origin

Interior surfaces of all metacarpal bones.

Insertion

- Base of the corresponding proximal phalanges.
- Dorsal digital expansion (extensor expansion) of fingers 2 to 4.

Action

- Abduction of fingers 2 to 4.
- Flexion of the metacarpophalangeal joints with extension of the proximal and distal interphalangeal joints of the fingers.

Innervation

Ulnar nerve (T1).

■ Palmar Interosseous Muscles

Origin

Metacarpal bones 2, 4, and 5.

Insertion

- Base of the corresponding proximal phalanges.
- Radiation into tendons of the extensor aponeurosis (dorsal digital expansion) of fingers 2, 4, and 5.
- Ulnar sesamoid bone of the thumb.

Action

- Adduction of fingers 2, 4, and 5.
- Flexion of metacarpophalangeal joints with extension of the proximal and distal interphalangeal joints of the fingers.

Innervation

Ulnar nerve (T1).

Trigger Point Location

Between the metacarpal bones.

Referred Pain Areas

- Index finger (maximum on the radial side) and dorsum of the hand (TP of the dorsal interosseous muscle of the index finger, a very frequent TP).
- Radial sides of the fingers.

Associated Inner Organs

None.

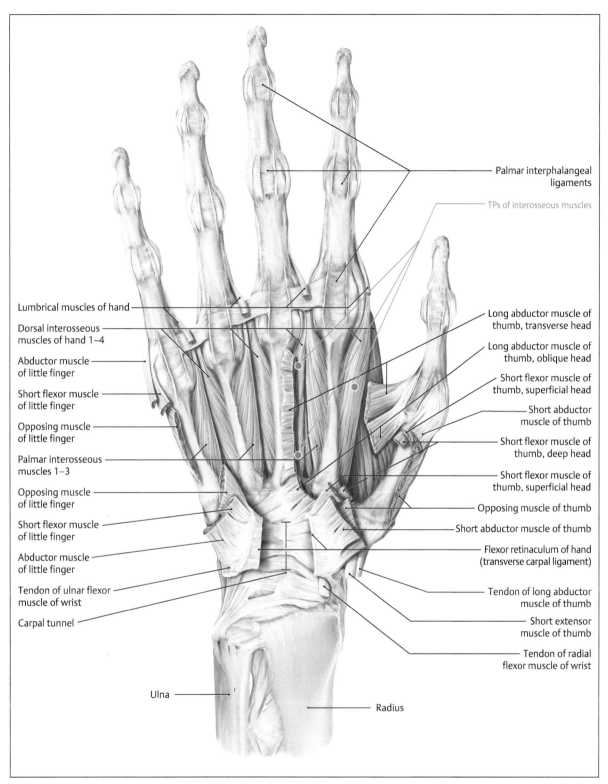

Palmar interphalangeal
ligaments

TPs of interosseous muscles

Lumbrical muscles of hand

Dorsal interosseous
muscles of hand 1–4

Abductor muscle
of little finger

Short flexor muscle
of little finger

Opposing muscle
of little finger

Palmar interosseous
muscles 1–3

Opposing muscle
of little finger

Short flexor muscle
of little finger

Abductor muscle
of little finger

Tendon of ulnar flexor
muscle of wrist

Carpal tunnel

Long abductor muscle of
thumb, transverse head

Long abductor muscle of
thumb, oblique head

Short flexor muscle of
thumb, superficial head

Short abductor
muscle of thumb

Short flexor muscle of
thumb, deep head

Short flexor muscle of
thumb, superficial head

Opposing muscle of thumb

Short abductor muscle of thumb

Flexor retinaculum of hand
(transverse carpal ligament)

Tendon of long abductor
muscle of thumb

Short extensor
muscle of thumb

Tendon of radial
flexor muscle of wrist

Ulna

Radius

▶ **Fig. 19.74**

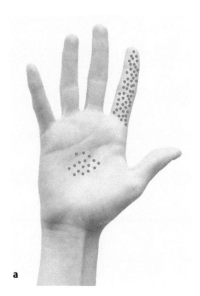

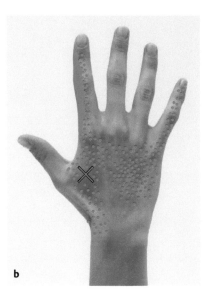

▶ **Fig. 19.75 (a–c)**

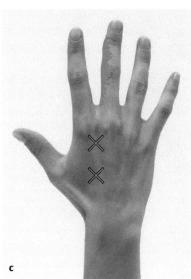

19.4 Upper Trunk Pain: Related Muscles

Greater Pectoral Muscle (▶Figs. 19.76, 19.77)

Origin

- Clavicular part:
  - Clavicle (sternal half).
- Sternocostal part:
  - Lateral at the manubrium and body of the sternum.
  - Rib cartilages 1 to 6.
  - Aponeurosis of the external oblique muscle of abdomen.

Insertion

- Crest of the lesser tubercle of the humerus.
- Deltoid tuberosity (anterior).

Action

- Clavicular part: flexion, adduction in the shoulder joint.
- Sternocostal part: adduction and internal rotation in the shoulder joint, inspiration muscle.

Innervation

Medial and lateral pectoral nerve (C6–C8).

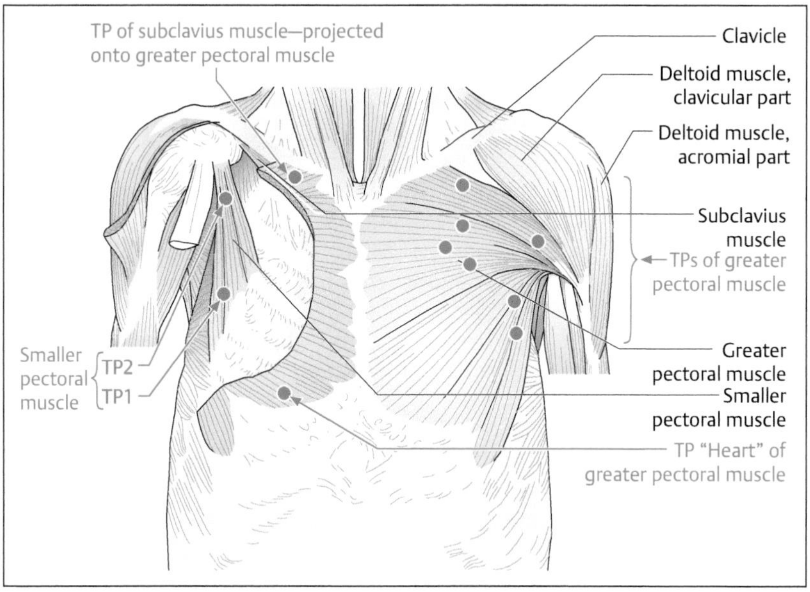

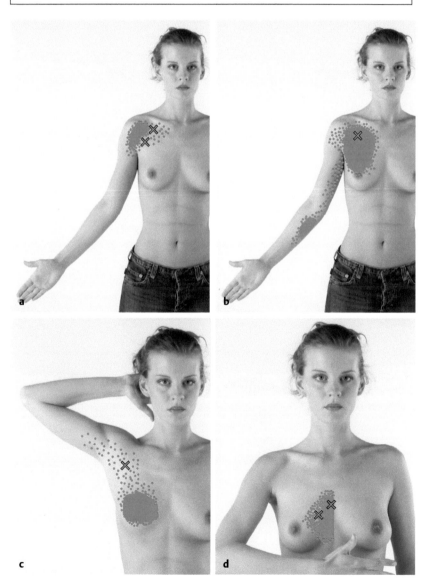

TP of subclavius muscle—projected onto greater pectoral muscle

Clavicle

Deltoid muscle, clavicular part

Deltoid muscle, acromial part

Subclavius muscle

TPs of greater pectoral muscle

Greater pectoral muscle

Smaller pectoral muscle

TP "Heart" of greater pectoral muscle

Smaller pectoral muscle
TP2
TP1

▶ **Fig. 19.76**

▶ **Fig. 19.77 (a–d)**

Trigger Point Location

TPs are distributed in the entire muscle. The TPs located more laterally and near the axillary fold are easily found using pincer palpation. The TPs located more sternally are easily found using flat palpation.

TP for "cardiac arrhythmia": This TP is located in a region defined by two vertical lines, one running through the mammilla and the other through the lateral border of the sternum. It can be palpated by searching in the intercostal space between the fifth and sixth ribs on the right side.

Referred Pain Areas

TP of the clavicular part:
- Anterior deltoid muscle area.
- Clavicular part itself.

TP of the lateral sternocostal part:
- Anterior breast area.
- Inner side of the upper arm.

Smaller Pectoral Muscle (▶Figs. 19.76, 19.78)

Origin

Third to fifth rib.

Insertion

Coracoid process (superomedial).

Action

- Draws scapula forward and down.
- Inspiration muscle with fixed scapula.

Innervation

Medial and lateral pectoral nerve (C6–C8).

Trigger Point Location

- TP1: Near the origin of the muscle at the fourth rib.
- TP2: At transition of the muscle belly and tendon, slightly inferior to the coracoid process of the scapula.

Referred Pain Areas

- Anterior deltoid muscle area.
- Breast region.
- Ulnar side of the upper arm, elbow, lower arm.
- Palm of the hand in the area of fingers 3 to 5.

The radiation pain pattern is very similar to that of the greater pectoral muscle.

- Medial epicondyle of the humerus.
- Anterior lower arm.
- Ulnar edge of the hand.
- Palm of the hand in the area of fingers 3 to 5.

TP in the medial sternocostal part:
- Sternum (without crossing the medial line) and adjacent area of the breast.

TP in the inferior sternocostal part:
- Anterior breast area, with hypersensibility of the mammilla and possibly of the entire breast (especially for women).

TP for "cardiac arrhythmia":
- This TP occurs with cardiac arrhythmia without causing pain.

Associated Inner Organs

Heart.

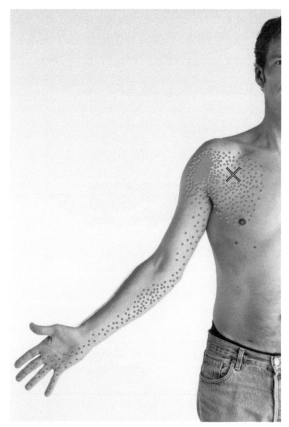

▶ **Fig. 19.78**

Associated Inner Organs

Heart.

Subclavius Muscle (▶Figs. 19.76, 19.79)

Origin

First rib (border between the cartilage and the bone).

Insertion

Middle third of the clavicle, on the lower surface.

Action

Draws the clavicle downward.

Innervation

Subclavian nerve (C5–C6).

Trigger Point Location

Near muscle insertion.

Referred Pain Areas

- Anterior region of the shoulder and upper arm.
- Radial side of the lower arm.
- Palmar and posterior area of the hand in the area of fingers 1 to 3.

Associated Inner Organs

The subclavius muscle is frequently innervated by a branch of the phrenic nerve. This results in connections with:
- Liver.
- Gallbladder.

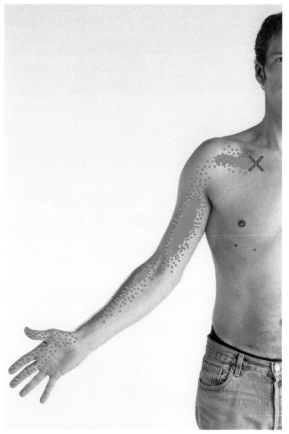

▶ **Fig. 19.79**

Stretching the Pectoral Muscles (▶Fig. 19.80a, b)

Starting Posture

The patient is standing in the gait posture facing a corner of the room.

Procedure

- The patient places both lower arms flat on opposite walls in the corner of the room. The upper arms are aligned horizontally (about 90-degree abduction). The upper body is upright and one foot is placed into the corner.

- Arms and upper body remain passive while the patient moves the upper body from the legs closer to the corner of the room. The arms will make an evasive motion into increased transversal abduction. The stretch is felt in the chest area.
- The patient holds the stretch for 30 seconds.

The arms can also be placed on the walls in more than 90-degree abduction. This results in increased stretching of other parts of the pectoral muscles. This stretch can also be performed on one side only.

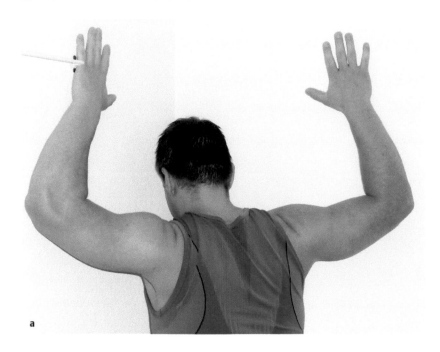

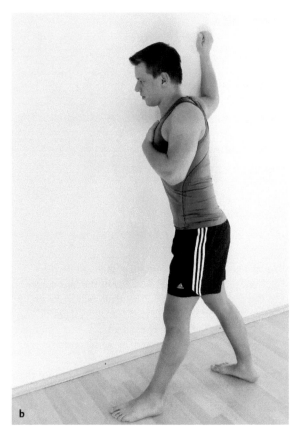

▶ **Fig. 19.80** Bilateral (**a**) and unilateral (**b**) stretching of the pectoral muscles.

Sternal Muscle (▶Figs. 19.76, 19.81)

Only present in 1 out of 20 people.

Origin

On one or both sides of the pectoral or sternocleidomastoid fasciae, with possible origins in the superior area of the sternum.

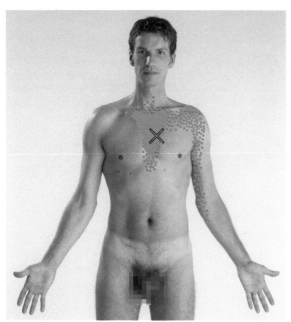

▶ **Fig. 19.81**

Insertion

Great variability, with possible insertions between the third to seventh costal cartilages, pectoral fascia, and fascia of the rectus abdominis muscle.

Action

Not known; possibly a fascia tensor.

Innervation

Medial pectoral nerve (C6–C8) or intercostal nerves.

Trigger Point Location

TPs can be located in the entire muscle belly, mostly in the middle area of the sternum.

Referred Pain Areas

- Entire sternum, sometimes also substernal.
- Upper chest area.
- Anterior upper arm and elbow.

> This referred pain mimics the pain experienced with cardiac infarction or angina pectoris.

Associated Inner Organs

Heart.

Superior Posterior Serratus Muscle (▶Figs. 19.82–19.84)

Origin

Spinous processes and supraspinal ligaments of CVB 7 to TVB 2.

Insertion

Exterior surface of ribs 2 to 5 (posterior).

Action

Inspiration muscle for deep inspiration.

Innervation

Anterior branches of spinal nerves T2–T5.

Trigger Point Location

In the neutral posture, this TP projects onto the posterior trunk wall at the level of the supraspinous fossa of the scapula, near the spine of the scapula. To palpate this TP, the shoulder must be protracted to reveal the TP.

Referred Pain Areas

- Below the scapula, in its upper half.
- Posterior deltoid muscle area.
- Posterior upper arm.
- Ulnar side of the lower arm.
- Posterior elbow.
- Anterior and posterior palm of the hand in the area of the hypothenar and finger 5.
- Pectoral area.

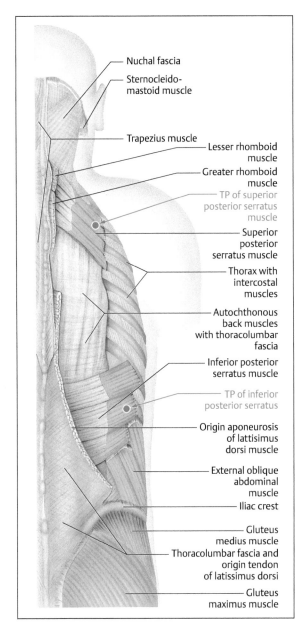

Nuchal fascia

Sternocleido-
mastoid muscle

Trapezius muscle

Lesser rhomboid
muscle

Greater rhomboid
muscle

TP of superior
posterior serratus
muscle

Superior
posterior
serratus muscle

Thorax with
intercostal
muscles

Autochthonous
back muscles
with thoracolumbar
fascia

Inferior posterior
serratus muscle

TP of inferior
posterior serratus

Origin aponeurosis
of lattisimus
dorsi muscle

External oblique
abdominal
muscle

Iliac crest

Gluteus
medius muscle

Thoracolumbar fascia and
origin tendon
of latissimus dorsi

Gluteus
maximus muscle

▶ **Fig. 19.82**

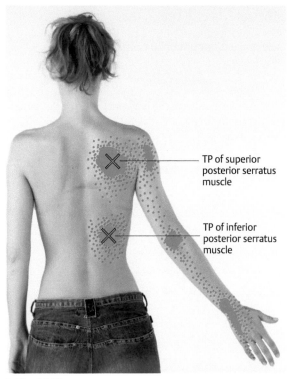

TP of superior
posterior serratus
muscle

TP of inferior
posterior serratus
muscle

▶ **Fig. 19.83**

Associated Inner Organs

- Heart.
- Lung.

Inferior Posterior Serratus Muscle (▶Figs. 19.82, 19.83)

Origin

Spinous processes and supraspinal ligaments of TVB 11 to LVB 2.

Insertion

Exterior surface of ribs 9 to 12 (posterior).

Action

Expiration muscle for deep expiration.

Innervation

Anterior branches of spinal nerves T9–T12.

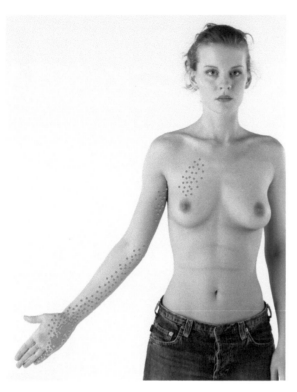

Trigger Point Location

In the muscle belly, near insertion at the ribs.

Referred Pain Areas

In the area of the muscle around the lower ribs.

Associated Inner Organs

- Kidney.
- Duodenum.
- Pancreas.
- Jejunum, ileum.
- Colon.
- Uterus.

▶ **Fig. 19.84**

Anterior Serratus Muscle (▶Figs. 19.85, 19.86)

Origin

Ribs 1 to 9 and intercostal spaces in the area of the mid-clavicular line.

Insertion

Medial border of the scapula.

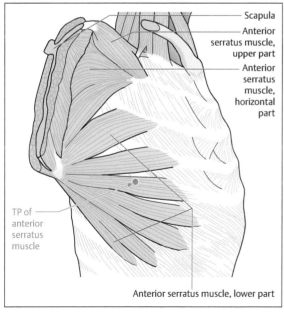

▶ **Fig. 19.85**

Action

- Draws scapula toward anterolateral.
- Inspiration accessory muscle.

Innervation

- Long thoracic nerve (C5–C7).
- Intercostal nerves.

Trigger Point Location

In muscle slip that arises from fifth or sixth rib, near the median axillary line.

Referred Pain Areas

- Anterolateral in the middle chest area.
- Medial of the lower angle of the scapula.
- Medial upper and lower arms.
- Palm of the hand with fingers 4 and 5.

Deep respiration, for example, during exercise, can cause side stitch pain (exercise-related transient abdominal pain [ETAP]).

Associated Inner Organs

Heart.

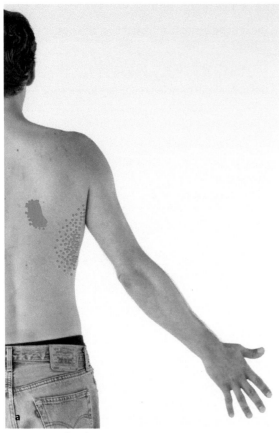

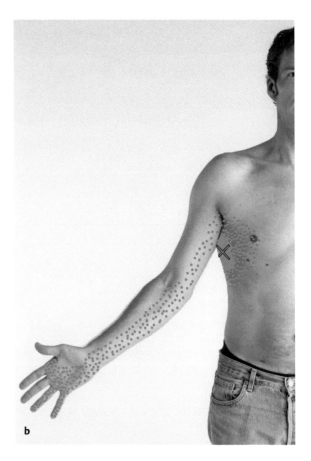

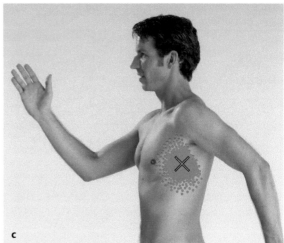

▶ **Fig. 19.86 (a–c)**

Erector Muscle of Spine (▶Figs. 19.87–19.89)

▪ Iliocostalis Muscle (▶Fig. 19.87)

Origin

- Sacrum.
- Iliac crest.
- Spinous processes of the lumbar spine (LSC).
- Thoracolumbar fascia.
- Costal angle.

Insertion

Superior and inferior at the transverse processes of the middle CSC or costal angle for the lumbar and thoracic areas.

Action

- Lateral flexion of the spine.
- Extension of the spine.

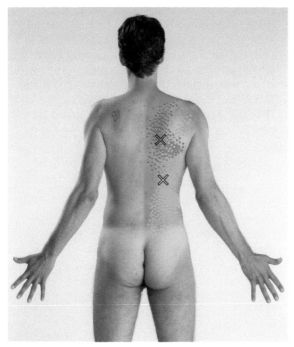

▶ **Fig. 19.87**

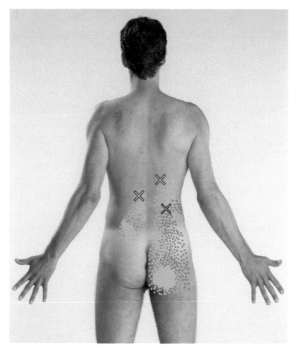

▶ **Fig. 19.88**

Innervation

Posterior branches of the segmental spinal nerves.

▪ Longissimus Muscle (Lumbar Part)
(▶ **Fig. 19.88**)

Origin

- Transverse processes.
- Sacrum.
- Iliac crest.
- Spinous processes and mammillary processes of the lumbar spine (LSC).

Insertion

- Transverse processes located superior to the origin.
- Mastoid process.
- Costal and accessory processes of ribs 2 to 12.

Action

Extension of the spine.

Innervation

Posterior branches of the segmental spinal nerves.

▪ Spinal Muscle (▶ **Fig. 19.89**)

Origin

Spinous processes of the spine.

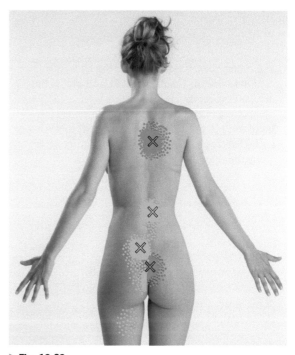

▶ **Fig. 19.89**

Insertion

Spinous processes of the six vertebrae located superior to the origin.

Action

Lateral flexion of spine.

Innervation

Posterior branches of the segmental spinal nerves.

Trigger Point Location

TPs can be distributed in the entire erector muscle of the spine. The following may be helpful in finding the TPs for the spinal muscle: the spinous processes may be hypersensible at the level where the TPs of the erector muscle of the spine are active.

Referred Pain Areas

- TP in the iliocostal muscle, middle thorax area: toward superior into the shoulder area and into the lateral chest wall.

- TP in the iliocostal muscle, lower thorax area: toward superior via the scapula, forward into the abdomen and into the upper lumbar spine (LSC).
- TP in the iliocostal muscle, lumbar part: toward inferior into the middle buttocks area.
- TP in the longissimus muscle, lumbar part: into the gluteal area and the sacroiliac joint region.
- TP in the spinal muscle: pain is concentrated around the TP.

Associated Inner Organs

- Jejunum, ileum.
- Colon.
- Kidney.
- Urinary bladder.
- Uterus.
- Ovary.
- Prostate.

Stretching the Autochthonous Back Muscles (▶Fig. 19.90)

Starting Posture

The patient is kneeling on the floor.

Procedure

- The patient bends forward, rolls the back into complete flexion, flexes the head, and places the head on the floor.
- The patient brings the arms in to the sides of the body and places them on the floor next to the lower legs. This creates a stretch along the entire spine.
- The patient holds the stretch for 30 seconds.

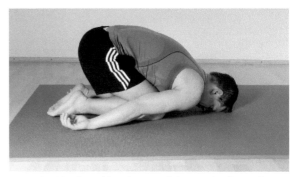

▶ **Fig. 19.90**   Stretching the autochthonous back muscles.

Rectus Abdominis Muscle, Internal and External Oblique Muscles of Abdomen, Transverse Abdominal Muscle, Pyramidal Muscle (▶Figs. 19.91–19.94)

▪ Rectus Abdominis Muscle

Origin

- Pubic crest.
- Pubic symphysis.

Insertion

- Fifth to seventh costal cartilage.
- Rib arch, medial area.
- Xiphoid process, posterior surface.

Action

- Trunk flexion.
- Abdominal press.
- Forced expiration.

Innervation

Anterior branches of spinal nerves T7–T12.

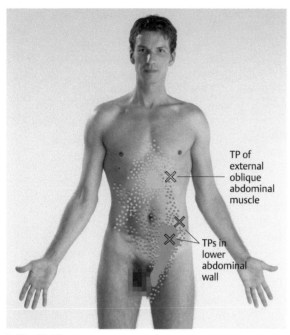

▶ **Fig. 19.91**

■ Internal Oblique Muscle of Abdomen

Origin

- Thoracolumbar fascia.
- Anterior two-thirds of the iliac crest.
- Lateral two-thirds of the inguinal ligament.

Insertion

- Rib arch.
- Anterior and posterior layer of the sheath of the rectus abdominis muscle.
- Conjoined tendon to pubic crest and pectineal line.

Action

- Trunk sidebend.
- Trunk rotation toward the ipsilateral side (together with the contralateral muscle).
- Abdominal press.
- Forced expiration.
- Strengthens inguinal canal.

Innervation

Anterior branches of spinal nerves T7–T12.

■ External Oblique Muscle of Abdomen

Origin

Anterior exterior surface of ribs 5 to 12.

Insertion

- Iliac crest.
- Inguinal ligament.
- Pubic tubercle.
- Pubic crest.
- White line.

Action

- Trunk sidebend.
- Trunk rotation toward the contralateral side (together with the contralateral muscle).
- Abdominal press.
- Forced expiration.

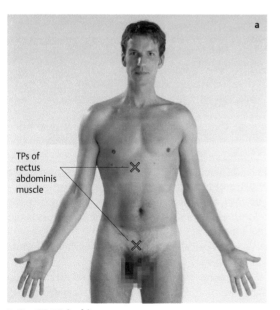

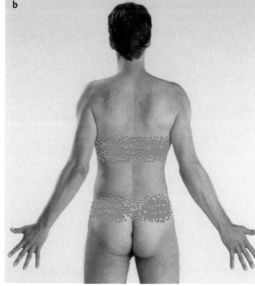

▶ **Fig. 19.92 (a, b)**

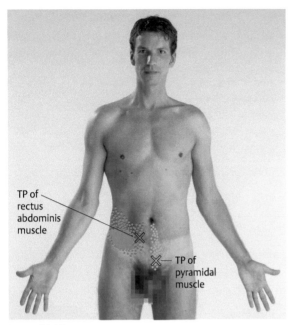

TP of rectus abdominis muscle

TP of pyramidal muscle

▶ **Fig. 19.93**

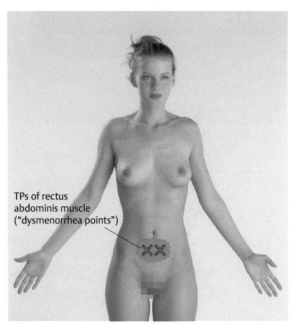

TPs of rectus abdominis muscle ("dysmenorrhea points")

▶ **Fig. 19.94**

Innervation

Anterior branches of spinal nerves T7–T12.

■ Transverse Abdominal Muscle

Origin

- Interior surface of the lower ribs.
- Thoracolumbar fascia.
- Anterior two-thirds of the iliac crest.
- Outer half of the inguinal ligament.

Insertion

- Anterior and posterior layers of the sheath of the rectus abdominis muscle.
- Pubic crest.
- Pectineal line (anterior border of the superior ramus of the pubis).

Action

- Abdominal press.
- Forced expiration.
- Strengthens inguinal canal.

Innervation

Anterior branches of spinal nerves T7–T12.

■ Pyramidal Muscle

Origin

Pubic crest, anterior of insertion of the rectus abdominis muscle.

Insertion

White line, distal.

Action

Strengthens the rectus sheath.

Innervation

Subcostal nerve (T12).

■ Abdominal Muscles

Trigger Point Location

TPs are distributed in the entire abdominal musculature. **Figs. 19.91** to **19.94** illustrate a selection of the more frequent TP locations.

Referred Pain Areas

In general, there are many TPs in the abdominal muscles and they share a common characteristic: they primarily produce pain locally in the area surrounding the TP. In addition, TPs in abdominal muscles also cause some visceral symptoms, for example, nausea, vomiting, or dysmenorrhea. Another special characteristic of abdominal TPs is that their referred pain crosses the median line.

Nevertheless, typical pain patterns for abdominal muscles are discussed below.

TPs of the **external oblique abdominal muscle**, rib section:

- "Heart pain."
- Symptoms resembling hiatal hernia.
- Epigastric pain extending to other abdominal areas.

TPs of the **lower abdominal** wall (all abdominal wall muscles):
- Pain in the groin and labia/testicles.
- Pain in other sections of the abdomen.

TPs along upper borders of the pubic bone and the lateral half of the inguinal ligament (**internal oblique abdominal and rectus abdominis muscles**):
- Pain in the area of urinary bladder, possibly urinary bladder spasms.
- Groin pain.
- Urinary retention.

TPs in the **transverse abdominal muscle**, near the insertion at the rib:
- Upper abdomen between the rib arches.

TPs in the **rectus abdominis muscle**, above the navel:
- Painful horizontal band across the back, at the level of the thoracolumbar junction.

TPs in the **rectus** abdominis, at the level of the navel, at lateral border of the muscle:
- Abdominal cramps and colic-like pain.
- Pain in the anterior abdominal wall without a fixed pattern.

TPs in the **rectus abdominis muscle**, below the navel:
- Dysmenorrhea.
- Painful horizontal band across the back, at the level of the sacrum.

TPs in **pyramidal muscle**:
- Between the symphysis and the navel, near the median line.

Associated Inner Organs

- Liver.
- Gallbladder.
- Stomach.
- Pancreas.
- Spleen.
- Duodenum.
- Jejunum, ileum.
- Colon.
- Kidneys.
- Uterus.
- Ovary.

The acute abdomen presents with induration of the abdominal wall. This can be explained as a segmental viscerosomatic reflex: the abdominal muscles develop hypertonicity as an immobilizing response to the peritoneal irritation of a segmentally associated organ.

TPs in the abdominal muscles regularly remain even after the organic disorder has healed.

Stretching the Abdominal Muscles (▶Fig. 19.95)

Starting Posture

The patient is supine.

Procedure

- A rolled-up towel is placed on the floor below the patient's lumbar spine.

- The patient lies on the towel with legs together and extended and arms extended and placed next to the head. This creates a stretch in the abdominal muscles.
- The patient holds the stretch for 30 seconds.

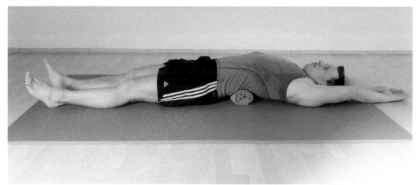

▶ **Fig. 19.95** Stretching the abdominal muscles.

19.5 Lower Trunk Pain: Related Muscles

Quadratus Lumborum Muscle (▶Figs. 19.96, 19.97)

Origin

Lower margin of the 12th rib.

Insertion

- Costal processes of LVB 1 to 4.
- Iliolumbar ligament.
- Posterior third of the iliac crest.

Action

- Lateral flexion of the trunk.
- Fixation of the 12th rib during respiration.

Innervation

Anterior branches of spinal nerves T12–L3.

Trigger Point Location

This TP can be more easily palpated if the patient is contralateral, with a rolled-up towel under the waist. This creates sidebending of the spine away from the muscle to be palpated. The superior arm is now placed in maximum abduction and the superior leg is partially flexed. This increases the desired sidebending.

The following muscle areas are palpated for TPs:
- In the angle above the iliac crest and lateral of the erector muscle of spine.
- Along the iliac crest.
- In the angle between the 12th rib and the erector muscle of spine.

The superficial TPs are found in the lateral areas of the muscle: one below the 12th rib and one above the iliac crest.

The deep TPs are found in two locations: one above the iliac crest, between the costal processes of the fourth and fifth lumbar vertebra and one at the level of the costal process of the third lumbar vertebra, in the medial areas of the muscle.

Referred Pain Areas

- Superior superficial TP: along the iliac crest, sometimes into the groin and lower lateral abdominal area.
- Inferior superficial TP: around the trochanter, partially radiating into the lateral upper leg.
- Superior deep TP: around the sacroiliac joint.
- Inferior deep TP: inferior buttocks.

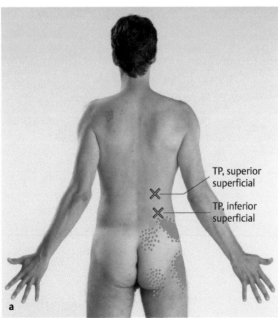

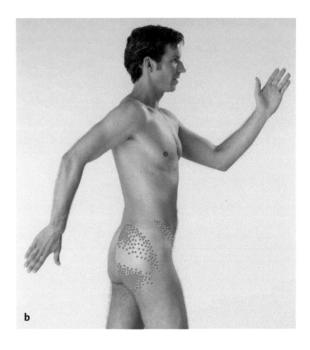

▶ **Fig. 19.96 (a, b)**

Associated Inner Organs

- Jejunum, ileum.
- Colon.
- Kidneys.
- Urinary bladder.
- Uterus, appendages, and prostate.

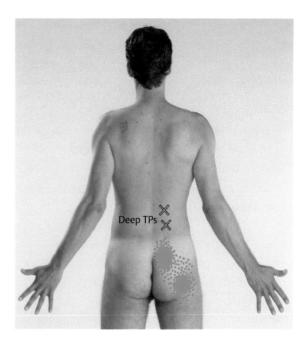

▶ **Fig. 19.97**

Stretching the Lateral Side of the Trunk (▶Fig. 19.98)

Starting Posture

The patient is in supine position.

Procedure

The side to be stretched is on the right.
- The patient bends the upper body toward the left and places the legs toward the left side: the left leg is abducted; the right leg is adducted. The area between the iliac crest and the 12th rib on the left side forms the pivot point.
- The patient flexes and adducts the right arm and places it below the head on the floor. This creates a stretch along the entire right side of the trunk, especially in the lower trunk area, between the iliac crest and the 12th rib on the right side.
- The patient holds the stretch for 30 seconds.

This procedure primarily stretches the latissimus dorsi, quadratus lumborum, and lateral abdominal muscles.

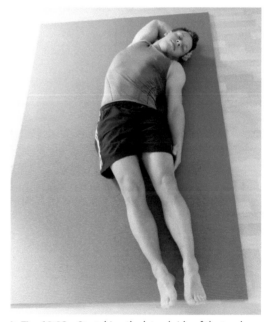

▶ **Fig. 19.98** Stretching the lateral side of the trunk.

Iliopsoas Muscle (▶Figs. 19.99, 19.100)

▪ Iliac Muscle

Origin

Iliac fossa.

Insertion

Lesser trochanter of the femur.

Action

- Flexion in the hip joint.
- External and internal rotation in the hip joint.

Innervation

Femoral nerve (L2–L3).

■ Greater Psoas Muscle

Origin

- Transverse processes of LVB 1 to 5.
- TVB 12–LVB 5 and intervertebral disks below TVB 12.

Insertion

Lesser trochanter of the femur.

Action

- Flexion in the hip joint.
- External and internal rotation in the hip joint.
- Abduction in the hip joint.
- Extension and lateral flexion of the LSC.

Innervation

Anterior branches of spinal nerves L1–L2.

■ Smaller Psoas Muscle

Origin

TVB 12 to LVB 1 including the intervertebral disk.

Insertion

Iliac fascia.

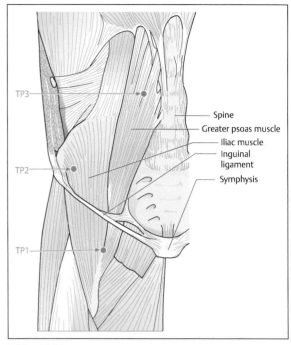

▶ **Fig. 19.99**

Action

Trunk flexion (weak).

Innervation

Anterior branch of spinal nerve L1.

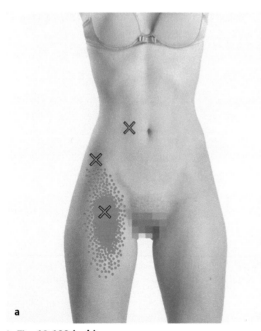

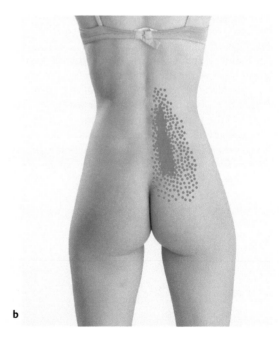

▶ **Fig. 19.100 (a, b)**

Trigger Point Locations for Iliac Muscle, Greater Psoas, and Smaller Psoas Muscles

- TP1: Lateral margin of the femoral triangle.
- TP2: In the iliac fossa at the level of the anterior superior iliac spine (ASIS).
- TP3: Carefully palpate lateral of rectus abdominis and below navel toward posterior and then toward medial to compress the greater psoas against the spine.

Referred Pain Areas

- Mainly in LSC, ipsilateral along the spine to the sacroiliac joint and to the upper/middle buttock area.
- Groin and anteromedial upper leg.

Associated Inner Organs

- Colon.
- Kidney.
- Urinary bladder.
- Uterus, appendages, and prostate.

Stretching the Hip Flexors and Gluteal Muscles (▶Fig. 19.101)

Starting Posture

The patient kneels in front of a stool or chair.

Procedure

- The patient places the knee of one leg on the floor as far away from the stool as possible.
- The patient places the foot of the other leg next to the stool.
- The patient places hands and lower arms for support on the stool and moves the abdomen as far away from the stool as possible. This creates a pronounced stretch in the anterior upper side of the leg that is kneeling on the floor (right leg in ▶**Fig. 19.101**). The buttocks of the other leg may also experience a stretch.
- The patient holds the stretch for 30 seconds.

Additional stretching may be experienced on the inside of the proximal upper leg in the leg placed next to the stool. This indicates stretching of the short adductors.

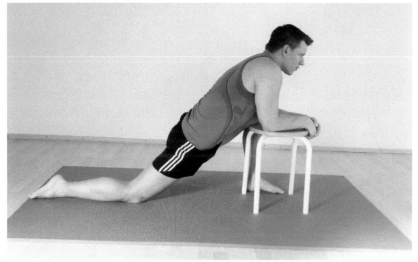

▶ **Fig. 19.101** Stretching the hip flexors and gluteal muscles.

Muscles of the Pelvic Floor (▶Fig. 19.102)

■ Internal Obturator Muscle

Origin

- Interior surface of the obturator membrane.
- Inferomedial bone margin of the obturator foramen.

Insertion

Trochanteric fossa.

Action

- Stabilization of the hip joint.
- External rotation in the hip joint.

Innervation

Obturator nerve (L5–S2).

■ External Anal Sphincter Muscle

Origin

Elliptical sphincter muscle.

Insertion

Perianal in subcutaneous, superficial, and deep connective tissues.

Action

Closes the anal canal (fecal continence).

Innervation

Pudendal nerve (S2–S4).

■ Levator Ani Muscle

Origin

- Posterior area of the pubic bone.
- Tendinous arch of the levator ani muscle.
- Spine of the ischium.

Insertion

- Anococcygeal ligament.
- Ansiform to the rectum.

Action

- Strengthens the pelvic floor.
- Maintains continence.

Innervation

Anterior branches of spinal nerves S3–S4.

■ Ischiococcygeal Muscle

Origin

- Sacrospinal ligament.
- Spine of the ischium.

Insertion

- Anococcygeal ligament.
- Coccygeal bone.

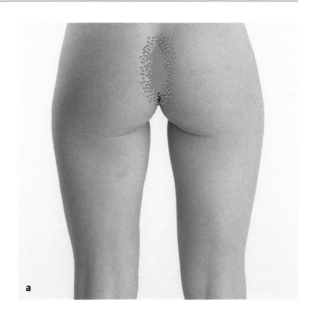

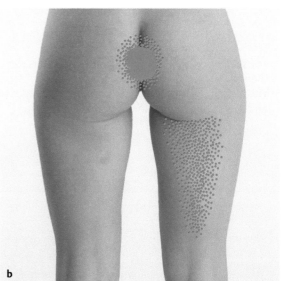

▶ **Fig. 19.102 (a, b)**

Action

Strengthens the pelvic floor.

Innervation

Anterior branches of spinal nerves S4–S5.

Trigger Point Location

Can be identified by rectal, vaginal, or pelvic floor palpation.

Referred Pain Areas

- Coccygeal bone.
- Inferior sacrum.
- Anus area.
- Posterior upper leg (internal obturator muscle).

Gluteus Maximus Muscle (▶Figs. 19.103–19.105)

Origin

- Exterior surface of the wing of the ilium behind the posterior gluteal line.
- Posterior third of the iliac crest.
- Thoracolumbar fascia.
- Sacrum.
- Sacrotuberal ligament.
- Coccygeal bone.

Insertion

- Gluteal tuberosity of the femur.
- Iliotibial tract (runs toward the lateral condyle of the tibia).

Action

- Extension in the hip joint.
- External rotation in the hip joint.

Innervation

Inferior gluteal nerve (L5–S2).

Associated Inner Organs

- Rectum.
- Urinary bladder.
- Uterus, appendages, and prostate.

Trigger Point Location

These TPs can be well palpated in patients lying on their side, with the side to be examined on top and legs slightly flexed.
- TP1: Approximately at the upper end of the gluteal fold, not far from insertion of muscle at the sacrum.
- TP2: Slightly superior to ischial tuberosity.
- TP3: At inferomedial border of muscle—at the inferior end of the gluteal fold—well palpable using pincer palpation.

Referred Pain Areas

- TP1: From the sacroiliac joint along the gluteal fold in the inferior muscle area and the beginning of the posterior upper leg.
- TP2: Along the entire muscle with emphasis on the inferior sacrum, lateral area below the iliac crest, and inferior buttocks. Pain is sometimes sensed in the deeper areas and feels like pain in the gluteus minimus muscles. No referred pain into the coccygeal bone.
- TP3: Coccygeal bone and inferomedial muscle area.

Associated Inner Organs

None.

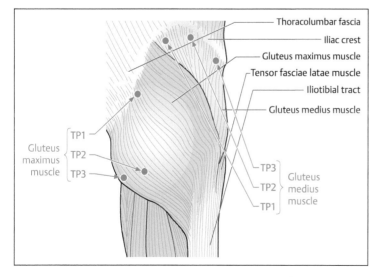

▶ **Fig. 19.103**

Thoracolumbar fascia
Iliac crest
Gluteus maximus muscle
Tensor fasciae latae muscle
Iliotibial tract
Gluteus medius muscle

Gluteus maximus muscle {TP1 TP2 TP3}

TP3 TP2 TP1 } Gluteus medius muscle

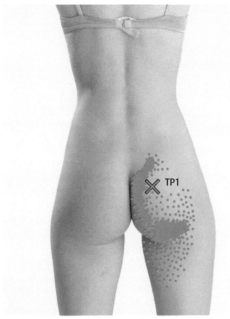

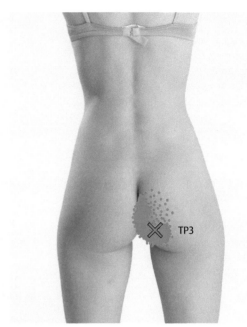

Gluteus Medius Muscle (▶Figs. 19.103, 19.106, 19.107)

Origin

Exterior surface of iliac bone (ilium; between the anterior and posterior gluteal lines).

Insertion

Greater trochanter (posterolateral).

Action

- Abduction in the hip joint.
- Internal rotation in the hip joint (anterior and lateral parts).
- External rotation in the hip joint (posterior and medial parts).
- Horizontal stabilization of the pelvis during the swing phase of gait.

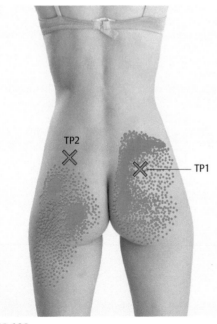

▶ **Fig. 19.106**

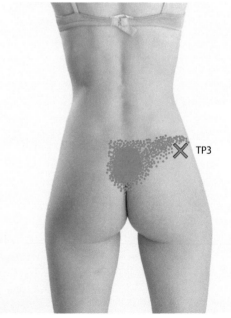

▶ **Fig. 19.107**

Innervation

Superior gluteal nerve (L4–S1).

Trigger Point Location

These TPs are palpated with patients lying on their side in a contralateral position, with legs flexed.
- TP1: In the posterior muscle belly, not far below the iliac crest and near the sacroiliac joint.
- TP2: Immediately below iliac crest, in about the middle of its course.
- TP3: Also located immediately below the iliac crest, but slightly further anterior, near the ASIS.

Referred Pain Areas

- TP1: Pain radiates from the posterior area of the iliac crest via the sacroiliac joint and sacrum into the entire buttock area.
- TP2: Pain radiates via the lateral and middle gluteal area to the posterior and lateral proximal upper leg.
- TP3: Pain radiates along the iliac crest and the lower lumbar area, especially into the sacrum.

Associated Inner Organs

None.

Gluteus Minimus Muscle (▶ Figs. 19.108–19.110)

Origin

Exterior surface of the iliac bone (between the anterior and posterior gluteal lines).

Insertion

Greater trochanter (anterior).

Action

- Abduction in the hip joint.
- Internal rotation in the hip joint (anterior and lateral parts).
- Horizontal stabilization of the pelvis in the swing phase of gait.

Innervation

Superior gluteal nerve (L4–S1).

Trigger Point Location

- Anterior TPs: at the level of ASIS, but slightly further below the iliac crest than with the gluteus medius muscle.
- Posterior TPs: in the entire muscle at the upper border of its origin.

Referred Pain Areas

- Anterior TPs: pain projects into the lower and lateral buttock, lateral upper leg, knee, and lower leg.
- Posterior TPs: pain projects across the entire buttock, especially inferomedial, and further into the posterior upper leg, popliteal cavity, and proximal third of the lower leg.

Associated Inner Organs

None.

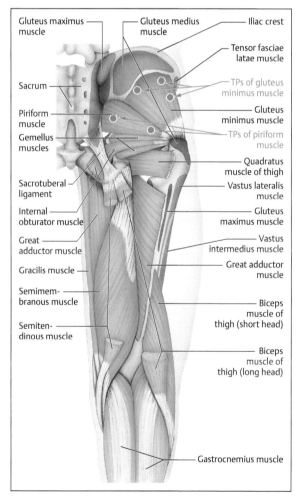

▶ **Fig. 19.108**

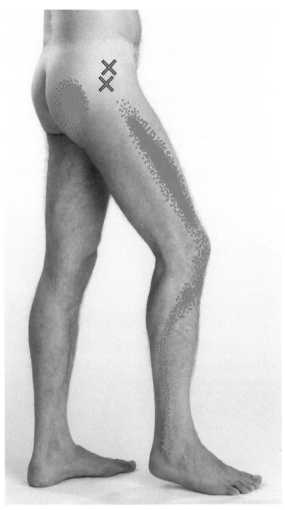

▶ **Fig. 19.109**

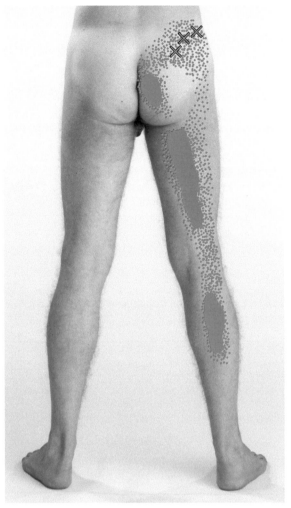

▶ **Fig. 19.110**

Piriform Muscle (▶Figs. 19.108, 19.111)

Origin

Pelvic surface of sacrum in the area of anterior sacral foramina 2 to 4.

Insertion

Greater trochanter.

Action

- External rotation in the hip joint.
- Internal rotation in the hip joint with hip flexed 90 degrees.
- Abduction in the hip joint with hip flexed 90 degrees.

Innervation

Anterior branches of spinal nerves S1–S2.

Trigger Point Location

To guide the localization of these TPs, a line is drawn between the proximal end of the greater trochanter and the point on the sacrum that corresponds to the ilium. The upper border of the piriformis muscle is located approximately on this line.

- TP1: If the guiding line described earlier is divided into thirds, this TP is slightly lateral to the transition from the middle to the lateral third.
- TP2: At the medial end of the guiding line.

Referred Pain Areas

- Sacroiliac joint.
- Entire gluteal area.
- Posterior two-thirds of the upper leg.

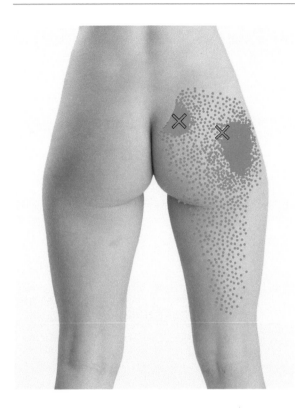

Associated Inner Organs

- Urinary bladder.
- Sigmoid.
- Rectum.
- Uterus, ovaries, appendages, and prostate.

▶ **Fig. 19.111**

Stretching the Piriform Muscle (▶ Fig. 19.112)

Starting Posture

The patient sits on the floor.

Procedure

The side to be stretched is on the right in this example.
- The patient sits upright, with the left leg extended.
- The patient flexes the right leg and places the right foot on the floor above the left knee.

- The patient uses the left hand to pull the right leg to the left side.
- The patient places the right hand on the floor behind the right buttock and rotates the upper body to the right, toward the right hand. This creates a stretch in the lower buttock area.
- The patient holds the stretch for 30 seconds.

▶ **Fig. 19.112** Stretching the piriform muscle.

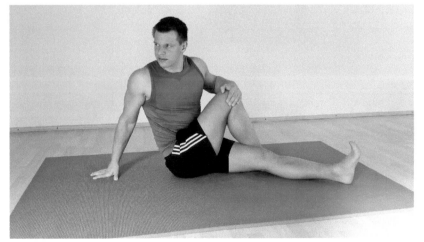

19.6 Hip, Upper Leg, and Knee Pain: Related Muscles

Tensor Fasciae Latae Muscle (▶Figs. 19.113, 19.114)

Origin

Iliac crest between the iliac tubercle and the ASIS (exterior surface).

Insertion

Via the iliotibial tract at the anterior surface of the lateral condyle of tibia.

Action

* Abduction in the hip joint.
* Stabilization of the knee in extension.

Innervation

Superior gluteal nerve (L4–S1).

Trigger Point Location

At the anterior border of the muscle, in the proximal third.

Referred Pain Areas

* Hip joint.
* Anterolateral upper leg, sometimes to the knee.

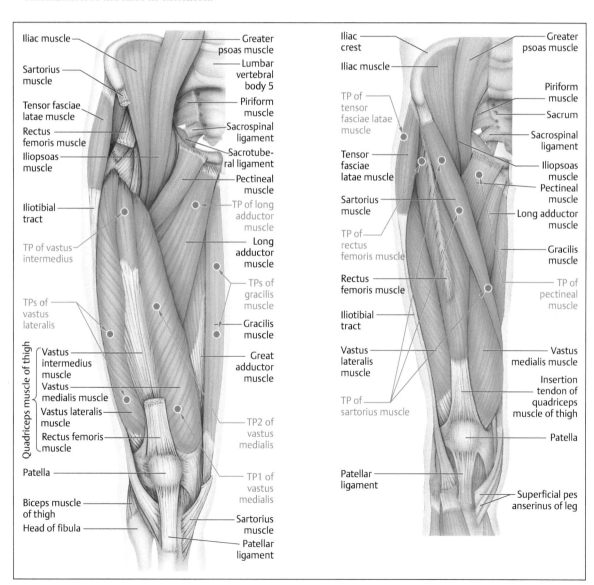

▶ **Fig. 19.113**

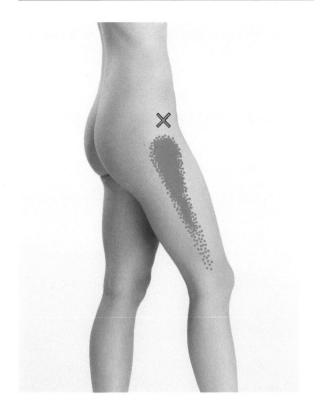

Associated Inner Organs

None.

▶ **Fig. 19.114**

Sartorius Muscle (▶Figs. 19.113, 19.115a–c)

Origin

Slightly below the ASIS.

Insertion

Tibial tuberosity, medial border.

Action

- Flexion in the hip joint.
- Abduction in the hip joint.
- External rotation in the hip joint.
- Flexion in the knee joint.
- Internal rotation in the knee joint.

Innervation

Femoral nerve (L3–L4).

Trigger Point Location

TP1 to 3 are located along the muscle, from proximal to distal.

Referred Pain Areas

Anterior and medial upper leg (along the muscle).

Associated Inner Organs

None.

Pectineal Muscle (▶Figs. 19.113, 19.115d)

Origin

- Pectineal line.
- Superior ramus of the pubic bone.

Insertion

Pectineal line, below the greater trochanter.

Action

- Flexion in the hip joint.
- Adduction in the hip joint.
- Internal rotation in the hip joint.

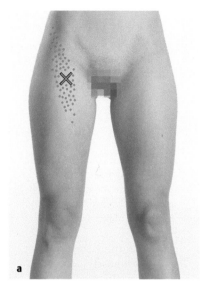

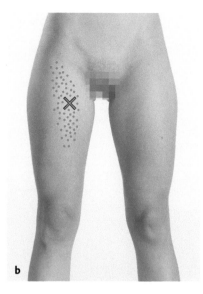

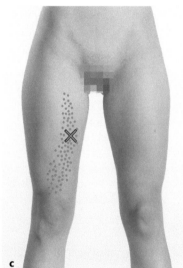

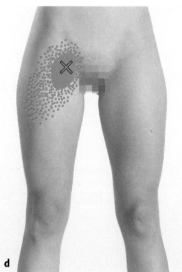

▶ **Fig. 19.115 (a–d)**

Innervation

- Femoral nerve (L2–L3).
- Sometimes also obturator nerve (L2–L3).

Trigger Point Location

Distal to the superior ramus of the pubic bone.

Referred Pain Areas

Deep groin pain immediately below the inguinal ligament.

Associated Inner Organs

- Urinary bladder.
- Uterus, appendages, and prostate.

Quadriceps Muscle of Thigh (▶Figs. 19.113, 19.116–19.118)

■ Rectus Femoris Muscle

Origin

- Anterior inferior iliac spine (AIIS).
- Iliac bone, superior to the acetabulum.
- Lateral lip of the rough line of the femur.
- Lateral supracondylar line.
- Lateral intermuscular septum of the thigh.

■ Vastus Medialis Muscle

Origin

- Lower section of the intertrochanteric line.
- Medial lip of the rough line of the femur.
- Spiral line of the femur.
- Medial intermuscular septum of the thigh.

■ Vastus Intermedius Muscle

Origin

Anterior and exterior surfaces of the femur (up to about a hand's width above the condyles).

■ Vastus Lateralis Muscle

Origin

- Upper section of the intertrochanteric line.
- Greater trochanter.

■ Rectus Femoris, Vastus Lateralis, Vastus Medialis, Vastus Intermedius Muscles

Insertion

- At the patella via the quadriceps tendon.
- At the tibial tuberosity via the patellar ligament.

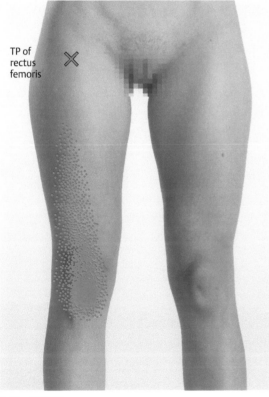

TP of rectus femoris

► **Fig. 19.116**

Action

- Extension in the knee joint.
- Rectus femoris also flexes hip.

Innervation

Femoral nerve (L3–L4).

Trigger Point Location

- TP of the **rectus femoris**: slightly inferior to the AIIS.
- TPs of the **vastus medialis**: at the medial border of the muscle. TP1 is located further distal, slightly above the patella; TP2 is located fairly precisely in the middle of the upper leg.
- TPs of the **vastus intermedius**: these TPs are difficult to palpate because the muscle is hard to examine digitally due to its deep location. The TPs are proximal in the muscle belly, but more distal than the TP of the rectus femoris. These TPs can be accessed by proximal palpation of the lateral borders of the rectus femoris and from there, deep palpation into the upper leg.
- TPs of the **vastus lateralis**: these TPs are very difficult to palpate because of the muscle's deep location inside the upper leg. They are distributed in the entire muscle belly and exhibit their typical referred pain only by compressing the muscle onto the femur.

Referred Pain Areas

- TP of the **rectus femoris**:
  - Knee joint.
  - Around patella.
  - Medial upper leg.
- TPs of the **vastus medialis**: anteromedial knee area (TP1) and upper leg area (TP2).
- TP of the **vastus intermedius**: in the entire anterior upper leg, with maximum in the middle of the upper leg.
- TPs of the **vastus lateralis**: lateral upper leg and knee area.

Associated Inner Organs

None.

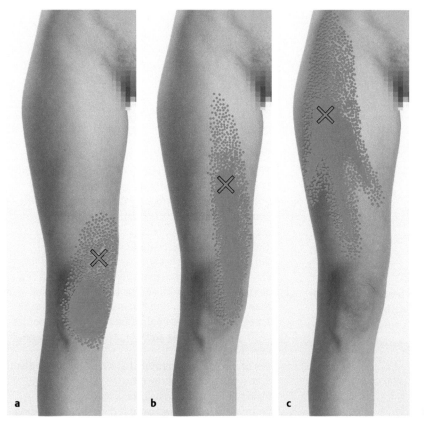

▶ **Fig. 19.117 (a–c)**

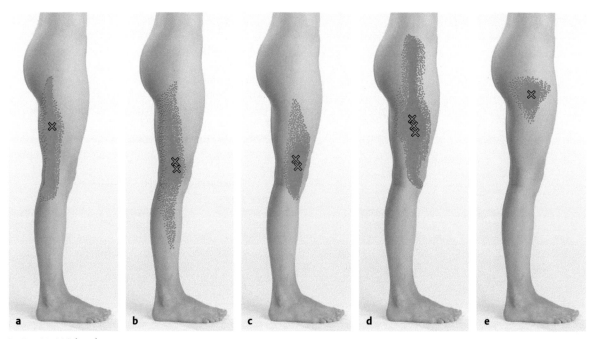

▶ **Fig. 19.118 (a–e)**

Stretching the Quadriceps Muscle of Thigh (▶Fig. 19.119)

Starting Posture

The patient is prone.

Procedure

- On the side to be stretched, the patient grasps the dorsum of the foot and pulls it toward the buttock. The other leg remains flat on the floor. This creates a stretch in the entire anterior upper leg of the side being held.
- The patient holds the stretch for 30 seconds.

If the patient is able to lie on a slightly raised treatment bench, the leg that is not being held can be positioned so that the foot is on the floor. This increases the stretch.

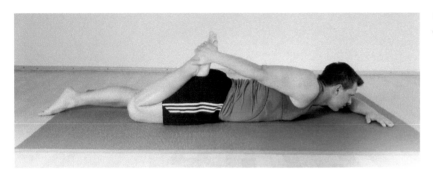

▶ **Fig. 19.119** Stretching the quadriceps muscle of thigh.

Gracilis Muscle (▶Figs. 19.113, 19.120)

Origin

Inferior ramus of the pubic bone (exterior surface).

Insertion

Anterior surface of the tibia (below the sartorius muscle).

Action

- Adduction in the hip joint.
- Flexion in the knee joint.
- Internal rotation in the knee joint (with flexed knee).

Innervation

Obturator nerve (L2–L3).

Trigger Point Location

In the middle third of the muscle belly.

Referred Pain Areas

Inner side of the upper leg.

Associated Inner Organs

- Uterus, appendages.
- Prostate.
- Urinary bladder.

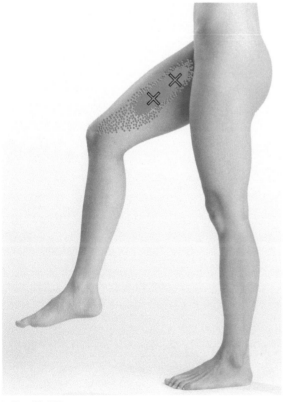

▶ **Fig. 19.120**

Long Adductor Muscle (▶Figs. 19.113, 19.121)

Origin

- Body of the pubic bone.
- Pubic tubercle (below and medial).

Insertion

Medial lip of the rough line of the femur (distal two-thirds).

Action

- Adduction in the hip joint.
- Internal rotation in the hip joint.

Innervation

Obturator nerve (L2–L3).

Short Adductor Muscle (▶Figs. 19.121, 19.122)

Origin

Inferior ramus and body of the pubic bone.

Insertion

Rough line of the femur (proximal third).

Action

Adduction in the hip joint.

Innervation

Obturator nerve (L2–L3).

Trigger Point Locations of Long and Short Adductor Muscles

These TPs can be well palpated by pretensing the muscles through hip flexion and abduction while patient is supine. The TPs are located in the proximal half of the muscles.

Referred Pain Areas of Long and Short Adductor Muscles

- Groin.
- Anteromedial upper leg.
- Suprapatellar.
- Along the edge of the tibia.

Associated Inner Organs

- Uterus, appendages.
- Prostate.
- Testicles.
- Urinary bladder.

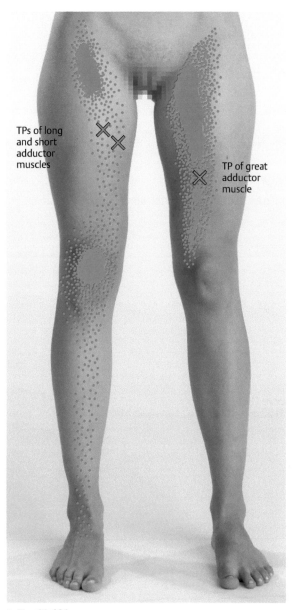

TPs of long and short adductor muscles

TP of great adductor muscle

▶ **Fig. 19.121**

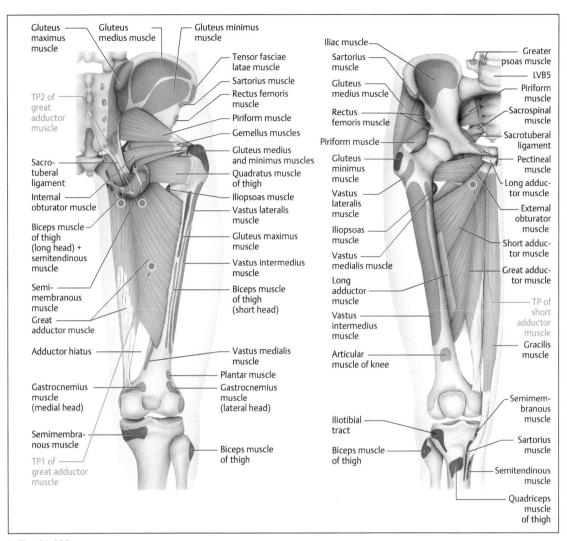

▶ **Fig. 19.122**

Great Adductor Muscle (▶Figs. 19.121, 19.122)

Origin

- Ramus of the ischium.
- Inferior ramus of the pubic bone.
- Ischial tuberosity.

Insertion

- Rough line of the femur up to the gluteal tuberosity.
- Adductor tubercle of the femur.

Action

- Extension in the hip joint.
- Adduction in the hip joint.
- Internal rotation in the hip joint.

Innervation

- Obturator nerve (L2–L4).
- Tibial nerve (L4–S3).

Trigger Point Location

- TP1: In the middle of the muscle, near insertion at the rough line of the femur.
- TP2: Near origin at the ischium and the pubic bone.

Referred Pain Areas

- TP1: Groin and anteromedial upper leg, not quite to the knee.
- TP2: Pubic bone, vagina, rectum, urinary bladder, or other diffuse pain in the lesser pelvis.

Associated Inner Organs

- Uterus, appendages.
- Prostate.
- Urinary bladder.

Stretching the Short Hip Adductors (▶ Fig. 19.123)

Starting Posture

The patient is seated on the floor.

Procedure

- The patient places soles of the feet together, holds the feet with the hands, and pushes the knees toward the floor using the lower arms and elbows. This creates a stretch in the proximal medial upper leg on both sides.
- The patient holds this stretch for 30 seconds.

Stretching the Long Hip Adductors (▶ Fig. 19.124)

Starting Posture

The patient is standing with legs apart in front of a stool or chair.

Procedure

- The patient flexes the knee of one leg while placing the lower arms on the stool/chair for support. The other leg remains extended on the floor. This creates a stretch of the entire medial upper leg on the extended side.
- The patient holds the stretch for 30 seconds.

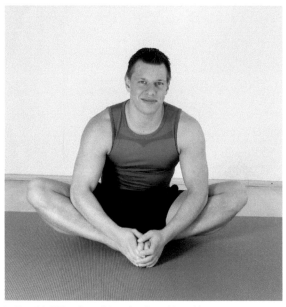

▶ **Fig. 19.123** Stretching the short hip adductors.

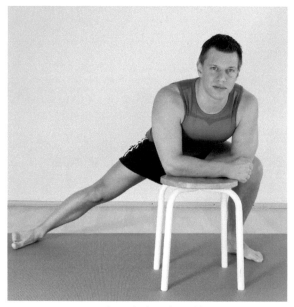

▶ **Fig. 19.124** Stretching the long hip adductors.

Biceps Muscle of Thigh (▶Figs. 19.125, 19.126)

Origin

- Ischial tuberosity (posterior surface).
- Lateral lip of the rough line of the femur (middle third).

Insertion

- Apex of the head of the fibula.
- Lateral supracondylar line of the femur.
- Fibular collateral ligament.
- Lateral condyle of the tibia.

Action

- Extension in the hip joint.
- Flexion in the knee joint.
- External rotation in the knee joint.

Innervation

Tibial and common peroneal nerve (L4–S3).

Trigger Point Location

Several TPs are found in the middle third of the postero-lateral upper leg.

Referred Pain Areas

- Popliteal cavity (main area of pain).
- Proximal posterolateral lower leg.
- Posterolateral upper leg, short of the gluteal fold.

Associated Inner Organs

None.

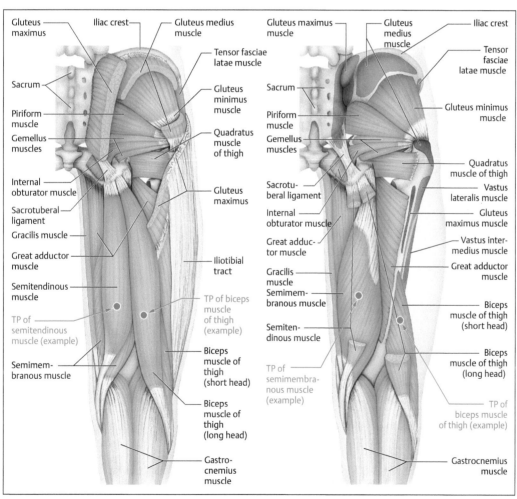

▶ **Fig. 19.125**

Semitendinous Muscle (▶Figs. 19.125, 19.126)

Origin

Ischial tuberosity (posterior area).

Insertion

Medial tibia surface (below the gracilis muscle).

Action

- Extension in the hip joint.
- Flexion in the knee joint.
- Internal rotation in the knee joint.

Innervation

Tibial nerve (L5–S1).

Semimembranous Muscle (▶Figs. 19.125, 19.126)

Origin

Ischial tuberosity (posterior surface).

Insertion

- Medial condyle of the tibia.
- Oblique popliteal ligament.
- Fascia of the popliteal muscle.

Action

- Extension in the hip joint.
- Flexion in the knee joint.
- Internal rotation in the knee joint.

Innervation

Tibial nerve (L5–S1).

Trigger Point Location

Several TPs are found in the middle third of the postero-medial upper leg.

Referred Pain Areas

- Inferior end of the buttock and the gluteal fold (main area of pain).
- Posteromedial upper leg.
- Medial half of the popliteal cavity and calf.

Associated Inner Organs

None.

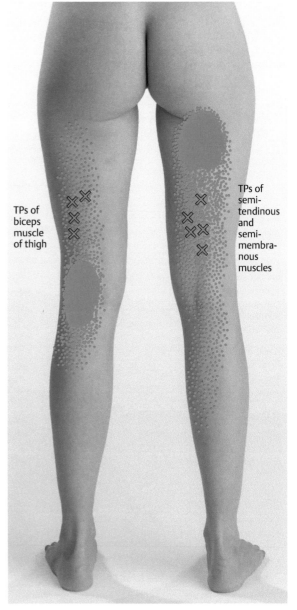

TPs of biceps muscle of thigh

TPs of semi-tendinous and semi-membra-nous muscles

▶ **Fig. 19.126**

Stretching the Ischiocrural Muscles (►Fig. 19.127)

Starting Posture

The patient is standing in the gait posture.

Procedure

- The patient places the leg of the side to be stretched forward and extends the knee joint.
- The patient places the arms on the back and bends the upper body forward. It is important that the upper body remains erect and extended, which is supported by the placement of the arms on the back. This creates a stretch on the posterior side of the upper leg.
- The patient holds the stretch for 30 seconds.

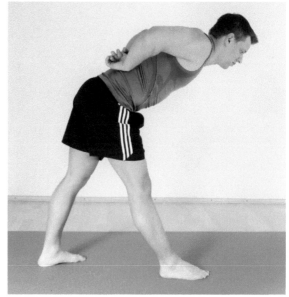

► **Fig. 19.127**   Stretching the ischiocrural muscles.

Popliteal Muscle (►Figs. 19.128, 19.129)

Origin

Posterior surface of the tibia (above the soleal line of the tibia and below the tibial condyles).

Insertion

- Lateral epicondyle of the femur.
- Radiates into the knee joint capsule.
- Connection to the lateral meniscus (posterior horn).

Action

- Internal rotation in the knee joint.
- Draws lateral meniscus backward.

Innervation

Tibial nerve (L5–S1).

Trigger Point Location

In the proximal half of the muscle origin, near the tibia.

Referred Pain Areas

Popliteal cavity.

Associated Inner Organs

None.

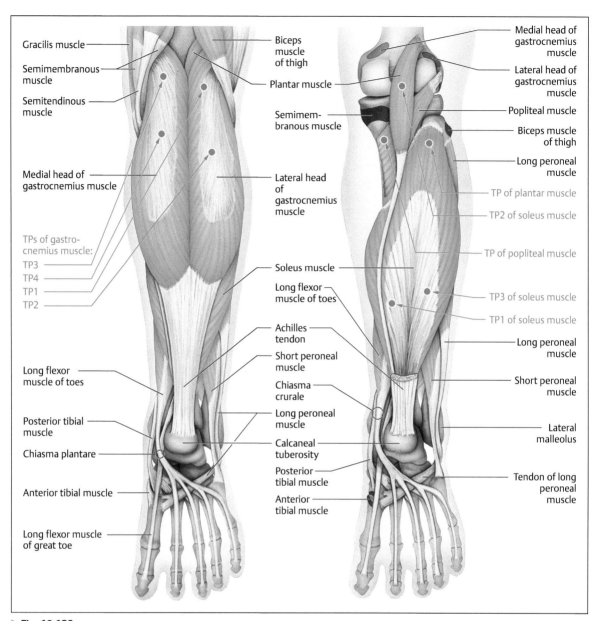

Gracilis muscle

Semimembranous muscle

Semitendinous muscle

Medial head of gastrocnemius muscle

TPs of gastro-
cnemius muscle:
TP3
TP4
TP1
TP2

Long flexor muscle of toes

Posterior tibial muscle

Chiasma plantare

Anterior tibial muscle

Long flexor muscle of great toe

Biceps muscle of thigh

Plantar muscle

Semimem-
branous muscle

Lateral head of gastrocnemius muscle

Soleus muscle

Long flexor muscle of toes

Achilles tendon

Short peroneal muscle

Chiasma crurale

Long peroneal muscle

Calcaneal tuberosity

Posterior tibial muscle

Anterior tibial muscle

Medial head of gastrocnemius muscle

Lateral head of gastrocnemius muscle

Popliteal muscle

Biceps muscle of thigh

Long peroneal muscle

TP of plantar muscle

TP2 of soleus muscle

TP of popliteal muscle

TP3 of soleus muscle

TP1 of soleus muscle

Long peroneal muscle

Short peroneal muscle

Lateral malleolus

Tendon of long peroneal muscle

▶ **Fig. 19.128**

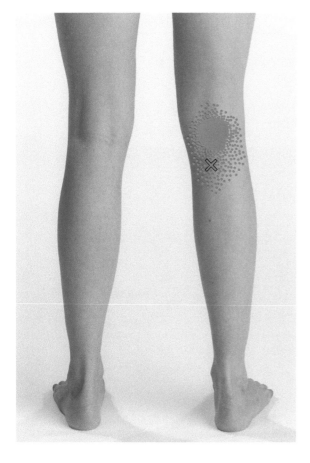

▶ **Fig. 19.129**

19.7 Lower Leg, Ankle, and Foot Pain: Related Muscles

Anterior Tibial Muscle (▶Figs. 19.130, 19.131)

Origin

- Lateral surface of the tibia (the proximal half).
- Interosseous membrane.

Insertion

- Medial cuneiform bone (plantar area).
- Base of the first metacarpal bone.

Action

- Posterior extension.
- Inversion of the foot.
- Stabilization of the longitudinal arch of the foot.

Innervation

Deep peroneal nerve (L4–L5).

Trigger Point Location

In the upper third of the muscle belly (transition from the proximal to the middle third of the lower leg).

Referred Pain Areas

- Anteromedial area of the upper ankle joint.
- Posterior and medial at the great toe.
- Narrowband radiating from TP anteromedial along the lower leg to the great toe.

Associated Inner Organs

None.

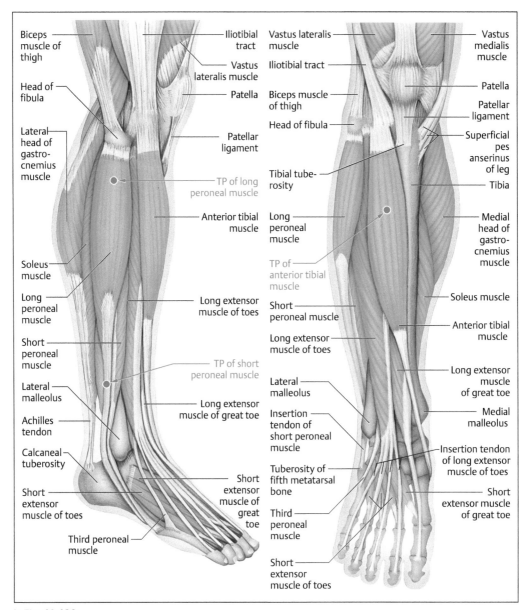

▶ **Fig. 19.130**

Posterior Tibial Muscle (Figs. 19.132, 19.133)

Origin

Posterior tibia and fibula surfaces (between the medial crest of the fibula, interosseous borders of the tibia and the fibula, and the interosseous membrane of the leg).

Insertion

- Tuberosity of the navicular bone.
- All tarsal bones (except talus).
- Medial tarsal ligaments (e.g., deltoid ligament of the ankle).

Action

- Plantar flexion.
- Inversion of foot.
- Stabilization of longitudinal arch of the foot.

Innervation

Tibial nerve (L4–L5).

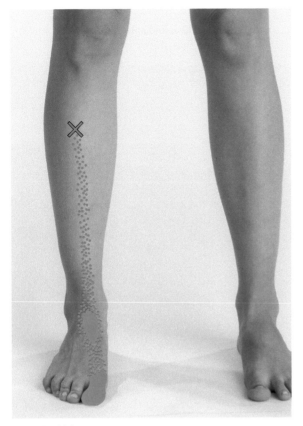

▶ **Fig. 19.131**

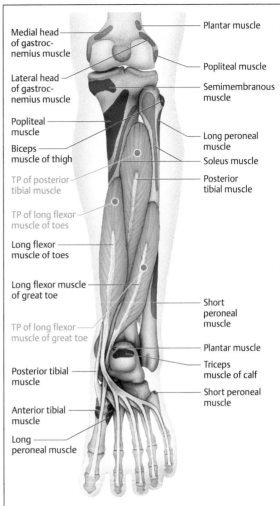

Medial head of gastrocnemius muscle

Lateral head of gastrocnemius muscle

Popliteal muscle

Biceps muscle of thigh

TP of posterior tibial muscle

TP of long flexor muscle of toes

Long flexor muscle of toes

Long flexor muscle of great toe

TP of long flexor muscle of great toe

Posterior tibial muscle

Anterior tibial muscle

Long peroneal muscle

Plantar muscle

Popliteal muscle

Semimembranous muscle

Long peroneal muscle

Soleus muscle

Posterior tibial muscle

Short peroneal muscle

Plantar muscle

Triceps muscle of calf

Short peroneal muscle

▶ **Fig. 19.132**

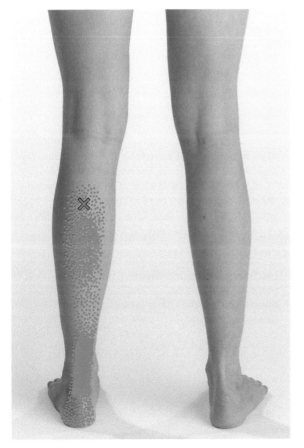

▶ **Fig. 19.133**

Trigger Point Location

Lateral to the posterior edge of the tibia and in the proximal quarter of the interosseous membrane. It can only be palpated through the soleus muscle.

Referred Pain Areas

- Calcaneal (Achilles) tendon (the main area of pain).

Long Peroneal Muscle (▶Figs. 19.130, 19.134)

Origin

- Lateral surface of the tibia (proximal two-thirds).
- Head of the fibula.
- Tibiofibular joint.

Insertion

- Base of the first metatarsal bone.
- Medial cuneiform bone.

Action

- Plantar flexion.
- Eversion of the foot.
- Stabilization of the transverse arch of the foot.

Innervation

Superficial peroneal nerve (L5–S1).

Short Peroneal Muscle (▶Figs. 19.130, 19.134)

Origin

Lateral surface of the tibia (distal two-thirds).

Insertion

Tuberosity of the fifth metatarsal bone.

Action

- Dorsiflexion.
- Eversion of the foot.
- Stabilization of the transverse arch of the foot.

Innervation

Superficial peroneal nerve (L5–S1).

- Radiating from TP to inferior in the middle of the lower leg via the heel and sole of foot to toes 1 to 5.

Associated Inner Organs

None.

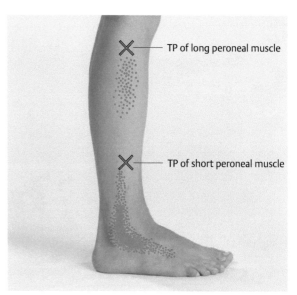

TP of long peroneal muscle

TP of short peroneal muscle

▶ **Fig. 19.134**

Trigger Point Locations for Long and Short Peroneal Muscles

- TP of **long peroneal muscle**: 2 to 4 cm distal to the head of the fibula above the body of the fibula.
- TP of **short peroneal muscle**: at the border between the middle and distal third of the lower leg, on both sides of the tendon of the long peroneal muscle.

Referred Pain Areas

- Lateral malleolus, also superior, inferior, and posterior to that area.
- Middle third of the lateral lower leg.
- Lateral on the foot.

Associated Inner Organs

None.

Third Peroneal Muscle (▶Fig. 19.135)

Origin

Anterior border of the fibula (distal third).

Insertion

Fifth metatarsal bone.

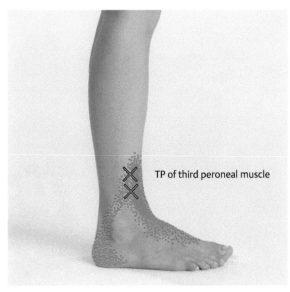

▶ **Fig. 19.135**

Action

- Dorsiflexion.
- Eversion of the foot.

Innervation

Deep peroneal nerve (L5–S1).

Trigger Point Location

Slightly distal and anterior to the TP for the short peroneal muscle.

Referred Pain Areas

- Anterolateral on the upper ankle joint and dorsum of the foot.
- Posterior of the lateral malleolus radiating toward the lateral heel.

Associated Inner Organs

None.

Gastrocnemius Muscle (▶Figs. 19.128, 19.136, 19.137)

Origin

Medial and lateral condyle of the femur.

Insertion

Calcaneal tuberosity (via the calcaneal tendon).

Action

- Plantar flexion.
- Knee flexion.

Innervation

Tibial nerve (S1–S2).

Trigger Point Location

- TPs 1 and 2: Slightly proximal of the middle of the muscle bellies: one TP each in the medial and lateral head of the gastrocnemius muscle.

- TPs 3 and 4: In the medial and lateral head of the gastrocnemius muscle, near the condyles.

Referred Pain Areas

- TP1:
  - Medial on sole of the foot.
  - Posteromedial lower leg.
  - Popliteal cavity and part of the posterior upper leg.
- TPs 2 to 4: Referred pain for these three TPs is found locally around the respective TP.

Associated Inner Organs

None.

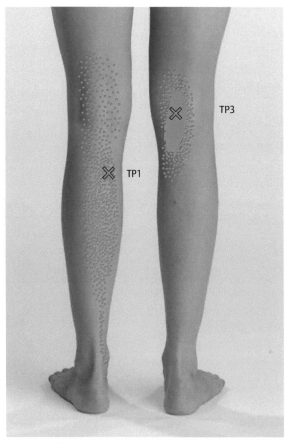

► **Fig. 19.136**

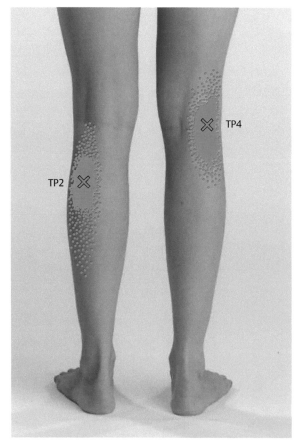

► **Fig. 19.137**

Soleus Muscle (►Figs. 19.128, 19.138)

Origin

- Soleal line of the tibia.
- Posterior surface of the tibia (middle third).
- Neck of the fibula and posterior surface of the fibula (proximal quarter).

Insertion

Calcaneal tuberosity (via the calcaneal tendon).

Action

Plantar flexion.

Innervation

Tibial nerve (S1–S2).

Trigger Point Location

- TP1: 2 to 3 cm distal to the heads of the gastrocnemius muscle and slightly medial to the median line.
- TP2: Near the head of the fibula (lateral in the calf).
- TP3: Further proximal than TP1 and lateral to the median line.

Referred Pain Areas

- TP1:
  - Calcaneal tendon.
  - Posterior and plantar heel.
  - Sole of the foot.
  - Slightly proximal of the TP.
- TP2: Upper half of the calf.
- TP3: Sacroiliac joint, ipsilateral.

Associated Inner Organs

None.

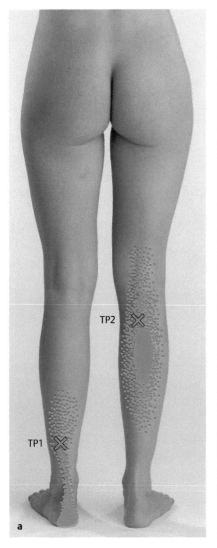
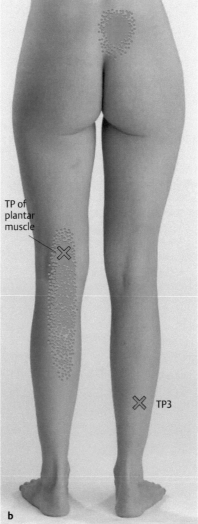

TP of
plantar
muscle

TP2

TP1

TP3

a

b

► **Fig. 19.138 (a, b)**

Plantar Muscle (►Figs. 19.128, 19.138b)

Origin

Lateral epicondyle of the femur (proximal to the head of the gastrocnemius muscle).

Insertion

Calcaneal tendon (medial, below the tendon of the gastrocnemius muscle).

Action

• Plantar flexion.
• Knee flexion.

Innervation

Tibial nerve (S1–S2).

Trigger Point Location

In the middle of the popliteal cavity.

Referred Pain Areas

Popliteal cavity and calf to about the middle of the lower leg.

Associated Inner Organs

None.

Stretching the Calf Muscles (▶Fig. 19.139)

Starting Posture

The patient is standing in the gait posture in front of stairs, a wall, or a cabinet.

Procedure

- The patient places both hands on the wall for support.
- The patient places the foot of the side to be stretched against the wall, with foot and toes flexed, heel firmly planted on the floor, and knee extended.
- The patient moves the upper body toward the wall. The heel should not move. This creates a stretch in the posterior lower leg.
- The patient holds the stretch for 30 seconds.

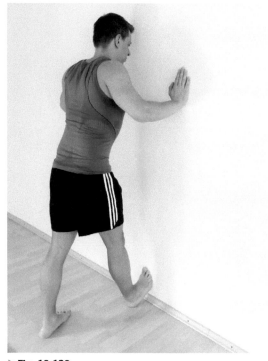

▶ **Fig. 19.139**

Long Extensor Muscle of Toes (▶Figs. 19.140, 19.141a)

Origin

- Fibula (anterior proximal two-thirds).
- Interosseous membrane.
- Tibiofibular joint.

Insertion

Dorsal digital expansion (extensor expansion) of toes 2 to 5.

Action

Posterior extension of the toes and foot.

Innervation

Deep peroneal nerve (L5–S1).

Trigger Point Location

About 8 cm distal to the head of the fibula, between the long peroneal muscle and the anterior tibial muscle.

Referred Pain Areas

- Dorsum of the foot, including toes 2 to 4.
- Anterior lower leg (inferior half).

Associated Inner Organs

None.

Long Extensor Muscle of Great Toe (▶Figs. 19.140, 19.141b)

Origin

Fibula (middle anterior area).

Insertion

Base of the distal phalanx of the great toe.

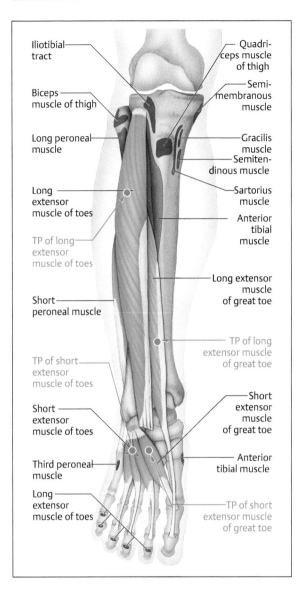

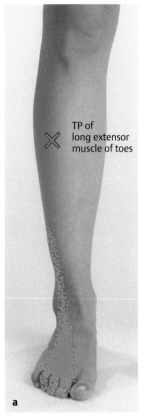
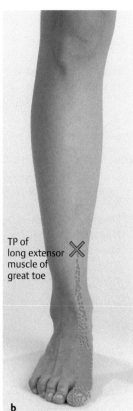

▶ **Fig. 19.141 (a, b)**

▶ **Fig. 19.140**

Action

- Posterior extension of the great toe and foot.
- Inversion of the foot.

Innervation

Deep peroneal nerve (L5–S1).

Trigger Point Location

Slightly distal to transition from the middle to the inferior third of the lower leg and anterior to the fibula. Located between long extensor muscles of the toes and the anterior tibial muscle.

Referred Pain Areas

Dorsum of the foot in the area of the first metatarsal bone and of the great toe, sometimes radiating in a narrow band up to the TP.

Associated Inner Organs

None.

Long Flexor Muscle of Toes (▶Figs. 19.132, 19.142, 19.143)

Origin

- Posterior surface of the tibia (distal to the soleal line of the tibia).
- Fibula (via the tendinous arch of the soleus muscle).

Insertion

Base of distal phalanges of toes 2 to 5.

Action

- Flexion of the distal phalanges of the toes.
- Plantar flexion.
- Stabilization of the longitudinal arch of the foot.

Innervation

Tibial nerve (S1–S2).

Trigger Point Location

This TP is palpated by displacing the medial belly of the gastrocnemius muscle. It is located on the posterior tibia surface, in the proximal third of the medial calf area.

Referred Pain Areas

- Sole of the foot (mediolateral) to toes 2 to 5 (main radiation).
- Lateral malleolus and lateral calf area up to TP.

Associated Inner Organs

None.

Long Flexor Muscle of Great Toe (▶Figs. 19.132, 19.142, 19.144)

Origin

- Posterior surface of the fibula (distal two-thirds).
- Intermuscular septum.
- Aponeurosis of the long flexor muscle of toes.

Insertion

- Base of the proximal phalanx of the great toe.
- Fibers to both medial tendons of the long flexor muscle of toes.

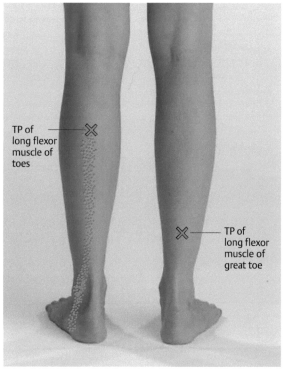

TP of long flexor muscle of toes

TP of long flexor muscle of great toe

▶ **Fig. 19.142**

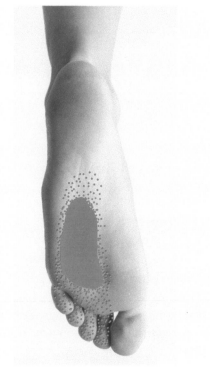

▶ **Fig. 19.143**

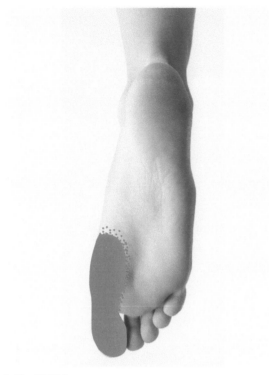

Action

- Flexion of the proximal phalanx of the great toe.
- Plantar flexion.
- Stabilization of the longitudinal arch of the foot.

Innervation

Tibial nerve (S2–S3).

Trigger Point Location

At transition from the middle to the inferior third of the lower leg and slightly lateral to the median line on the posterior fibula surface. This TP is palpated through the superficial calf muscles.

Referred Pain Areas

Plantar area of the great toe and the first metatarsal bone.

Associated Inner Organs

None.

Short Extensor Muscle of Toes (▶Figs. 19.140, 19.145)

Origin

Calcaneus (posterior surface).

Insertion

- Proximal phalanx of the great toe.
- Toes 2 to 4 (via the long extensor tendons).

Action

Toe extensor.

Innervation

Deep peroneal nerve (L5–S1).

Trigger Point Location

In the first third of the muscle bellies.

Referred Pain Areas

Area of the medial dorsum of the foot near the ankle.

Associated Inner Organs

None.

Short Extensor Muscle of Great Toe (▶Figs. 19.140, 19.145)

Origin

Posterior area of the calcaneus.

Insertion

- Dorsal digital expansion (extensor expansion) of the great toe.
- Base of the proximal phalanx of the great toe.

Action

Posterior extension in the metatarsophalangeal joint of the great toe.

Innervation

Deep peroneal nerve (L5–S1).

Trigger Point Location

In the first third of the muscle belly.

Referred Pain Areas

Area of medial dorsum of the foot near the ankle joint.

Associated Inner Organs

None.

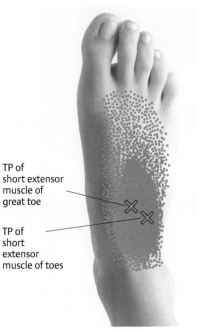

TP of
short extensor
muscle of
great toe

TP of
short
extensor
muscle of toes

▶ **Fig. 19.145**

Abductor Muscle of Great Toe (▶Figs. 19.146, 19.147)

Origin

- Medial process of the calcaneal tuberosity.
- Flexor retinaculum of the foot.

Insertion

Proximal phalanx of the great toe (medial).

Action

- Abduction of the great toe.
- Plantar flexion.

Innervation

Medial plantar nerve (S1–S2).

Trigger Point Location

In the muscle belly, distributed at the inner edge of the foot.

Referred Pain Areas

Inner side of the heel and inner edge of the foot.

Associated Inner Organs

None.

Short Flexor Muscle of Toes (▶Figs. 19.146, 19.148)

Origin

Calcaneal tuberosity (plantar).

Insertion

Middle phalanges of toes 2 to 5 (split tendons).

Action

- Flexion of toes 2 to 5.
- Stabilization of arch of foot.

Innervation

Medial plantar nerve (S1–S2).

Trigger Point Location

In muscle belly, in proximal middle area of the sole of the foot.

Referred Pain Areas

Metatarsal heads 2 to 4 with only minor tendency to radiate further.

Associated Inner Organs

None.

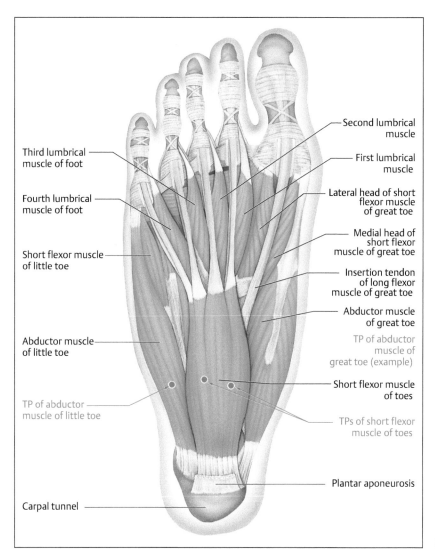

Third lumbrical
muscle of foot

Fourth lumbrical
muscle of foot

Short flexor muscle
of little toe

Abductor muscle
of little toe

TP of abductor
muscle of little toe

Carpal tunnel

Second lumbrical
muscle

First lumbrical
muscle

Lateral head of short
flexor muscle
of great toe

Medial head of
short flexor
muscle of great toe

Insertion tendon
of long flexor
muscle of great toe

Abductor muscle
of great toe

TP of abductor
muscle of
great toe (example)

Short flexor muscle
of toes

TPs of short flexor
muscle of toes

Plantar aponeurosis

▶ **Fig. 19.146**

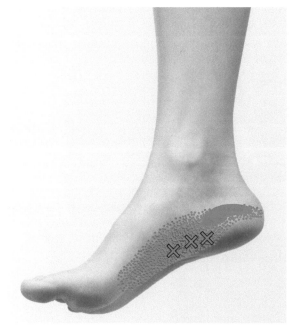

▶ **Fig. 19.147**

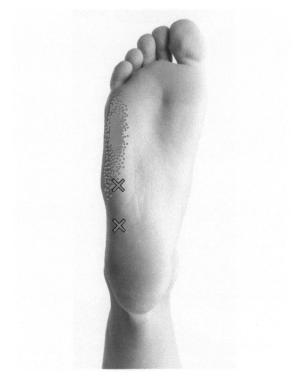

▶ **Fig. 19.148**   ▶ **Fig. 19.149**

Abductor Muscle of Little Toe (▶ Figs. 19.146, 19.149)

Origin

Medial and lateral processes of the calcaneal tuberosity.

Insertion

- Base of the proximal phalanx of toe 5 (lateral).
- Fifth metatarsal bone.

Action

- Flexion of toe 5.
- Abduction of toe 5.
- Stabilization of the longitudinal arch of the foot.

Innervation

Lateral plantar nerve (S2–S3).

Trigger Point Location

In the muscle belly, distributed at the outer edge of the sole of the foot.

Referred Pain Areas

Fifth metatarsal head, with only minor tendency toward radiating into the lateral area of the sole of the foot.

Associated Inner Organs

None.

Quadratus Plantae Muscle (▶ Figs. 19.150, 19.151)

Origin

Two-headed from the margins of the calcaneus.

Insertion

Tendon of the long flexor muscle of the toes.

Action

Helps with flexion of toes 2 to 5.

Innervation

Lateral plantar nerve (S2–S3).

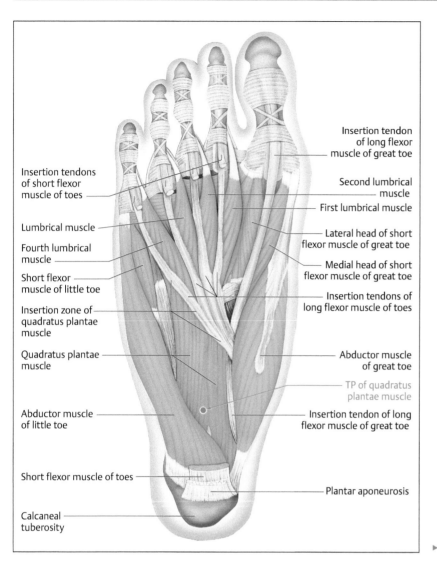

Insertion tendon of long flexor muscle of great toe

Insertion tendons of short flexor muscle of toes

Second lumbrical muscle

First lumbrical muscle

Lumbrical muscle

Lateral head of short flexor muscle of great toe

Fourth lumbrical muscle

Medial head of short flexor muscle of great toe

Short flexor muscle of little toe

Insertion tendons of long flexor muscle of toes

Insertion zone of quadratus plantae muscle

Quadratus plantae muscle

Abductor muscle of great toe

TP of quadratus plantae muscle

Abductor muscle of little toe

Insertion tendon of long flexor muscle of great toe

Short flexor muscle of toes

Plantar aponeurosis

Calcaneal tuberosity

▶ **Fig. 19.150**

Trigger Point Location

Palpable immediately in front of the heel through the plantar aponeurosis.

Referred Pain Areas

Plantar area of the heel.

Associated Inner Organs

None.

Dorsal Interosseous Muscles of Foot (▶Figs. 19.151, 19.152)

Origin

Two-headed from the interior surfaces of all the metatarsal bones.

Insertion

- Base of the proximal phalanges (toe 2: medial side; toes 2 to 4: lateral side).
- Dorsal digital expansion (extensor expansion) of the toes.

Action

Abduction of toes 2 to 4.

Innervation

Lateral plantar nerve (S2–S3).

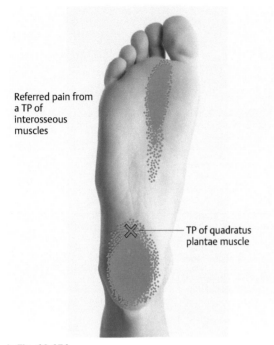

Referred pain from a TP of interosseous muscles

TP of quadratus plantae muscle

▶ **Fig. 19.151**

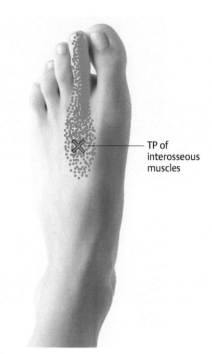

TP of interosseous muscles

▶ **Fig. 19.152**

Plantar Interosseous Muscles (▶Figs. 19.151–19.153)

Origin

One-headed from metatarsal bones 3 to 5.

Insertion

* Base of proximal phalanges of toes 3 to 5.
* Dorsal digital expansion (extensor expansion) of the toes.

Action

Adduction of toes 3 to 5.

Innervation

Lateral plantar nerve (S2–S3).

Trigger Point Location

Palpable between the metatarsal bones from plantar and posterior.

Referred Pain Areas

Referred pain from these TPs is found along the side of the toe where the muscle tendon inserts. Pain can project toward posterior as well as toward plantar.

Associated Inner Organs

None.

Adductor Muscle of Great Toe (▶Figs. 19.153, 19.154)

Origin

* Oblique head: base of metatarsal bones 2 to 4.
* Transverse head: capsular ligaments of metatarsophalangeal joints 3 to 5 and deep transverse metatarsal ligament.

Insertion

* Lateral sesamoid bone.
* Proximal phalanx of the great toe (lateral).

Action

* Adduction of the great toe.
* Flexion of the great toe.
* Stabilization of transverse and longitudinal arches of the foot.

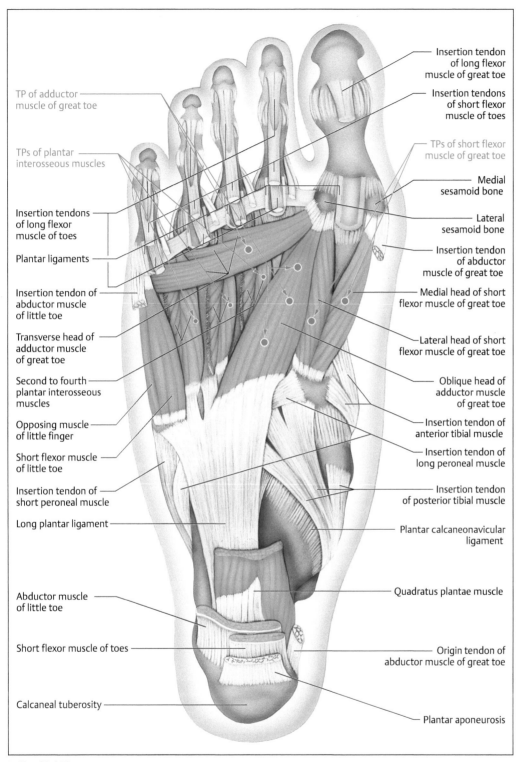

TP of adductor
muscle of great toe

TPs of plantar
interosseous muscles

Insertion tendons
of long flexor
muscle of toes

Plantar ligaments

Insertion tendon of
abductor muscle
of little toe

Transverse head of
adductor muscle
of great toe

Second to fourth
plantar interosseous
muscles

Opposing muscle
of little finger

Short flexor muscle
of little toe

Insertion tendon of
short peroneal muscle

Long plantar ligament

Abductor muscle
of little toe

Short flexor muscle of toes

Calcaneal tuberosity

Insertion tendon
of long flexor
muscle of great toe

Insertion tendons
of short flexor
muscle of toes

TPs of short flexor
muscle of great toe

Medial
sesamoid bone

Lateral
sesamoid bone

Insertion tendon
of abductor
muscle of great toe

Medial head of short
flexor muscle of great toe

Lateral head of short
flexor muscle of great toe

Oblique head of
adductor muscle
of great toe

Insertion tendon of
anterior tibial muscle

Insertion tendon of
long peroneal muscle

Insertion tendon
of posterior tibial muscle

Plantar calcaneonavicular
ligament

Quadratus plantae muscle

Origin tendon of
abductor muscle of great toe

Plantar aponeurosis

▶ **Fig. 19.153**

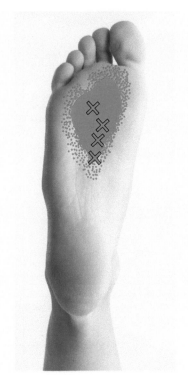

▶ **Fig. 19.154**

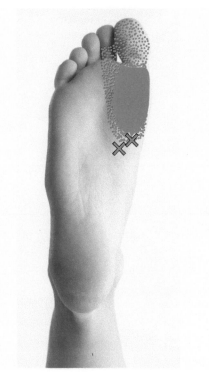

▶ **Fig. 19.155**

Innervation

Lateral plantar nerve (S2–S3).

Referred Pain Areas

In area around metatarsal heads 1 to 4.

Trigger Point Location

Palpable in the area of the metatarsal heads 1 to 4 through the aponeurosis.

Associated Inner Organs

None.

Short Flexor Muscle of Great Toe (▶Figs. 19.153, 19.155, 19.156)

Origin

- Cuboid bone.
- Cuneiform bones 1 to 3.

Insertion

Base of metatarsophalangeal joint of the great toe (running with one tendon, respectively, lateral and medial across the sesamoid bones).

Action

- Flexion of the great toe.
- Stabilization of the arch of the foot.

Innervation

Tibial nerve (S2–S3).

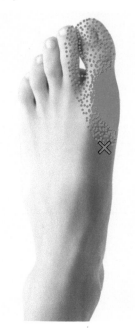

▶ **Fig. 19.156**

Trigger Point Location

At the medial inner edge of the foot, slightly proximal to the metatarsal head 1.

Referred Pain Areas

Plantar and medial around metatarsal head 1 and involving toes 1 and 2.

Associated Inner Organs

None.

20 Bibliography

Muscle Chains (Richter)

1. Ahonen J, Lathinen T, Sandström M, Pogliani G, Wirhed R. Sportmedizin und Trainingslehre. Stuttgart: Schattauer; 1999
2. American Academy of Osteopathy. 52 AAO Yearbooks from 1938–1998. Indianapolis, IN: AAO; 2001
3. Amigues J. Osteopathie-Kompendium. Stuttgart: Sonntag; 2004
4. Arbuckle BG. The Selected Writings. Indianapolis, IN: AAO; 1994
5. Barral J. Le Thorax. Paris: Maloine; 1989
6. Barral J. Manipulations Uro-Genitales. Paris: Maloine; 1984
7. Barral JP, Croibier A. Trauma. Ein Osteopathischer Ansatz. Bad Kötzting: Verlag f. Ganzheitl. Med.; 2003
8. Becker RE. Life in Motion. Fort Worth, TX: Stillness Press; 1997
9. Becker RE. The Stillness of Life. Fort Worth, TX: Stillness Press; 2000
10. Beckers D, Deckers J. Ganganalyse und Gangschulung. Berlin: Springer; 1997
11. Benichou A. Os clés, os suspendus. Paris: Ed. SPEK; 2001
12. van den Berg F. Angewandte Physiologie. Stuttgart: Thieme; 2002
13. Bobath B. Hémiplegie de l'adulte bilans et traitement. Paris: Masson; 1978
14. Bogduk N. Klinische Anatomie von Lendenwirbelsäule und Sakrum. Berlin: Springer; 2000
15. Boland U. Logiques de pathologies orthopédiques en chaînes ascendantes et descendantes et la méthode exploratoire des "Delta Pondéral". Paris: Ed. Frison-Roche; 1996
16. Bouchet A. Cuilleret J. Anatomie, Tome I–IV. Paris: SIMEP; 1983
17. Bourdiol RJ. Pied et statique. Paris: Maisonneuve; 1980
18. Bricot B. La Reprogrammation Posturale Globale. Montpellier: Sauramps Medical; 1996
19. Brokmeier A. Manuelle Therapie. 3rd ed. Stuttgart: Hippokrates; 2001
20. Brügger A. Die Erkrankungen des Bewegungsapparates und seines Nervensystems. Stuttgart: G. Fischer; 1997
21. Buck M, Beckers D, Adler SS. PNF in der Praxis. Berlin: Springer; 2001
22. Buekens J. Osteopathische Diagnose und Behandlung. Stuttgart: Hippokrates; 1997
23. van Buskirk RL. The Still Technique. Indianapolis, IN: AAO; 2000
24. Busquet L, Gabarel B. Ophtalmologie et osteopathie. Paris: Maloine; 1988
25. Busquet L. Les chaines musculaires du tronc et de la colonne cervicale. 2ième édition. Paris: Maloine; 1985
26. Busquet L. Les chaînes musculaires traitement crâne. Paris: Ed. Frison-Roche; 2004
27. Busquet L. Les chaînes musculaires, Tome II. Lordosecyphoses- scolioses et déformations thoraciques. Paris: Ed. Frison-Roche; 1992
28. Busquet L. Les chaînes musculaires, Tome III. La pubalgie. Paris: Ed. Frison-Roche; 1993
29. Busquet L. Les chaînes musculaires, Tome IV. Membres inférieurs. Paris: Ed. Frison-Roche; 1995
30. Busquet-Vanderheyden M. Les chaines musculaires la chaine viscérale. Paris: Ed. Busquet; 2004
31. Butler DS. Rehabilitation und Prävention. Berlin: Springer; 1998
32. Calais-Germain B. Anatomie pour le mouvement. Méolans-Revel: Editions Désiris; 1991
33. Calais-Germain B. Le périnée feminin. Arques: Prodim; 1997
34. Cambier J, Dehen H, Poirier J, Ribadeau-Dimas JL. Propédeutique neurologique. Paris: Masson; 1976
35. Cathie AG. The Writings and Lectures of A.G. Cathie. Indianapolis, IN: AAO; 1974
36. Ceccaldi A, Favre JF. Les pivots ostéopathiques. Paris: Masson; 1986
37. Chaitow L. Cranial Manipulation Theory and Practice. Edinburgh: Churchill Livingstone; 2000
38. Chaitow L. Fibromyalgia Syndrom. Edinburgh: Churchill Livingstone; 2000
39. Chaitow L. Maintaining Body Balance Flexibility and Stability. Edinburgh: Churchill Livingstone; 2004
40. Chaitow L. Modern Neuromuscular Techniques. Edinburgh: Churchill Livingstone; 1997
41. Chaitow L. Muscle Energy Techniques. Edinburgh: Churchill Livingstone; 2001
42. Chaitow L. Palpation Skills. Edinburgh: Churchill Livingstone; 2000
43. Chaitow L. Positional Release Techniques. Edinburgh: Churchill Livingstone; 2002
44. Chapman F. An Endocrine Interpretation of Chapman's Reflexes. Indianapolis, IN: American Academy of Osteopathy; 1937
45. Chauffour P, Guillot JM. Le lien mécanique ostéopathique. Paris: Maloine; 1985
46. Cole WV. The Cole Book. Indianapolis, IN: AAO; o.J
47. Colot T, Verheyen M. Manuel pratique de manipulations ostéopathiques. Paris: Maisonneuve; 1996
48. De Wolf AN. Het sacroiliacale Gewricht, Huidige inzichten Symposium 1.4.1989. Utrecht: Smith Kline & French; 1990
49. DiGiovanna E, Schiowitz S. An Osteopathic Approach to Diagnosis and Treatment. 2nd ed. Philadelphia, PA: Lippincott-Raven; 1997
50. Downing CH. Osteopathic Principles in Disease. Indianapolis, IN: AAO; 1988
51. Dummer T. A Textbook of Osteopathy. Vol. 1. Move Sussex: Jotom Publications; 1999
52. Dummer T. A Textbook of Osteopathy. Vol. 2. Move Sussex: Jotom Publications; 1999

53. Dummer T. Specific Adjusting Technique. Move Sussex: Jotom Publications; 1995
54. Feely RA. Clinique osteopathique dans le champ crânien traduction française. Louwette HO, Paris: Ed. Frison-Roche; 1988
55. Finet G, Williame CH. Biométrie de la dynamique viscérale et nouvelles normalisations ostéopathiques. Paris: Ed. Jollois; 1992
56. Fryette HH. Principes de la technique ostéopathique. Traduction par Abehsera A. et Burty F. Paris: Frison-Roche; 1983
57. Frymann VM. The Collected Papers of Viola Frymann. Indianapolis, IN: AAO; 1998
58. Füeßl HS, Middeke M. Duale Reihe Anamnese und klinische Untersuchung. 4th ed. Stuttgart: Thieme; 2010
59. Gesret JR. Asthme. Paris: Editions de Verlaque; 1996
60. Giammatteo T, Weiselfish-Giammatteo S. Integrative Manual Therapy for the Autonomic Nervous System and Related Disorders. Berkeley, CA: North Atlantic Books; 1997
61. Gleditsch JM. Reflexzonen und Somatotopien. Schorndorf: WBV; 1983
62. Gray H. Gray's Anatomie. London: Pamajon; 1995
63. Greenman P. Lehrbuch der osteopathischen Medizin. 3rd ed. Stuttgart: Haug; 2005
64. Grieve GP. Common Vertebral Joint Problems. Edinburgh: Churchill Livingstone; 1988
65. Grieve GP. Mobilisation of the Spine. Edinburgh: Churchill Livingstone; 1991
66. Habermann-Horstmeier L. Anatomie, Physiologie und Pathologie. Stuttgart: Schattauer; 1992
67. Handoll N. Die Anatomie der Potency. Pähl: Jolandos; 2004
68. Hebgen E. Vizeralosteopathie. 3rd ed. Stuttgart: Hippokrates; 2008
69. Helsmoortel J. Lehrbuch der viszeralen Osteopathie. Stuttgart: Thieme; 2002
70. Hepp R, Debrunner H. Orthopädisches Diagnostikum. 7th ed. Stuttgart: Thieme; 2004
71. Hoppenfeld S. Examen clinique des membres et du rachis. Paris: Masson; 1984
72. Jealous JS. The Biodynamics of Osteopathy. CD-ROMs. Farmington, CT: Biodynamics/Biobasics Program; 2002–2003
73. Johnston WL. Scientific Contributions of William L. Johnson. Indianapolis, IN: AAO; 1998
74. Kapandji IA. Physiologie articulaire, Tome I–III. Paris, Maloine; 1977
75. Kimberly PE. Outline of Osteopathic Manipulative Procedures, 3rd ed. Kirksville, MO: Kirksville College of Osteopathic Medicine; 1980
76. Kissling R. Das Sacroiliacalgelenk. Stuttgart: Enke; 1997
77. Klein P, Sommerfeld P. Biomechanik der menschlichen Gelenke. München: Urban und Fischer; 2004
78. Klinke R, Pape H-C, Kurtz A, Silbernagl S. Physiologie. 6th ed. Stuttgart: Thieme; 2009
79. Korr IM. The Collected Papers of Irvin M. Korr. Vols. I and II. Indianapolis, IN: AAO; 1979, 1997
80. Kramer J. Bandscheibenbedingte Erkrankungen. Stuttgart: Thieme; 1994
81. Kuchera WA, Kuchera ML. Osteopathic Considerations in Systemic Dysfunction. Rev. 2nd ed. Columbus, OH: Greyden Press; 1994
82. Kuchera WA, Kuchera ML. Osteopathic Principles in Practice. Rev. 2nd ed. Columbus, OH: Greyden Press; 1993
83. Landouzy JM. Les ATM Evaluation. Traitement Odontologiques et Osteopathiques. Paris: Editions de Verlaque; 1993
84. Lee D. The Pelvic Girdle. Edinburgh: Churchill Livingstone; 1999
85. Leonhardt M, Tillmann B, Tördury G, Zilles K. Anatomie des Menschen. Lehrbuch und Atlas. Stuttgart: Thieme; 2002
86. Lewit K. Lewit Manuelle Medizin. 7th ed. Heidelberg: Barth; 1997
87. Liebenson C. Rehabilitation of the Spine. Philadelphia, PA: William and Wilkins; 1996
88. Liem T, Dobler TK. Leitfaden Osteopathie. München: Urban und Fischer; 2002
89. Liem T. Kraniosakrale Osteopathie. 5th ed. Stuttgart: Hippokrates; 2009
90. Liem T. Praxis der Kraniosakralen Osteopathie. 3rd ed. Stuttgart: Haug; 2010
91. Lignon A. Le puzzle crânien. Paris: Ed. De Verlaque; 1989
92. Lignon A. Schématisation neurovégétative en ostéopathie. Paris: Ed. de Verlaque; 1987
93. Lipincott RC, Lipincott HA. A Manual of Cranial Technique. Fort Worth, TX: The Cranial Academy Inc.; 1995
94. Littlejohn JM. Classical Osteopathy. Reprinted lectures from the archives of the Osteopathic Institute of Applied Technique. Maidstone: The John Wernham College of Classical Osteopathy; n.d.
95. Littlejohn JM. Lesionology. Maidstone: Maidstone College of Osteopathy; n.d.
96. Littlejohn JM. The Fundamentals of Osteopathic Technique. London: BSO; n.d.
97. Littlejohn JM. The Littlejohn Lectures. Vol. I. Maidstone: Maidstone College of Osteopathy; n.d.
98. Littlejohn JM. The Pathology of the Osteopathic Lesion. Maidstone College of Osteopathy. Indianapolis, IN: AAO Yearbook; 1977
99. McKenzie RA. Die lumbale Wirbelsäule. Waikanae, New Zealand: Spinal Publications; 1986
100. McKone WL. Osteopathic Athletic Healthcare. London: Chapman & Hall; 1997
101. Magoun H. Osteopathy in the Cranial Field. Original edition, Fort Worth, TX: SCTF, 2nd reprint; 1997
102. Magoun H. Osteopathy in the Cranial Field. Fort Worth, TX: SCTF; 1976
103. Meallet S, Peyrière J. L'ostéopathie tissulaire. Paris: Editions de Verlaque; 1987
104. Meert G. Das Becken aus osteopathischer Sicht. München: Urban und Fischer; 2003
105. Milne M. The Heart of Listening 1. Berkeley, CA: North Atlantic Books; 1995
106. Milne M. The Heart of Listening 2. Berkeley, CA: North Atlantic Books; 1995
107. Mitchell FL Jr. Handbuch der MuskelEnergieTechniken. Bände 1–3. Stuttgart. Hippokrates 2004–2005
108. Myers TW. Anatomy Trains. München: Urban & Fischer; 2004
109. Netter F. Farbatlanten der Medizin. Band 5 Nervensystem I, Neuroanatomie und Physiologie. Stuttgart: Thieme; 1987
110. Niethard F, Pfeil J, Biberthaler P. Duale Reihe Orthopädie und Unfallchirurgie. 6th ed. Stuttgart: Thieme; 2009
111. O'Connell JA. Bioelectric Fascial Activation and Release. Indianapolis, IN: AAO; 1998

112. Patterson MM, Howell JN. The Central Connection: Somatovisceral/Viscerosomatic Interaction. Indianapolis, IN: AAO; 1992
113. Peterson B. Postural Balance and Imbalance. Indianapolis, IN: AAO; 1983
114. von Piekartz H. Kraniofasziale Dysfunktionen und Schmerzen. Stuttgart: Thieme; 2000
115. Pschyrembel Klinisches Wörterbuch. Berlin: Walter de Gruyter; 2002
116. von Leonhardt H, Tillmann B, Töndury G, Zilles K. Rauber/Kopsch. Anatomie des Menschen. 3rd ed. Band I–IV. Stuttgart: Thieme; 2003
117. Reibaud P. Potentiel ostéopathique crânien, Mobilité crânienne, Techniques crâniennes. Paris: Editions de Verlaque; 1990
118. Ricard F, Thiebault P. Les techniques osteopathiques chiropractiques américaines. Paris: Frison Roche; 1991
119. Ricard F. Traitement Osteopathique des Douleurs d'origine Lombo-Pelvienne, Tome 1. Paris: Atman; 1988
120. Ricard F. Traitement Osteopathique des Douleurs d'origine Lombo-Pelvienne, Tome 2. Paris: Atman; 1988
121. Richard JP. La colonne vertébrale en ostéopathie, Tome 1. Paris: Editions de Verlaque; 1987
122. Richard R. Lésions ostéopathiques du membre inférieur. Paris: Maloine; 1980
123. Richard R. Lésions ostéopathiques du sacrum. Paris: Maloine; 1978
124. Richard R. Lésions ostéopathiques iliaques. Paris: Maloine; 1979
125. Richard R. Lésions ostéopathiques vertébrales, Tome 1. Paris: Maloine; 1982
126. Richard R. Lésions ostéopathiques vertébrales, Tome 2. Paris: Maloine; 1982
127. Rohen J. Funktionelle Anatomie des Menschen. Stuttgart: Schattauer; 1998
128. Rohen J. Funktionelle Anatomie des Nervensystems. Stuttgart: Schattauer; 1994
129. Rohen J. Topographische Anatomie. Stuttgart: Schattauer; 1992
130. Rolf I. Re-establishing the Natural Alignment and Structural Integration of the Human Body for Vitality and Well-Being. Rochester, VT: Healing Arts Press; 1989
131. Sammut E, Searle-Barnes P. Osteopathische Diagnose. München: Pflaum; 2000
132. Schultz RL, Feitis R. The Endless Web. Berkeley, CA: North Atlantic Books; 1996
133. Sergueef N. Die Kraniosakrale Osteopathie bei Kindern. Bad Kötzting: Verl. f. Osteopathie; 1995
134. Silbernagl S, Despopoulos A. Taschenatlas Physiologie. 7th ed. Stuttgart: Thieme; 2007
135. Sills F. Craniosacral Biodynamics. Vols. I and II. Berkeley, CA: North Atlantic Books; 2004
136. Solano R. Le nourisson, l'enfant et l'osteopathie crânium. Paris: Maloine; 1986
137. Speece C, Crow W. Osteopathische Körpertechniken nach W.G. Sutherland. Ligamentous Articular Strain (LAS). Stuttgart: Hippokrates; 2003
138. Spencer H. Die ersten Prinzipien der Philosophie. Pähl: Jolandos; 2004
139. Steinrücken H. Die Differentialdiagnose des Lumbalsyndroms mit klinischen Untersuchungstechniken. Berlin: Springer; 1998
140. Still AT. Das große Still-Kompendium. Pähl: Jolandos; 2002

141. Denys-Struyf G. Les chaines musculaires et articulaires. Paris: ICTGDS; 1979
142. Sutherland WG. Contributions of Thought. Fort Worth, TX: Rudra Press; 1998
143. Sutherland WG. Teachings in the Science of Osteopathy. Fort Worth, TX: Sutherland Cranial Teaching Foundation; 1990
144. Sutherland WG. The Cranial Bowl. 1st ed. Reprint. Fort Worth, TX: Free Press Co.; 1994
145. Travell J, Simons DG. Myofascial Pain and Dysfunction: The Trigger Point Manual. Vols. I–II. 2nd ed. Philadelphia, PA: Lippincott Williams & Wilkins; 1999
146. Tucker C. The Mechanics of Sports Injuries. Oxford: Blackwell; 1990
147. Typaldos S. Orthopathische Medizin. Bad Kötzting: Verlag f. Ganzh. Med.; 1999
148. Upledger JE, Vredevoogd JD. Lehrbuch der CranioSacralen Therapie I. 6th ed. Stuttgart: Haug; 2009
149. Upledger JE. Die Entwicklung des menschlichen Gehirns und ZNS: A Brain Is Born. Stuttgart: Haug; 2004
150. Upledger JE. Lehrbuch der CranioSacralen Therapie II Beyond the Dura. Stuttgart: Haug; 2002
151. Vannier L. La Typologie et ses applications therapeutiques. Boiron; 1989
152. Villeneuve P, Weber B. Pied, équilibre & mouvement. Paris: Masson; 2000
153. Villeneuve P. Pied équilibre & rachis. Paris: Ed. Frison-Roche; 1998
154. Villeneuve P. Pied, équilibre & posture. Paris: Ed. Frison-Roche; 1996
155. Vleeming A, Mooney V, Dorman T, Snijders C, Stoeckart R. Movement, Stability and Low Back Pain. Edinburgh: Churchill Livingstone; 1999
156. Ward RC. Foundations of Osteopathic Medicine. Philadelphia, PA: Williams & Wilkins; 1997
157. Wernham J. Osteopathy, Notes on the Technique and Practice. Maidstone: Maidstone Osteopathic Clinic; 1975
158. Willard FH, Patterson MM. Nociception and the Neuroendocrine-Immune Connection. Indianapolis, IN: AAO; 1994
159. Wodall P. Principes et pratique osteopathiques en gynécologie. Paris: Maloine; 1983
160. Wright S. Physiologie. Appliqué à la médecine. Paris: Flammarion; 1980
161. Piret S, Béziers MM. La Coordination Motrice, Masson 1971
162. The Integrative Action of the Nervous System. New Haven, CT: Yale University Press; 1947
163. Burns L. Osteopathic Sciences. Cincinnatti; 1911
164. Mac Conail MA, Basmajian JV. Muscles and Movements: A Basis for Human Kinesiology. Baltimore, Williams & Wilkins Comp.; 1969
165. Wahrig-Burfeind R. Wahrig deutsches Wörterbuch. Wissen Media Verlag; 2006
166. Wernham J. Mechanics of the spine and pelvis. Maidstone; 1955

Posture (Richter)

1. American Osteopathic Association. Foundations for Osteopathic Medicine. 2nd ed. Philadelphia, PA: Lippincott Williams & Wilkins; 2003
2. Boland U. Logiques de pathologies orthopédiques en chaînes ascendantes et descendantes et la méthode

exploratoire des "delta pondéral". Paris: Frison-Roche; 1996

3. Bourdiol RJ. Pied et statique. Paris: Maisonneuve; 1980
4. Bricot B. La reprogrammation posturale globale. Montpellier: Sauramps Medical; 1996
5. Busquet L. Les chaînes musculaires du tronc et de la colonne cervicale. 2nd ed. Paris: Maloine; 1985
6. Busquet L. Les chaînes musculaires, Tome II. Lordoses, Cyphoses, Scolioses et Déformations thoraciques. Paris: Frison-Roche; 1992
7. Busquet L. Les chaînes musculaires, Tome IV. Membres inférieurs. Paris: Frison-Roche; 1995
8. Drake RL, Vogl W, Mitchell AWM. Gray's Anatomie für Studenten. München: Elsevier/Urban & Fischer; 2007
9. Fryette HH. Principes de la technique ostéopathique. Traduction par Abehsera A et Butry F. Paris: Frison-Roche; 1983
10. Korr IM. The Collected Papers of Irvin M. Korr. Vols. 1 and 2. Indianapolis, IN: AAO; 1979, 1997
11. Kuchera WA, Kuchera ML. Osteopathic Considerations in Systemic Dysfunction. 2nd ed. Columbus, OH: Greydon Press; 1994
12. Kuchera WA, Kuchera ML. Osteopathic Principles in Practice. 2nd ed. Columbus, OH: Greydon Press; 1993
13. Landouzy JM. Les ATM Evaluation. Traitement odontologiques et osteopathiques. Paris: Editions de Verlaque; 1993
14. Littlejohn JM. Classical Osteopathy. Reprinted Lectures from the Archives of the Osteopathic Institute of Applied Technique. Maidstone: The John Wernham College of Classical Osteopathy; 1999
15. Magee DJ. Orthopedic Physical Assessment. 5th ed. Philadelphia, PA: Saunders; 2008
16. Magee DJ, Zachazewski JE, Quillen WS. Scientific Foundations and Principles in Musculoskeletal Rehabilitation. Philadelphia, PA: Saunders; 2007
17. Magee DJ, Zachazewski JE, Quillen WS. Pathology and Intervention in Musculoskeletal Rehabilitation. Philadelphia, PA: Saunders; 2009
18. McArdle D, Katch VL. Exercise Physiology. 6th ed. Philadelphia, PA: Lippincott Williams & Wilkins; 2007
19. McMahon PJ. Current Diagnosis and Treatment in Sports Medicine. New York, NY: McGraw-Hill; 2007
20. Neumann DA. Kinesiology of the Musculoskeletal System. Philadelphia, PA: Mosby; 2000
21. O'Connell JA. Bioelectric Fascial Activation and Release. Indianapolis, IN: AAO; 1998
22. Oschmann JL. Energiemedizin. München: Elsevier/Urban & Fischer; 2006
23. Peterson B. Postural Balance and Imbalance. Indianapolis, IN: AAO; 1983
24. Rohen J. Funktionelle Anatomie des Nervensystems. Stuttgart: Schattauer; 1994
25. Silbernagl S, Despopoulos A. Taschenatlas Physiologie. 7th ed. Stuttgart: Thieme; 2007
26. Still AT. Das große Still-Kompendium. Pähl: Jolandos; 2002
27. Travell J, Simons DG. Myofascial Pain and Dysfunction. The Trigger Point Manual. Vols. I–II. 2nd ed. Philadelphia, PA: Lippincott Williams & Wilkins; 1999
28. Trepel M. Neuroanatomie. 3rd ed. München: Elsevier/Urban & Fischer; 2004
29. Vleeming A, Mooney V, Dorman T, Snijders C, Stoeckart R. Movement, Stability and Low Back Pain. Edinburgh: Churchill Livingston; 1999

Trigger Points and How to Treat Them (Hebgen)

1. Baldry P. Akupunktur, Triggerpunkte und muskuloskelettale Schmerzen. 1st ed. Uelzen: Medizinisch Literarische Verlagsgesellschaft; 1993
2. Dvorak J. Manuelle Medizin: Diagnostik. 4th ed. Stuttgart: Thieme 2001
3. Fleischhauer K, ed. Benninghoff Anatomie: Makroskopische und mikroskopische Anatomie des Menschen – Band 2. 13th/14th ed. München: Urban & Schwarzenberg; 1985
4. Klinke R, Pape H-C, Kurtz A, Silbernagl S, eds. Physiologie. 6th ed. Stuttgart: Thieme; 2009
5. Kostopoulos D, Rizopoulos K. The Manual of Trigger Point and Myofascial Therapy. 1st ed. Thorofare, NJ: Slack Incorporated; 2001
6. Kuchera ML. Integrating Trigger Points into Osteopathic Approaches. Berlin: IFAO-Fortbildung; 2004
7. Kuchera ML, Kuchera WA. Osteopathic Considerations in Systemic Dysfunction. 2nd ed. Columbus, OH: Greyden Press; 1994
8. Lang F. Pathophysiologie: Pathobiochemie. 3rd ed. Stuttgart: Enke; 1987
9. Netter FH. Atlas der Anatomie des Menschen. 2nd ed. Basel: Ciba-Geigy AG; 1994
10. Pöntinen P, Gleditsch J, Pothmann R. Triggerpunkte und Triggermechanismen. 4th ed. Stuttgart: Hippokrates; 2007
11. Putz R, Pabst R, eds. Sobotta: Atlas der Anatomie des Menschen – Band 2. 20th ed. München: Urban & Schwarzenberg; 1993
12. Schmidt RF, Thews G, eds. Physiologie des Menschen. 29th ed. Berlin: Springer; 2004
13. Schünke M, Schulte E, Schumacher U. Prometheus—Lern-Atlas der Anatomie. Allgemeine Anatomie und Bewegungssystem. 2nd ed. Stuttgart: Thieme; 2007
14. Schünke M. Topographie und Funktion des Bewegungssystems. 1st ed. Stuttgart: Thieme; 2000
15. Schwegler J. Der Mensch: Anatomie und Physiologie. 4th ed. Stuttgart: Thieme; 2006
16. Silbernagl S, Despopoulos A. Taschenatlas Physiologie. 7th ed. Stuttgart: Thieme; 2007
17. Simons D. Myofascial Pain Syndrome due to Trigger Points. 1st ed. Cleveland, OH: Gebauer Company; 1987
18. Staubesand J, ed. Benninghoff Anatomie: Makroskopische und mikroskopische Anatomie des Menschen – Band 1. 13th ed. München: Urban & Schwarzenberg; 1985
19. Staubesand J, ed. Sobotta: Atlas der Anatomie des Menschen—Band 1. 19th ed. München: Urban & Schwarzenberg; 1988
20. Travell J, Simons D. Myofascial Pain and Dysfunction: The Trigger Point Manual. Vol. 2. 1st ed. Baltimore, MD: Williams & Wilkins; 1992
21. Travell J, Simons D. Myofascial Pain and Dysfunction: The Trigger Point Manual. Vol. 1. 1st ed. Baltimore, MD: Williams & Wilkins; 1983
22. Whitaker RH, Borley NR. Anatomiekompaß: Taschenatlas der anatomischen Leitungsbahnen. 1st ed. Stuttgart: Thieme; 1997
23. Zenker W, ed. Benninghoff Anatomie: Makroskopische und mikroskopische Anatomie des Menschen—Band 3. 13th/14th ed. München: Urban & Schwarzenberg; 1985

21 Illustration Credits

Fig. 3.1 From Hüter-Becker A, Hrsg. Das Neue Denkmodell in der Physiotherapie. Bd.1: Bewegungssystem. 2nd ed. Stuttgart: Thieme; 2006:294

Fig. 3.4 (a–f) From Brokmeier AA. Kursbuch Manuelle Therapie. Biomechanik, Neurologie, Funktionen. 3rd ed. Stuttgart: Hippokrates; 2001:86

Fig. 3.5 From Brokmeier AA. Kursbuch Manuelle Therapie. Biomechanik, Neurologie, Funktionen. 3rd ed. Stuttgart: Hippokrates; 2001:114–116

Fig. 4.2 From Liem T. Kraniosakrale Osteopathie. Ein praktisches Lehrbuch. 5th ed. Stuttgart: Hippokrates; 2010:233

Fig. 4.8 (a, b) From Liem T. Kraniosakrale Osteopathie. Ein praktisches Lehrbuch. 5th ed. Stuttgart: Hippokrates; 2010: 576

Fig. 4.8 (c) From Liem T. Kraniosakrale Osteopathie. Ein praktisches Lehrbuch. 5th ed. Stuttgart: Hippokrates; 2010:578

Fig. 4.9 (a, b) From Liem T. Kraniosakrale Osteopathie. Ein praktisches Lehrbuch. 5th ed. Stuttgart: Hippokrates; 2010:579

Fig. 4.11 (a) From Liem T. Kraniosakrale Osteopathie. Ein praktisches Lehrbuch. 5th ed. Stuttgart: Hippokrates; 2010:92

Fig. 5.7 (a) From Hermanns W. GOT: Ganzheitliche Osteopathische Therapie. 2nd ed. Stuttgart: Hippokrates; 2009:53

Fig. 5.7 (b) From Hermanns W. GOT: Ganzheitliche Osteopathische Therapie. 2nd ed. Stuttgart: Hippokrates; 2009:52

Fig. 9.4 – Fig. 9.14: Photographs by Annick Greven, Burg Reuland, Belgium

Fig. 10.1 – Fig. 10.11: Photographs by Eric Hebgen, Königswinter, Germany

Fig. 14.1 From Schmidt RF, Thews G, eds. Physiologie des Menschen. 29th ed. Berlin: Springer; 2004

Fig. 14.3 From Silbernagl S, Despopoulos A. Taschenatlas Physiologie. 7th ed. Stuttgart: Thieme; 2007:67

Fig. 14.4 From Simons D. Myofascial pain syndrome due to trigger points. In: Goodgold J, ed. Rehabilitation Medicine. St. Louis, MO: Mosby Year Book; 1988:686–723

The anatomical illustrations in **Part B – Trigger Points: Diagnosis and Treatment** – are taken from Schünke M. Topographie und Funktion des Bewegungssystems. Stuttgart: Thieme; 2000, Schünke M, Schulte E, Schumacher U. Prometheus LernAtlas der Anatomie. Allgemeine Anatomie und Bewegungssystem. Illustrations by Wesker K and Voll M. 2nd ed. Stuttgart: Thieme; 2007, and Schwegler J. Der Mensch – Anatomie und Physiologie. 3rd ed. Stuttgart: Thieme; 2002.

Photographs in **chapter 9:** Ullrich + Company, Renningen, Germany.

Photographs of the stretching exercises in **chapter 19:** Eric Hebgen, Königswinter, Germany.

22 List of Abbreviations

ABD	Abduction
ADD	Adduction
AIIS	Anterior inferior iliac spine
AL chain	Anterolateral chain
ANS	Autonomic nervous system
AP chain	Anteroposterior chain
ASIS	Anterior superior iliac spine
ATP	Adenosine triphosphate
CCP	Common compensatory pattern
CNS	Central nervous system
COJ	Cervico-occipital junction
CSC	Cervical spinal column
CSF	Cerebrospinal fluid
CTJ	Cervicothoracic junction
CV joint	Costovertebral joint
CVB	Cervical vertebral body
EMG	Electromyography
ERS	Extension–rotation–sidebending
FRS	Flexion–rotation–sidebending
GAG	Glycosaminoglycans
GDS	Godelieve Denys-Struyf (method)
H.I.O.	"Hole-in-one"
HPA	Hypothalamus–pituitary–adrenal (axis)
ILA	Inferior lateral angle
LSC	Lumbar spinal column
LSJ	Lumbosacral junction
LTA	Lower thoracic aperture
LTR	Local twitch response
LVB	Lumbar vertebral body
MET	Muscle energy technique
MTP	Metatarsophalangeal joint
NCP	Noncompensated pattern
NMT	Neuromuscular therapy
NSR	Neutral–sidebending–rotation
OA joint	Occipitoatlantal joint
OAA	Occipitoatlantoaxial complex
OM	Occipitomastoid suture
PA	Posteroanterior chain
PE	Pelvis
PIR	Postisometric relaxation
PL	Posterolateral chain
PNF	Proprioceptive neuromuscular facilitation
PNS	Parasympathetic nervous system
PRM	Primary respirator mechanism
PRT	Positional release therapy
PSIS	Posterior superior iliac spine
SAT	Specific adjusting technique as per Dummer
SBL	Superficial back line
SBS	Sphenobasilar synchondrosis
SC	Spinal column
SCM	Sternocleidomastoid (muscle)
SCS	Strain–counterstrain (technique)
SFL	Superficial front line
SIJ	Sacroiliac joint
SNS	Sympathetic nervous system
TFL	Tensor fasciae latae (muscle)
TLJ	Thoracolumbar junction
TP	Trigger point
TSC	Thoracic spinal column
TVB	Thoracic vertebral bodies
UAJ	Upper ankle joint
UCCP	Uncommon compensatory pattern
UTA	Upper thoracic aperture

Index

Note: *f* refers to information contained *within* a figure.